THE LOCK AND KEY OF MEDICINE

LARA V. MARKS

The Lock and Key of Medicine

Monoclonal Antibodies and the

Transformation of Healthcare

Yale UNIVERSITY PRESS

NEW HAVEN AND LONDON

Yale University Press books may be purchased in quantity for educational, business, or promotional use. For information, please e-mail sales.press@yale.edu (U.S. office) or sales@yaleup.co.uk (U.K. office).

Set in Scala and Scala Sans types by Westchester Book Group.
Printed in the United States of America.

Library of Congress Control Number: 2015930850
ISBN 978-0-300-16773-3 (cloth : alk. paper)

A catalogue record for this book is available from the British Library.

This paper meets the requirements of ANSI/NISO Z39.48–1992 (Permanence of Paper).

10 9 8 7 6 5 4 3 2 1

To my two children, Daniel and Anna, and to the memory of César Milstein, Hubert Schoemaker, and Michael Neuberger, each of whom played a vital part in the development of Mabs, and to the memory of my mentor Irvine Loudon

CONTENTS

ILLUSTRATIONS

TABLES

We purchase them through catalogs and online suppliers; we mail them in polypropylene tubes; we pass them surreptitiously from hand to pocket at scientific meetings; we borrow (with or without permission) a drop from a labmate for a crucial assay; we add microliter amounts to cultures of cells to activate, isolate, kill, block, blot, immunoprecipitate, and stain; we inject them into experimental animals to inhibit or elicit responses or to track specific cell populations; and we introduce them into our patients in an effort to view or destroy their tumors. As scientists, we imagine the one that will define a new molecule, a new cell type, a new signaling pathway. As clinicians, we visualize a better therapy, a complete cure. We hope for the one that will answer the central question, make us famous, or make us rich. Each one is different, yet all are the same. No single class of reagents stirs our creativity, or propels our successes, even in our dreams, with as much excitement as do monoclonal antibodies, or Mabs.

D. Margulies, "Monoclonal Antibodies," 2005

EVERYWHERE AROUND US today imperceptibly small "magic bullets" called Mabs are quietly affecting our lives. Six out of ten of the best-selling drugs in the world are Mabs. In 2013 the global sales of the ten blockbuster Mabs were estimated to be worth over $58.1 billion. The Mabs market was estimated to be approximately $78 billion for the year 2012, and it is predicted to grow around 15 percent between 2012 and 2018.

Mabs are not only successful drugs but also powerful tools for a wide range of medical applications. In industry, they are critical to the purification of drugs. Elsewhere they are essential research probes for determining the pathological pathway and cause of diseases such as cancer and autoimmune and neurological disorders. They are used on a routine basis in hospitals to type blood and tissue, a process vital to ensuring safe blood transfusion and organ transplantation. On the diagnostic front,

Mabs are intrinsic components in home-testing kits for detecting ovulation, pregnancy, or menopause. They are used for the analysis of body fluids for medical diagnosis, and to determine whether a heart attack has occurred. They are at the forefront of public health efforts, helping, for example, to identify hospital infections such as methicillin-resistant *Staphylococcus aureus* (MRSA). At a global level, governments also depend on Mab-based tests to contain the spread of infectious diseases such as AIDS and pandemic flu, or to detect the potential release of anthrax or smallpox by bioterrorists.

Mabs are indispensable not only to health, but also to many other aspects of modern life: they help identify viruses in animal livestock or plants, prevent food poisoning, and are used to investigate environmental pollution. Yet, despite their ubiquity and significance, most people have never heard of Mabs or how they have both transformed healthcare and spawned an entire new industry.

Produced in the laboratory, Mabs are derived from the billions of tiny antibodies made every day by our immune systems to combat substances, known as antigens, that are regarded as foreign or potentially dangerous. Millions of different types of antibodies can be found in the blood of humans and other mammals. Made by white blood cells known as B lymphocytes, each antibody is highly specific, that is, it has the ability to bind to only one particular antigen, which may be derived from bacteria, viruses, fungi, parasites, pollen, or nonliving substances such as toxins, chemicals, drugs, or foreign particles considered alien to the body. Once antibodies have marked their particular antigen, they and other types of cells produced by the immune system can attack it.

The story of Mabs started when an Argentinian émigré, César Milstein, arrived at the Laboratory of Molecular Biology (LMB) in Cambridge, England. It was here—where Francis Crick and James Watson had unraveled the structure of DNA in 1953—that Milstein, together with Georges Köhler, a German biologist, would pioneer in 1975 the seminal technique for the production of Mabs and demonstrate their clinical application. The procedure for producing Mabs involves injecting a mouse with a specific antigen to stimulate its production of antibodies. These antibodies are then harvested from the mouse's spleen and fused with an immortal myeloma cancer cell to make what is called a hybrid cell, or hybridoma, which secretes Mabs. Each Mab is identical and can be reproduced endlessly either by injecting the hybridoma into the abdominal cavity of mice, or, as is increasingly the case today, by its artificial growth in a culture medium.

Armed with the technique to produce unlimited quantities of Mabs and at minimum cost, scientists have developed a vast array of uses for the technology since 1975. In the diagnostics field, Mabs have opened the means to detect numerous diseases previously impossible to identify until they had reached an advanced stage. Similarly, diagnostic tests, which took days if not weeks before the arrival of Mabs, now take just minutes to complete and have also greatly enhanced the accuracy of diagnostics and reduced their cost.

On the therapeutic front, Mabs have radically altered the treatment of more than fifty major diseases, many considered untreatable before. Mab therapies are used for a broad range of conditions today, including organ transplants, cancer, inflammatory and autoimmune diseases, cardiovascular and infectious diseases, allergies, and ophthalmic disorders. In addition to offering a host of new drugs to fight disease, Mabs have provided the means to monitor a patient's response to therapy and helped lead the way in personalized medicine.

Despite the prevalence of Mabs, few know of their existence outside the scientific and medical community. Their emergence is often overshadowed by the 1973 discovery in the United States of recombinant DNA, or gene cloning, which inspired the creation of Genentech, the world's first company dedicated to biotechnology. Although recombinant DNA set the stage for a major breakthrough in manufacturing and production techniques that enabled the development of cheaper and more effective treatments for disease, I argue in this book that Mabs have had just as much, if not more, of a far-reaching effect on our society and daily life. The history of Mabs provides fresh insight into the beginnings of the biotechnology revolution usually missed by previous studies of the biotechnology industry. Looking back, perhaps this historical oversight is not surprising. Mabs did not transform healthcare overnight or with major fanfare. Instead they quietly brought about new understandings of the pathways of disease and slipped unobserved into routine clinical diagnostics on a large scale. Unnoticed at the time, Mabs brought with them new treatment possibilities often taken for granted and considered mundane today.

This book is very much a tale of the complexities and difficulties inherent in science and its practical application. Milstein and Köhler's breakthrough in 1975 was rooted in scientists' quest from the late nineteenth century to unravel the mechanism behind the diversity of antibodies made by the body's immune system and to find new treatments to fight infectious diseases. Their work was not a linear process, and it was subject to both controversy and intense national rivalry. What helped galvanize the field was a theory put forward in the 1890s by Paul Ehrlich, a German physician. Ehrlich conceptualized all cells as having a wide variety of special receptors that acted as gatekeepers or locks, permitting entry only to substances like antibodies whose structure matched such receptors. He was convinced that antibodies bind to specific receptors found on antigens in the same way as a key fits a lock and that one day scientists would be able to create antibodies that could act as magic bullets, seeking out and destroying specific disease-causing microorganisms without harming the rest of the body.

Ehrlich's theory came under attack in the ensuing decades. Many scientists found it puzzling how the immune system could produce antibodies with such high levels of specific affinity to match the wide diversity of antigens. The debate about antibody formation twisted and turned for many years as scientists worked to see how antibodies might be applied clinically. Diphtheria was one of the first diseases to be successfully treated with antibodies. The treatment, developed in the 1890s, entailed injecting patients with blood serum taken from animals immunized against diphtheria. This serum, known as antisera, contained highly potent antibodies which targeted diphtheria and helped boost the immune system to fight the disease. By the 1930s serum therapy had become a common treatment for many infectious diseases, and antisera had become an important agent in immunobased tests. Such diagnostics exploited the lock and key mechanism, in which antibodies attached to specific cell receptors, facilitated the analysis and identification of different cell types. (The antibodies acted as markers for locating and measuring cells in biological samples.) The first immunobased test developed was for typhoid in 1896.

Despite their utility for therapeutics and diagnostics, antisera had major limitations. The supply of antisera depended on an individual animal's lifetime and varied between batches, which made it difficult to standardize. Consequently, some scientists looked for ways to create artificial antibodies to specific antigens. Although they had come close to achieving this by 1970, artificial antisera were difficult to reproduce so were limited in quantity and had a short half-life. Milstein and Köhler's innovation in 1975 heralded a new era by introducing the means to produce unlimited quantities of standardized antibodies specific to any antigen.

Milstein and Köhler's procedure, however, was not adopted overnight. Many scientists failed to grasp its significance at first, and the technique was not patented by the British National Research Development Corporation, which could not foresee its having any commercial application. Transforming Mabs, which had started life as a laboratory tool, into something that could be of use to the outside world was neither straightforward or inevitable. Yet within a few years many scientists had become interested in the technology. This interest was in part fueled by Milstein, who collaborated with researchers in disciplines different from his own to demonstrate the utility of Mabs. One of his first collaborators was Claudio Cuello, a fellow Argentinian émigré. Together Milstein and Cuello proved the validity of Mabs for immunobased tests that by the 1970s were being routinely used for diagnosis in parasitology, virology, immunology, cancer, and other fields. Their work marked a major breakthrough for scientists who previously had struggled to reproduce (and compare) the results of their diagnostic tests that relied on antisera. Moreover, Milstein and Cuello extended the reach of immunobased diagnostics by demonstrating how Mabs, used as probes, could enhance the pathological investigation of the brain and the central nervous system.

In addition to Cuello, Milstein launched projects with many other scientists. Foremost among these was a partnership with Alan Williams and Andrew McMichael, two immunologists based at Oxford University. Together the collaborators discovered the potency of Mabs for identifying and distinguishing different markers found on the surface of cells. By laying the basis for a whole new field of investigation into immune cells and the immune response's regulatory network, their work opened up new targets for diagnostic and therapeutic intervention.

As the interest in Mabs began to gain momentum outside the confines of Cambridge, Milstein found it increasingly difficult to satisfy the avalanche of demands for his cells. Fortunately in February 1977 he received an unexpected visit from David Murray, founder of Sera-Lab, a British company producing and marketing antisera as reagents for the scientific community. Learning of Milstein's difficulties, Murray quickly agreed to distribute Milstein's cells through Sera-Lab, an arrangement that marked the first commercialization of Mabs. How Sera-Lab came to be a pioneer in the market is an unusual tale. Unlike American startups, which dominate the traditional histories told of the commercialization of biotechnology, Sera-Lab was founded with no venture capital funding or outside support.

That a British company spearheaded the first marketing of Mabs, a technology devised in a British laboratory by an émigré Argentinian scientist with his German colleague, highlights the international nature of biotechnology commercialization. Sera-Lab's venture to sell Mabs took place in the midst of the excitement generated by the founding of Genentech in 1976. The emergence of Genentech, which had been set up to market recombinant DNA products, galvanized numerous alliances among academics, entrepreneurs, and venture capitalists to launch new companies to commercialize biotechnology. Most of the early enterprises set up in the wake of Genentech's birth were dedicated to exploiting recombinant DNA for the mass production of natural products such as interferon and insulin for drugs. But the early germination of the modern biotechnology industry did not rest solely on recombinant DNA. By the 1970s a number of pioneering companies were developing Mab products, including Sera-Lab and two startups: Hybritech in San Diego and Centocor in Philadelphia. Entrepreneurs who risked entry into the field had no guarantee of success and were entering totally uncharted territory. Such individuals faced major financial, personal, professional, and regulatory challenges as well as a great deal of hostility, pessimism, and litigation.

Among the stories told in this book is that of David Murray, who set up Sera-Lab to earn his living after being forced to abandon his position as general manager of his father's cabaret club, a place notorious as a result of the part played by one of its dancers, Christine Keeler, in the British political scandal known as the Profumo affair. Murray's endeavors are told alongside those of Hubert Schoemaker, a young Dutch immigrant who, after completing a biochemistry doctorate at Massachusetts

Institute of Technology, became involved in commercializing Mabs out of his desire to relieve the suffering of the sick, a passion awakened by the birth of his profoundly disabled daughter. At much the same time Ivor Royston, a British immigrant who had settled in America as a child, began hunting for a more effective treatment for his cancer patients when he attained a clinical position in oncology at Stanford University. Risk-taking was part of the bloodline for these men. During World War II, Murray had been a saboteur in occupied Europe, Schoemaker's father had participated in the Dutch underground resistance, and Royston's father had fought with the Polish army and then alongside Field Marshall Montgomery in Italy.

When starting on their adventure, little did these intrepid individuals realize how much Mabs would change the world. For example, Mabs played a critical role in the purification of recombinant interferon, which is often hailed as one of early successes of modern biotechnology. After this success with interferon, Mabs were used to purify many other commercial drug products. Mabs were also soon adopted as a means to improve blood typing and grouping. Mabs critically helped shift the process of blood typing away from its dependency on human blood, providing a reagent that was easier to standardize, cheaper to produce, and suitable for use in automated blood-grouping machines.

The use of Mabs for blood typing and the purification of drugs was just the start of medical applications explored for the technology. By the late 1970s, many clinicians had great expectations that Mabs could transform cancer therapy. Yet Mabs proved more difficult to deploy in cancer diagnostics and therapeutics than originally anticipated. The first marketed Mab drug was not for cancer, but for the prevention of acute kidney rejection in transplant patients in 1986. No more Mab drugs were approved over the next seven years. Indeed, by the early 1990s many had become despondent about its therapeutic potential. The downfall of Centoxin in 1992 is illustrative of some of the difficulties that entrepreneurs faced in bringing Mab therapeutics to market. Not only did they encounter the difficulties inherent in the science of drug development, but they also had to satisfy financial stakeholders. Centocor's failure to win U.S. regulatory approval for Centoxin not only brought its developer to the brink of bankruptcy, but also cast a long shadow over the viability of Mab therapeutics as a whole.

Although much of the optimism surrounding Mab therapeutics of the early 1980s had dissipated by the end of the decade, new protein engineering techniques developed in these years helped improve the efficacy and safety of Mabs and stimulated a renaissance of Mab therapeutics in the 1990s. In 1993, Abciximab (ReoPro), developed by Centocor for reducing blood clots in heart attack patients, was approved and became the first reengineered Mab to reach market, marking a significant breakthrough. Other reengineered Mabs soon followed suit, and gained momentum from 1996. Many of these drugs started as treatments for rare diseases where profit margins were minimal, but were then soon approved for more common conditions, bringing the possibility of $1 million in revenue. The rise of blockbuster drugs shows how far reengineering had improved the safety and efficacy of Mabs and how much the knowledge of the immune system and the utility of Mabs had advanced since the early days.

Mabs have had their strongest therapeutic impact in the field of cancer. The first Mab to reach the market for cancer was edrecolomab (Panorex), which was granted German regulatory approval in 1995 for the treatment of postoperative colorectal cancer. Developed by Centocor in partnership with the Wistar Institute, it was withdrawn in 2001 because of its poor efficacy in comparison with other drugs. Since 1997, however, the U.S. Food and Drug Administration (FDA) has approved twelve Mab drugs for cancer treatment, including rituximab (Rituxan), approved in 1998 for the treatment of non-Hodgkin's lymphoma. By 2012 there were over 160 candidates in clinical trials for cancer, with seventy of them in phase III trials, the stage before a drug is submitted for regulatory approval.

One of the advantages of Mab drugs is that they can specifically target cancer cells while avoiding healthy cells. This means they cause fewer debilitating side effects than more conventional chemotherapy or radiotherapy. In addition, Mabs have enabled the identification and characterization of cancerous tumors previously difficult to detect and differentiate from other tumors, thereby providing a better understanding of cancer. They have also opened a path to more personalized medical treatment. Trastuzumab (Herceptin), for example, was specifically developed to target HER2/neu, a protein overexpressed by tumors found in 25 percent of newly diagnosed breast-cancer patients. Tumors expressing HER2/neu are known to grow more aggressively and therefore to have more fatal outcomes. Trastuzumab was explicitly approved in 2000 together with a companion diagnostic to detect HER2/neu.

Aside from cancer, Mabs have aided the treatment of other previously untreatable diseases, most notably autoimmune and inflammatory diseases. The first Mab marketed for the treatment of such disorders was infiliximab (Remicade). Initially approved for Crohn's disease (gut wall disorder) in 1998, the drug rapidly became a blockbuster drug, being used for chronic inflammatory conditions such as psoriasis (a noncontagious skin disease), rheumatoid arthritis (a joint disease), ulcerative colitis (a large intestine disorder), and ankylosing spondylitis (a spine disease). Overall, Mabs have shifted the treatment paradigm for autoimmune disorders away from merely ameliorating their painful symptoms to targeting and disrupting their cause.

Mabs are now marketed not only for cancer and autoimmune disorders, but also for a range of other diseases, including allergic conditions such as asthma, age-related macular degeneration (an eye disorder), multiple sclerosis (a neurological disorder), and osteoporosis (brittle bones). They are also being investigated for central nervous system disorders such as Alzheimer's disease (a degenerative brain disease), metabolic diseases such as diabetes, and the prevention of migraines. Today, the growth and profitability of Mabs are outstripping those of earlier types of biotechnology drugs and more traditional pharmaceutical ones. Indeed their expansion is among the fastest in the global pharmaceutical world. In part this reflects the sectors' embrace of Mabs as an answer to dwindling drugs in the pipeline and reduced revenue streams in the face of the expiration of key patents and the growth of generic medicines.

Although Mab drugs have brought untold relief to patients with previously untreatable illnesses, they are not a total elixir. Such therapies do not offer a total cure and can cause complications. Moreover, they come with a very high price tag, which since the 1990s has raised important questions about the cost-effectiveness of Mab therapeutics and has put them at the heart of debates over the rising cost of healthcare provision and whether and how innovative drugs should be made universally available.

Mabs have come a long way since their development as a tool to answer a basic scientific research question. Indeed, as the possible uses of

Mabs continue to unfold and their dominance in healthcare continues to strengthen, it is easy to forget scientists' initial struggle to produce sustainable and reproducible antibodies in the laboratory—and how the ability to produce antibodies was just the first chapter in how this technology continues to transform health care. Today we are on the brink of exciting new engineering discoveries which will enhance the potency and safety of Mab therapeutics and may make it possible to lower the dose given to patients and reduce costs. In no area are these developments more important than in the fight against infectious diseases, which to date has gained little traction in the Mab therapeutic sector. Because Mabs boost a host's immune response rather than kill microbes directly, they could provide a pivotal tool in the fight against the rising tide of drug resistance ushered in with the antibiotic era.

ACKNOWLEDGMENTS

THIS BOOK WAS BORN out of work I began while a research consultant at Silico Research, where I became involved in analyzing alliances between pharmaceutical and biotechnology companies. My attention was soon drawn to the large number of alliances being signed between companies for various monoclonal antibodies (Mabs), which launched my quest to understand the history of this technology and its influence on healthcare. Conversations with Paul Martin and Soraya de Chadarevian inspired me to study the subject in earnest. What struck me upon starting my research was how little most people outside the medical and scientific community knew about Mabs compared with other forms of biotechnology such as gene cloning. This knowledge gap even led, initially, to some difficulties in getting research council support for my work. The book was finally made possible by a charitable donation from Centocor OrthoBiotech (a subsidiary of Johnson & Johnson), as well as funding from the Medical Research Council and Michael Clark and Geoff Hale for two website exhibitions on the life and work of César Milstein and the development and testing of alemtuzumab, the first humanized Mab drug. These can be found on www.whatisbiotechnology.org. Some of the research was also supported by small travel grants from the Wellcome Trust and Roche Diagnostics GmbH. This book is also indebted to Jean Thomson Black and Samantha Ostrowski at Yale University Press, who championed the project and oversaw it through to completion, and to my friend Rosemary Sassoon, who urged on my writing. Many thanks also go to Julie Carlson for her rigorous editing of the final manuscript.

The starting point for my research was Alberto Cambrosio and Peter Keating's book *Exquisite Specificity* (1995), which provides a detailed description of scientists' adoption of Mabs in the laboratory until the early 1990s. My research was immeasurably helped thereafter by Anne Faulkner Schoemaker, the widow of Hubert Schoemaker, a cofounder of Centocor, which was one of the first companies to commercialize Mab diagnostics and therapeutics. Anne not only gave me access to her husband's personal papers, but also generously put me in touch with other key industry executives and scientists to interview. Subsequently, I was kindly helped by Celia Milstein, the widow of César Milstein, the co-developer of Mabs, as well as Allen Packwood and his team of archivists at the Churchill Archives Centre and Annette Faux at the Laboratory of Molecular Biology who guided me through Milstein's papers. The material not only provided insight into the early development of Mabs in Milstein's laboratory, but also gave me leads to others active in the field. One of these was Jenny Murray, the widow of David Murray who had helped her husband build Sera-Lab, the first company to ever commercialize Mabs. Jenny both plied me with stories of the early days and gave me contacts of many others who were involved.

I also am indebted to many others who generously agreed to be interviewed and share their papers, and whose names are listed in full in the Bibliography. Special thanks go to Roy Calne, Michael Clark, James Christie, Claudio Cuello, Don Drakeman, Martin Glennie, Geoff Hale, David Holveck, Masamichi Koike, Ivan Leftkovits, Ron Levy, Nils Lonberg, Richard McCloskey, Michael Neuberger, Steven Sacks, David Secher, Theophil Staehelin, Pedro Tetteroo, Ján Vilček, Herman Waldmann, and Greg Winter. I am very grateful to them for their patience and for the time they devoted to the project both in interviews and by reading through various chapter drafts.

Much appreciation goes to the following individuals for their editorial comments on various parts of my book: Norberto Serpente, Alison Kraft, David Lawrence, Roger Cooter, Janice Reichert, Malcolm Nicolson, Ilana Löwy, and Dmitriy Myelnikov. I was also touched by the interest my Open University colleagues and students showed in my research. I am indebted as well to David Armstrong and Nik Rose at King's College London for providing me with an academic base to conduct my research and to my colleagues in the Department of History and Philosophy of Science at Cambridge University. Thanks too go to Sabrina Fernandez, Lucy Brown, Susan Chandler, and other staff in the Department of Social Science, Health and Medicine at King's College London for their administrative support. I am also grateful to Barbara Prainsack in the department for her help with proofreading, her collegial encouragement, and her warm support in the final stages of completing the book, and to Sylvia Camporesi for her help in proofreading.

This book could not have been completed without the help of my mother, Shula Marks, and Anne Summers, who undertook the time-consuming and painstaking task of editing the final manuscript—a task I found difficult to complete in the last stages due to a cerebral hemorrhage I suffered in March 2013. The episode left me very thankful to be alive to enjoy the fun and laughter of my children, Daniel and Anna, and to be surrounded by my loving family and supportive friends. I am also grateful to my father, Yitz Marks, for his help in proofreading some of the book. Last, but not least, it could not have been seen through to the end without the steadfast love, care, and optimism of my husband, Emmett Power, who has been a pillar of strength throughout.

ALL	acute lymphocytic leukemia
BII	Basel Institute of Immunology
BMT	bone marrow transplant
CAT	Cambridge Antibody Technology
CD	cluster of differentiation
CDR	complementarity-determining region
CHO	Chinese hamster ovary
CLL	Chronic lymphocytic leukemia
ELISA	enzyme-linked immunosorbent assays
FACS	fluorescence-activated cell sorter
FDA	Food and Drug Administration
GVHD	graft-versus-host disease
HLA	human leukocyte antigens
HLDA	human leukocyte differentiation antigens
Ig	Immunoglobulin
LMB	Laboratory of Molecular Biology
Mab	monoclonal antibody
MRC	Medical Research Council
NCI	National Cancer Institute
NHL	non-Hodgkin's lymphoma
NHS	National Health Service
NIH	National Institutes of Health
NRDC	National Research Development Corporation
PCR	polymerase chain reaction
RIA	radioimmunoassay
RA	rheumatoid arthritis
rDNA	recombinant DNA
SRBC	sheep red blood cell
TNF	tumor necrosis factor

THE LOCK AND KEY OF MEDICINE

CHAPTER ONE

Hunting for the Elusive "Magic Bullet"

IN THE CLOSING DECADES of the nineteenth century, medical researchers, searching for a cure for infectious diseases, uncovered natural substances in the blood that seemed to act as very precise weapons against disease. Labeled "antibodies," these substances aroused the hope that one day scientists would be able to harness their power and use them as "magic bullets" to fight these diseases without damaging healthy parts of the body.

The process of transforming antibodies into magic bullets was, however, beset with difficulties. For much of the twentieth century progress was slow, hampered not only by scientists' inability to understand the immune system and how it produced antibodies, but also by their inability to isolate and purify individual antibodies from the billions produced by the body's defense system. All of this changed in 1975 with the development of monoclonal antibodies (Mabs), a breakthrough discovery made possible by the coming together of knowledge and techniques developed in many different geographic locations, laboratories, and disciplines, as well as at the bedside. The process was far from linear not only because of these logistical obstacles, but also because the evolving science was subject to the personal and theoretical rivalries among scientists. In many ways, the history of Mabs is as much about how substances, originally invisible to the naked eye, were imagined and then transformed into material entities.

The discovery of antibodies was built on years of medical and scientific inquiry into the nature of immunity and the development of techniques to fight infectious disease. Keen observers of epidemic diseases, such as pestilence and plague, had long noticed that individuals who suffered and survived one outbreak of disease appeared unscathed when it recurred.[1] Such knowledge underpinned the development of vaccination against smallpox, and by the late nineteenth century doctors were using artificially weakened forms of a disease organism to confer immunity to that disease.[2]

Much of the early development of vaccines took place with little understanding of the immune mechanism that underlay their success. Until the late nineteenth century, most explanations rested on the belief that immunity stemmed not from a defense mechanism within the host, but from the infective agent itself. In 1883, however, Élie Metchnikoff, a Ukrainian biologist working at the Pasteur Institute, Paris, posited a new theory of immunity. He suggested that immunity occurred when white blood cells, known as phagocytes, sought out and ingested foreign invaders. This startled his contemporaries, particularly pathologists, who had hitherto believed that phagocytes contributed to the spread of disease by transporting foreign matter around the body. Nonetheless, Metchinkoff's theory, later called "cellular immunity," transformed our understanding of immunity, as scientists came to understand that immunity occurred due to processes taking place within the body, not outside of it.[3]

In the 1890s, this understanding of immunity took a new turn with the work of the German bacteriologist Hans Buchner, who discovered soluble components capable of destroying bacteria in blood serum. As a result, he argued that immunity was mediated by cell-free components, later defined as "complements," floating in the blood, which he labeled "humoral immunity." Buchner's work set off an intense battle over whether cells or other blood-borne factors were more important in conferring immunity. As the immunologist and historian Arthur Silverstein has commented, the dividing line at times reflected the Franco-Prussian War, with French scientists defending Metchnikoff and German scientists promoting Buchner.[4]

While these tensions continued into the early twentieth century, the newly emerging discipline of bacteriology began to provide another perspective on the disease process. For centuries, disease was thought to be caused by poisons from slimes and miasmas. In the late nineteenth century, however, bacteriologists began to discover poisons produced by bacteria, labeled toxins, that remained in the body even after the bacteria had died. Toxins were now seen as the cause of disease, and therapy moved from the destruction of bacteria to a concern with toxins. This approach took on a new importance following the work conducted by Henry Sewall, an American physiologist, and Albert Calmette, a French bacteriologist in the 1880s, who discovered that pigeons became resistant to relatively large amounts of rattlesnake poison if given gradually increasing amounts of the toxin beforehand.[5]

New ideas arose from the work of Emil von Behring, a German physician and physiologist. Steeped in military medicine and concerned with the treatment of wounds, Behring began to experiment with disinfectants, using iodoform on infections in animals. He discovered that while iodoform was incapable of killing pathogenic germs, animals exposed to it developed resistance to germs. Soon afterward, he noticed that anthrax bacteria could be destroyed in test tubes by adding serum taken from rats, animals known to be resistant to anthrax. This could not be repeated with blood serum from animals without anthrax resistance. Moreover, rat serum was ineffective against bacteria other than anthrax. Behring also found that blood taken from an animal previously exposed to a pathogen was more effective than blood taken from an unexposed animal.[6]

These observations led Behring to wonder whether something unknown in the organism was responsible for destroying bacteria while leaving other body tissues and organs unaffected. With this in mind, he and Kitasato Shibasaburō, a Japanese physician and bacteriologist, conducted further animal experiments at the Koch Institute in the summer of 1890, and discovered that blood serum taken from animals that had survived diphtheria or tetanus provided some protection when injected into animals with no previous exposure to such diseases. The serum also cured animals with diphtheria and tetanus. This evidence led them to hypothesize the presence of "forces" in the blood of the exposed animals, but not in those uninfected.[7] Additional research indicated that toxins injected into nonimmune animals remained in the animals' blood and other bodily fluids long after their death. These findings confirmed the newly emerging theory of "humoral immunity" and opened up a radically new path for therapy.[8]

Soon after Behring and Shibasaburō's findings were publicized, Paul Ehrlich, a German physician with expertise in structural chemistry, detected in blood a substance he called antibodies that seemed to confer immunity against plant toxins.[9] He discovered that these antibodies were very specific—antibodies against ricin offered no protection against abrin. He observed that ricin and abrin toxins could not be distinguished by their toxicity but by the antibodies they generated, and noticed that antibodies responded in this way not just to bacterial toxins but to other toxins as well. Furthermore, he noted that large quantities of antibodies could be produced by only small amounts of toxin, and found that immunity developed six days after exposure to the toxin, but then remained for a long time.[10]

In 1897 Ehrlich published a theory that would transform understandings of the mechanism behind the body's immune system and production of antibodies. Drawing on knowledge gained from his earlier investigation of dyes, he hypothesized that all cells possessed a wide variety of special receptors, which he termed "side chains," and that these functioned like gatekeepers or locks for each cell. Each side chain, he argued, permitted entry of substances only with structures matching their own. Such side chains served two purposes. The first and primary one was to let nutrients into the cell; the second was to act as a defense mechanism when a cell was attacked by foreign substances, or "antigens."[11] Cells would also generate additional side chains when they encountered an antigen and these would break off to become antibodies that bound and neutralized free-floating antigens. He argued that each antibody possessed receptors designed to match specific antigens in the way that a key fits a particular lock. Ehrlich borrowed this metaphor from Hermann Emil Fischer, a German chemist and former colleague, to explain the specific binding of enzymes to substrates (Figure 1.1).[12]

Ehrlich's theory was not without critics.[13] One of the strongest was Jules Bordet, a Belgian immunologist and microbiologist based at the Pasteur Institute, Paris, who detected the presence of another substance when heating fresh serum containing antibacterial antibodies during the 1890s.

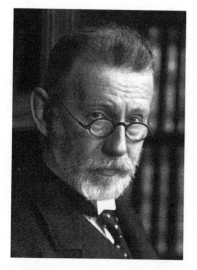 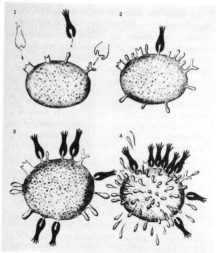

FIGURE 1.1. Paul Ehrlich, ca. 1908, with his depiction of his side-chain theory of immunity. Ehrlich believed that immune cells had a vast array of receptors (1), each specific to a particular substance (2). When a toxin interacted with the relevant receptor (3), the cell would be activated and would react by producing more receptors, which would then be released into the bloodstream as antibodies to neutralize the toxin (4). (Photograph from Bildarchiv Bayerische Staatsbibliothek, Porträt- und Ansichtensammlung, Bild-Nr. Port-003494; illustration from P. Ehrlich, "Croonian Lecture: On Immunity with Special Reference to Cell Life," *Proceedings of the Royal Society of London* 66 [1899]: 424–48)

Initially called "alexin" and later renamed "complement," this substance appeared to act as an accessory to antibodies in destroying antigens. Bordet's finding sparked an intense debate over the nature of the interaction between antibodies and their complements.[14]

The accuracy of the details of Ehrlich's theory was debated well into the twentieth century. Nonetheless, Ehrlich had laid the basis for a new understanding of immunity. His hypothesis not only explained the origin of protective antibodies, but also powerfully depicted, in words and later in diagrams, how antibodies functioned. Their ability to target precisely certain chemical groups on specific molecules led Ehrlich to prophesy that one day antibodies would be developed that, like "magic bullets," could seek out and destroy specific disease-causing microorganisms without harming the rest of the body. The term "magic bullets" came from Weber's romantic opera *Der Freischütz* (The marksman), in which a man sells his soul to the devil in exchange for magic bullets with which he hoped to win a marksmanship contest to gain a lady's hand.[15] Although Ehrlich soon turned to organic arsenic compounds for therapeutics, his dream about antibodies was to inspire other scientists. In 1901, Behring was awarded a Nobel Prize, followed by Ehrlich and Metchnikoff in 1908. Many mysteries about antibodies, however, lingered.[16]

A key question was when and how antibodies formed in the body and acquired their ability to bind to particular antigens. For much of the early twentieth century there were two competing schools of thought on this question, neither of which appreciated the importance of the other's work. Each view was shaped by a scientist's particular discipline training and outlook. On one side were the biologists who were interested in unraveling the interaction of the antigen with the cell and the implications this had for understanding the biological phenomenon behind the antibody response. On the other were the chemists, whose preoccupation with structural and quantitative relationships made them keen to determine the size of the antibody repertoire and the mechanism which established the specificity of antibodies.[17]

During the early twentieth century Ehrlich's side-chain hypothesis held center stage. According to this view, antibodies existed in the body independently of any exposure to antigens. Each antibody, Ehrlich argued, had a unique three-dimensional configuration with certain functional domains and affinity. This hypothesis, later known as the "selection theory," suggested that antigens selected antibodies with compatible receptors. Ehrlich's idea was soon challenged, however, by the "instruction theory," which portrayed antibodies as completely new entities, formed as the result of some form of an antigen template. Antigens were thought to interact and impress their specificity on normal substances, which in turn became antibodies. Champions of this idea were Karl Landsteiner, an Austrian biologist and physician based initially in Holland and then New York, and Oskar Bail, a German hygienist, bacteriologist, and immunologist at the German University in Prague. Doubts about Ehrlich's notion of a preexisting repertoire of antibodies strengthened after 1917 as a result of Landsteiner's experiments, which demonstrated that the body could produce antibodies against new synthetic antigens. Scientists wondered how, if Ehrlich's model were true, the body could prepare in advance effective antibodies to these novel antigens, as well as the wide diversity of antigens encountered during a lifetime.[18]

A vehement critic of Ehrlich's theory was Ludwick Fleck, a Polish microbiologist and immunologist. During the 1930s he rejected the then growing consensus that antibodies were chemical substances, arguing that a body's defense did not rest with any individual type of molecule like an antibody, but was inherent in the global property of serum. He was particularly dismissive of the "lock and key" concept, believing it oversimplified the host-pathogen interaction. From his perspective, the interaction between host and parasite was not to be considered as "attack" and "defense," but rather as a process "akin to development, ageing or cyclic fluctuations in life cycles of parasites and bacteria."[19]

Debates about antibodies and their purpose entered a new phase during the 1930s, spurred on by new quantitative analytical methods and new biochemical techniques, notably the introduction of ultra-centrifugation and electrophoresis. These helped shift the concept of antibodies from an "ill-defined set of serum activities" to definable protein molecules. It now became possible to describe the chemical structure of antibodies and antigens, and to establish how they bound to each other in molecular terms.[20]

At the forefront of the new research was Linus Pauling, an American chemist at the California Institute of Technology (Caltech). In 1940 he postulated that the binding of an antibody to an antigen was determined by the molecules' shape rather than their chemical composition. Echoing Ehrlich's earlier notion that antibodies and antigens worked together like a lock and a key, Pauling suggested that the structure and specificity of an antibody was molded by its physical interaction with a particular antigen rather than by its chemical composition.[21]

By the 1950s many scientists had become dissatisfied with the theories so far proposed because none adequately accounted for the simultaneous diversity and specificity of antibodies. In 1955 Niels Jerne, a Danish physician and immunologist then involved in serum measurement and standardization at the Danish National Serum Institute and for the World Health Organization, published a new theory. Reflecting his strong mathematical grounding, Jerne questioned the supposition underlying many contemporary theories: that there existed an infinite number of antibodies and antigens. He argued instead that initially mammals possess a small repertoire of antibodies in their blood, and that copies of antibodies are produced as a result of the successful binding of an antibody to an antigen. Jerne developed this idea, which he called the "natural selection theory," as a result of his exploration of the differential binding between antibodies and antigens, which had revealed that a single antibody could bind to many antigens. Borrowing the lock and key metaphor, he explained that keys did not have to fit 100 percent perfectly to open a lock.[22]

Initially, Jerne's hypothesis attracted little support because scientists could not see how a protein such as an antibody could replicate itself. Within two years, however, Jerne's insights provided the foundation for what was later known as "clonal selection theory." This theory was formulated independently by David Talmage at the University of Colorado and Frank Macfarlane Burnet at the Walter and Eliza Hall Institute of Medical Research in Melbourne. Like Jerne, Talmage argued that a small number of antibodies could distinguish between a larger number of antigen determinants, and stressed the importance of differentiating between an antiserum containing many different specificities and the individual antibodies it contained. Overall, clonal selection theory showed that the cell provided the mechanism for multiplying antibodies. Awarded a Nobel Prize in 1960 for his part in the formulation of clonal selection, Burnet surmised that the body possessed certain cells dedicated to making antibodies, and that these cells were where antibody diversity was generated, stored, and expressed. In this context, the antibody repertoire was produced by cells naturally, without any dependence on external antigens, and this repertoire was encoded by a small number of genes that were in place during the fetal stage of development and could expand through somatic mutation.[23]

The principle underlying clonal selection theory was soon supported experimentally. In 1958 two scientists, the molecular geneticist Joshua Lederberg and the biologist Gustav Nossal, published results of an experiment, originally launched to disprove the theory, that instead confirmed that one cell was responsible for the production of just one type of antibody.[24] The following year Lederberg elaborated the genetic framework described by Burnet, and showed the existence of a specific antibody gene that could mutate rapidly to a full repertoire, a process that took place not only during fetal development but throughout life.[25]

The clonal theory echoed the earlier findings of Astrid Fagreaus, a Swedish immunologist who had discovered in 1948 that antibodies were generated by B cells, a type of white blood cell in bone marrow.[26] Further research by Jacques Miller and Graham Mitchell in the early 1960s confirmed the view that bone marrow generates antibody cells (bone marrow lymphocyte B cells), with help from cells in the thymus (thymus lymphocyte T cells).[27]

Clonal selection explained not only antibody formation, but also observations made since the early twentieth century that antibody responses to a particular antigen were exponentially higher and faster after the initial encounter. Additionally, it appeared to provide a clue to immunodeficiency diseases as well as the mechanisms underlying auto-immunity and self-tolerance that had been puzzling scientists since the early twentieth century.[28] Overall the theory helped bring together the humoral and cellular theories used to explain the function of the immune system as a whole.

As theories about antibody formation twisted and turned, the application of antibodies to clinical problems was taking on a life of its own. By the mid-twentieth century antibodies had become a major tool in medical treatment in the form of serum therapy. The foundation for this work went back to Behring, who had started to apply his antibody discoveries to find a cure for diphtheria in the 1890s. Known colloquially as "the strangler of children," diphtheria was a pressing concern, claiming the lives of around fifty thousand German children annually. By the summer of 1891, Behring had demonstrated the therapeutic possibilities of blood serum taken from animals immunized against diphtheria, but was unable to develop a supply of strong enough serum in high enough quantities to treat humans. To resolve this problem Behring entered a partnership in 1893 with Ehrlich and the pharmaceutical manufacturer Farbwerke Hoechst. Within a year they had developed a standardized, potent serum from horses that proved clinically safe for use in humans. Their success was based on Ehrlich's observation that a toxin needed to be injected over a long period and in steadily increasing doses to secure a high potency of antibodies in animal serum, and that this potency varied over time. The trick was to capture an animal's serum when the antibodies had reached their maximum strength.[29]

The new serum therapy helped to decrease diphtheria mortality from 50 to 25 percent after its introduction to Paris, offering great hope in eliminating a much feared disease. Next Behring turned his attention to developing similar therapies for tetanus and streptococcal infections. By 1896 Hoechst was marketing tetanus serum for immunizing humans and animals. Yet demand for the therapy remained small, reflecting the low incidence of tetanus. Efforts to develop serum therapies against streptococcal infections and tuberculosis also had little success.[30]

Optimism about serum therapy was reignited with the successful emergence of a treatment for meningococcal meningitis, an epidemic disease that was taking lives across the world in the early twentieth century. The treatment, which reduced mortality by half, resulted from the separate efforts of the German physician Georg Jochmann and the American physician and pathologist Simon Flexner. By the late 1920s antipneumococcal sera had also become a central component of pneumonia control in six U.S. states. This was facilitated by a precipitation technique developed by Lloyd Felton, a scientist at Harvard Medical School, which enabled greater purification of antibodies in serum.[31]

By the 1930s serum therapy had become the choice treatment for many infectious diseases. In addition to those already mentioned, it included treatments for erysipelas, scarlet fever, whooping cough, anthrax, botulism, gas gangrene, brucellosis, dysentery, tularemia, measles, poliomyelitis, mumps, influenza meningitis, and chickenpox. Serum therapy was not without its side effects, however. Labeled "serum sickness," symptoms included fever, rashes, joint pains, and sometimes anaphylactic complications. Behring observed such problems as early as 1893. Almost all patients receiving serum therapy manifested some form of adverse reaction, even if mild. These were attributed to the fact that serum preparations were drawn from animals, so contained proteins foreign to humans.[32]

Over the years, scientists tried various solutions. Early on, Behring discovered that water, salts, proteins, and ferments could break down diphtheria serum, and developed a fractionation technique that separated the antibodies found in the serum. This method enriched the antibodies in the serum, thus lowering the dosage needed and decreasing the frequency of side effects. Reactions in patients were also significantly reduced with the introduction of Felton's precipitation technique in 1924 and the application of ultra-centrifugation and electrophoresis from 1939, all of which provided more purified antibodies.[33]

While preparations from animal serum were being improved, human serum also began to be investigated. By the second decade of the twentieth century, two French physicians, Charles Nicolle and Ernest Conseil, had shown that it was possible to induce immunity against infectious diseases like typhus and measles by using serum taken from patients convalescing from these diseases. In 1920 it was found that patients who recovered from diseases like measles retained protective antibodies into adult life. Use of human serum for treatment nonetheless remained constrained because large quantities of serum were required. In 1933, however, Charles McKhann and his colleagues at Harvard devised a new technique of obtaining purified antibodies from human placentas. This not only ensured greater purity, but also a more highly concentrated source of antibodies than before. The development of new fractionation methods deployed by Edwin Cohn in 1944 for military blood supplies led to further progress. It enabled the production of concentrated gamma-globulin, a class of proteins discovered in 1939 to contain most of the antibodies in human blood. Cohn's approach made it possible to give much smaller doses of human serum, which reduced the risk of serum sickness. His method was adopted quickly for the prevention and treatment of measles.[34]

Alongside efforts to improve the purification of animal and human serum, artificial antibodies were explored. As early as 1894 Behring hypothesized that it might be possible one day to produce antibodies "without the aid of an animal body." Many scientists subsequently attempted to make antibodies in vitro. By 1929 at least ten successful attempts to create artificial antibodies had been reported, and a hundred clinics and research laboratories were thought to be active in this area. An application for a patent for an artificial diphtheria antibody was also filed in Germany during this period.[35]

The drive to make artificial antibodies gathered momentum in the 1940s with the work of Pauling, who established a research program at Caltech in 1941 for this purpose, funded by the Rockefeller Foundation. Within a year he had announced the successful production of an artificial antibody and applied for a patent, establishing its commercial exploitation with Lederle Laboratories. Excitement for the project soon dissipated, however, when other scientists, notably Landsteiner, found it impossible to reproduce Pauling's results.[36]

The inability to make artificial antibodies was particularly disappointing given the difficulties of standardizing animal and human serum and the expense of serum production. Because animals and humans cannot be stimulated to produce specific antibodies, their serum contains thousands of different antibodies, each differing in affinity and specificity. Serum varies not only batch to batch, but between the particular animals or humans, because of the wide differences in exposures to toxins over a lifetime. These variables mean that each new batch requires extensive characterization and testing. Furthermore, serum preparations required intravenous injection, demanding considerable expertise from the physician. Not surprisingly, then, interest in serum therapy dwindled with the arrival of sulphonamides in the 1930s and then penicillin in the 1940s. These medications proved not only easier and cheaper to produce but also more straightforward to administer and less toxic. They were also far more effective against infectious diseases.[37]

More success was to be had in the use of antisera for diagnostics. Scientists had begun to investigate the use of antibody-containing sera for diagnostic tests since the late nineteenth century based on the observation that antibodies could disintegrate (lyse), separate (precipitate), or clump together (agglutinate) bacteria within a solution. With antigens and antibodies found to have predictable biochemical reactions, physicians soon deployed antisera as diagnostic probes to define, isolate, and measure a wide variety of immunological molecules. The first was the Widal test, which was introduced in 1896 for the diagnosis of typhoid. This was followed by the Landsteiner test for blood grouping (1900–1901), and the Wasserman test for detecting syphilis (1906). Many others followed, one of the most important being the Coombs anti-globulin test developed in 1945, which was used to detect antibodies causing the premature destruction of red blood cells. It proved important for both blood transfusions and detecting Rh incompatibility between mother and fetus. By the 1960s, the use of antisera for diagnostics was widespread in clinics and hospitals, aided in part by the emergence of electrophoresis and labeling techniques, which employed first enzymes and then radioisotopes.[38]

Despite the success of serological diagnostics, in the years after the Second World War many clinicians perceived immunology and its application as an auxiliary medical discipline of little relevance. During the 1950s, however, a deepening knowledge of the chemical structure of antibodies and the mechanism behind their diversity provided a new avenue for improving the clinical utility of antibodies for diagnosis and therapy. A key to the antibody enigma came from an unexpected source: myeloma cell lines (also known as plasmacytomas). As early as 1951, while studying the blood of patients with myeloma (a type of cancer that develops from plasma cells in the bone marrow), Henry Kunkel, an American immunologist based at the Rockefeller Institute, New York, unexpectedly discovered that myeloma proteins resembled normal antibodies and that malignant plasma cells of multiple myeloma produced just one abnormal antibody. This contrasted with normal plasma cells, which produce a large array of antibodies. His observation, and the fact that each myeloma cell was identical and fairly easy to obtain in large quantities from blood or urine taken from multiple myeloma patients, led him to investigate myelomas as a model for normal antibodies. Soon Kunkel and his colleagues had unraveled the chain structure of myeloma proteins and divided them into different classes and subclasses.[39]

The use of myeloma cells for investigating normal antibodies spread beyond Kunkel's laboratory, following a major advance in the production of such cells by the molecular biologist Michael Potter and colleagues at the National Cancer Institute in Bethesda from the late 1950s. Potter had found, serendipitously, that an injection of mineral oil into the peritoneal cavity of BALB/c mice, a particular strain of laboratory mice, induced the growth of myeloma cells. The method provided for the indefinite growth of myeloma cells in mice on an unprecedented scale. By 1962 Potter and his team had established a collection of myeloma cell lines for distribution to researchers around the world. Access to these cells was enhanced by various researchers, most notably Kengo Horibata and A. W. Harris under the supervision of Melvin Cohn at the Salk Institute in San Diego, who adapted Potter's mouse myelomas to grow in tissue culture. With a ready supply of myeloma cells, scientists could much more easily investigate the normal immune response.[40]

Research into the immune system was further enhanced by the appearance of another tool in 1963: a plaque assay that helped scientists to see and count the antibody-producing cells with their naked eye. Devised by Niels Jerne at the University of Pittsburgh, with his postdoctoral researcher Albert Nordin, this technique provided a means to determine how many antibody cells were involved in the antibody response.[41]

Theo Staehelin, a fellow colleague of Jerne and Nordin at Pittsburgh, who witnessed the test in its formative stage, recalled Niels walking "one day in November 1962 into our lab. He held a beaker with a turbid, dilute suspension of sheep erythrocytes in his hand and asked . . . [rhetorically] whether one might see the difference upon lysis of the cells. On the bench, I had a bottle of the detergent sodium desoxycholate (10%) which we used to solubilize rat liver microsomal membranes in order to liberate membrane-bound polysomes. With a pipette, I added a few drops to the red cell suspension under slight stirring. Within seconds, the turbid solution turned transparent like a light red wine. Niels looked quite pleased. . . . Just a few weeks later, Niels and Al Nordin announced and showed around in the department the result of a single experiment whose simplicity, beauty, and significance excited everyone. It was the "Plaque Formation in Agar by Single Antibody-Producing Cells."[42] The technique for viewing the antibodies spread rapidly to laboratories all over the world, and during the next two decades was cited in publications more than four thousand times.[43]

During the 1960s antibody research entered a new era as a result of the work of two scientists: Gerald Edelman, an American biologist and former student of Kunkel based at the Rockefeller Institute for Medical Research in New York City, and Rodney Porter, an English biochemist working initially at the National Institute for Medical Research in Mill Hill, London, and then at St. Mary's Hospital in London. Each scientist was interested in deciphering the structure of antibodies to answer the long-standing question of how a group of antibody proteins that seemed almost identical could simultaneously target any one of a multitude of antigens. By early 1962 they had independently shown that the structure of antibodies consisted of heavy and light protein chains, which joined together to form three sections yielding a molecule shaped like the letter "Y."[44]

The work of Edelman and Porter, which led to their being awarded a Nobel Prize in 1972, inspired further investigations into antibody structure across the world. By 1969 the amino-acid sequence of human antibodies had been unraveled, a detailed picture of how the antibody worked had been built up, and its composition of both constant and highly varying regions had been revealed. Central to these developments was the collaborative analysis of amino-acid sequences carried out by a young German

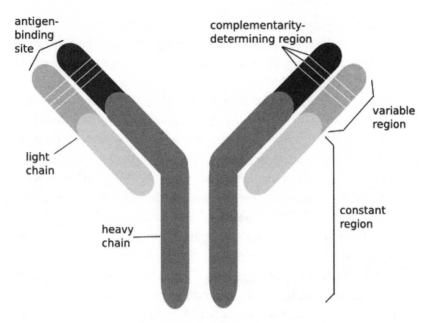

FIGURE 1.2. Basic structure of an antibody

postdoctoral fellow Norbert Hilschman, together with Kunkel and the American chemist Lyman Craig at the Rockefeller Institute. By the end of the 1960s, they had determined that while the upper regions of the "Y," each made up of a light chain paired with a long chain, varied between antibodies, the stem region of the "Y" shape, which is composed of the two long heavy chains, was constant (Figure 1.2). The top arms of the "Y" provided unique binding sites designed for each specific antigen, whereas the stem bound together other components required for attacking such targets. Finally scientists had an explanation for what had puzzled them so long. Variations in the amino-acid sequence of individual antibodies in the upper regions of their "Y" shape was responsible for their multiple binding shapes, which in turn enabled their attachment to different antigens.[45]

The foundation in 1969 of what was to become the world's largest institute of immunological research in the 1970s, the Basel Institute of Immunology (BII), led to the further investigation of antibodies. The BII was one of a number of basic research institutes established and funded by the multinational pharmaceutical company F. Hoffmann–La Roche in this period to keep the company abreast of developments in biology, cell biology, and biochemistry. Championed by Alfred Pletscher, the company's director of medical research, the BII officially opened its doors in 1971.

By this time, scientists already knew a great deal about the immune system and how it worked, but questions remained. The BII's overall objective was to conduct basic research into immunology, with a particular emphasis on the "molecular, cellular, genetic and regulatory problems of antibody formation and antibody structure and function."[46] Directed by Jerne, a major founding member, the institute rapidly became an international hub of collaborative research. Its turnover of scientists was kept deliberately high in order to keep research and ideas flowing. Theo Staehelin, one of BII's first permanent members, described the institute as "the mecca of immunology." Its influence extended well beyond its physical boundaries. Its *Annual Reports* soon provided the largest circulation of immunology news in the world, and many of its visitors, who spent their formative scientific years there, later became internationally renowned immunologists.[47]

In 1974, Jerne electrified immunological research with the publication of his "idiotypic network theory." Jerne aimed to provide a blueprint for understanding the regulatory mechanism governing the immune system, looking specifically at how stimulatory and suppressive factors were balanced. His central tenet was that there was "a vast number of immune responses [in the body that were] . . . going on all the time, even in the absence of a foreign antigen." This meant that antibodies primarily responded to each other, and treated external antigens as subordinate, merely disturbing the equilibrium normally existing between "idiotypes," a term first coined by the French immunologist Jacques Oudin in 1966 to describe the unique antigenic regions of individual antibodies that elicit an antibody response. Importantly, Jerne argued that antibodies reacted not only to foreign antigens, but also to self-constituent antibodies, which could explain the paucity of autoimmune responses.[48]

Not everyone was convinced by Jerne's theory. Many doubted whether it could indeed be tested empirically. In time, regulatory elements other than the idiotypes highlighted by Jerne proved to have a more prominent role in immune regulation, diminishing his theory's relevance. Nonetheless, it immediately galvanized research, setting off the equivalent of what the historian Anne-Marie Moulin has called a "Copernican revolution" in the field of immunology. Critically, it stimulated new experimental research dedicated to unraveling the nature and consequences of network regulation and to exploring antibody diversity.[49]

While the immunological community was impressed by Jerne's new theory, the emergence of a more practical development excited them even more. This was the development of a technique to create hybrid cells capable of secreting monoclonal antibodies, each identical (clones) and derived from a single (mono) kind of lymphocyte B cell.

Scientists had experimented for years with antibodies taken from antibody-containing blood sera, using them as highly selective and sensitive reagents for the structural analysis of a wide variety of antigens. The information gained from these experiments was limited, however, by the inherent heterogeneity of antisera, which could result in cross-reactions during the testing process. Devising single antibodies with known specificity to particular antigens was therefore a highly significant goal. The idea that someday it might be possible to adapt the myeloma line to secrete limitless amounts of antibody was first put forward in 1967 by Melvin Cohn. The task was not easy. One of the difficulties was finding a way of isolating an individual antibody from the billions produced by the immune system. The closest scientists had come to realizing this ambition was through the use of myeloma cells. But while myeloma cells provided an abundant source of single antibodies, it was not known which antigens they targeted. Part of the problem is that myeloma cells are triggered by malignancy, a process that hits cells at random. Attempts to induce tumors to produce antibodies to an injected antigen had also so far failed. Myeloma cells on their own were therefore unsuitable for experimental studies exploring the molecular basis of antibody specificity.[50]

Methods to create individual antibodies with known specificity were to be given a boost by new techniques for the fusion of cells developed in the 1960s. Cellular fusion had been of interest ever since the nineteenth century to both cellular biologists and geneticists. Research in this area took off in a new direction in 1960 when Georges Barski and colleagues at the Institut Gustave Roussy in Villejuif, France, spotted cellular fusion between two different tumor cell lines that had been taken from two different inbred strains of mice and grown as a cell mixture in tissue cultures. This research quickly attracted international attention because it raised the hope that a new technique for cellular fusion could now be devised to replace time-consuming breeding methods. Crucially, the technique opened the way for more genetic analyses in mammals, particularly the investigation of mutated genes responsible for heritable human diseases. Inducing cellular fusion initially proved difficult. From 1962, however, the process became easier through the introduction of the Sendai virus to promote fusion, the use of myeloma cells, and the adoption of the selective hypoxanthine-aminopterin-thymidine (HAT) medium to separate the fused cells. Soon cellular fusion was being undertaken by scientists on a large scale, with many of them successfully fusing two different mammalian species: human and mouse.[51]

One of the earliest scientists to exploit the new methods to produce single antibodies with known specificity was Joseph Sinkovics, a Hungarian clinical pathologist and laboratory clinical virologist based at the M.D. Anderson Hospital in Houston. Starting his research in the mid-1960s, he successfully developed a cell line of antibodies with known specificity that could be grown indefinitely by fusing antibody-producing plasma cells with lymphoma cells. Such antibodies could be grown in continuous cultures in spinner bottles or as ascites tumors in mice.

Sinkovics and his team were unable to take his research further, however, due to a lack of funding. At the same time, in the early 1970s, at the National Institute of Medical Research in Mill Hill, London, Brigitte Ita Askonas, an Austrian-Canadian biochemist who had just spent a year at the BII, and the immunologists Alan Williamson and Brian Wright found a way to clone B cells (single antibodies with known specificity) in vivo, using spleen cells from mice immunized with haptenated carrier antigens.[52] Their work was part of a wider project to understand the process underlying the generation of B cells and antibody diversity. While their work revealed many aspects of B cells, the antibodies had a major drawback—they survived for only a short time.[53]

The successful development of antibodies in Texas and London was largely ignored. What attracted greater interest was a splenic fragments culture technique devised by Norman Klinman, an American immunologist based at the University of Pennsylvania with an attachment to the Wistar Institute, an independent research institution internationally renowned for its development of vaccines against polio, rabies, and rubella.

Klinman's technique, which was published in 1969, provided a powerful tool for the isolation of single B lymphocytes secreting a single type of antibody. The method involved irradiating mice spleens, thereby destroying their antibody-producing capability, then injecting them with new antibody-producing cells, some of which lodged in the spleen. Cubes of the spleen were then grown individually in tissue culture with an added antigen. If a given fragment had an antibody-producing cell, it would produce antibodies, called "monofocal" antibodies, that were very specific to that particular antigen.[54]

One of the first to adopt Klinman's technique was Walter Gerhard, a Swiss-trained physician who moved from the BII to take up postdoctoral research under Klinman in the early 1970s. He was trying to develop antisera as a tool to understand the antigenic structure of hemagglutinin, a glycoprotein found on the surface of influenza viruses that was considered an important mechanism in the recurrence of influenza in man. Frustrated by the heterogeneity of the antisera he was using, Gerhard was looking for a means to improve them. Klinman's technique offered him a major way forward.[55]

By 1975 Gerhard had successfully cultivated monofocal antibodies with known specificity against influenza viruses. Some of his best hybrid cells produced between two hundred and three hundred nanograms of monofocal antibodies. This was a sufficient quantity to test different strains of the influenza virus and to determine immune responses to influenza. Disappointingly, however, Gerhard's hybrid cells began to decrease their secretion of antibodies after thirty to forty days and usually petered out altogether after ninety days.[56]

At the same time, Ron Levy, an oncologist at Stanford University and former colleague of Klinman, deployed the method to produce tumor antigens in order to find a way of improving cancer diagnostics and treatment. With Klinman's technique, Levy recounted, "We got really high-quality antibodies but only for a short period of time. The cells would die, and then we would have to make them again." Overall, too, the technique yielded very few antibodies, so it was unsuitable for use as a long-term diagnostic and therapeutic tool.[57]

More progress was made at the Laboratory of Molecular Biology (LMB) in Cambridge, England, by the Argentinian-born British immunologist César Milstein and the German postdoctoral biologist Georges Köhler who joined him from the BII in 1974. Both were interested in finding mutant genes in the variable region of antibodies that bind to antigens, and they shared the belief that this approach was important to understanding the process of somatic mutation (the genetic alteration of cells after conception), which they believed underlay the diversity of antibodies. Milstein and researchers elsewhere had already carried out some groundwork for this research. But they faced a laborious hunt for the mutant genes because they lacked an antibody with defined specificity. Given that an antibody with clearly defined specificity to a target would provide the most effective means of detecting the slight differences caused by such mutations, Milstein and Köhler quickly turned their attention to devising one.[58]

To achieve their goal they decided to use tissue culturing and a hybrid cell line that Milstein had created with his postdoctoral researcher Dick Cotton by fusing a human lymphocyte with two myelomas (one from a mouse and the other from a rat). The significance of the cell line was that it could express antibodies to the parental cells. Milstein and Köhler also drew from the work of Jerrold Schwaber and Edward Cohen based at the University of Chicago, who in 1973 had produced a hybrid cell line able to secrete both myeloma and lymphoctye-derived antibodies through the fusion of human lymphocytes and mouse myeloma cells.[59]

In order to overcome some of the drawbacks of previous efforts, Milstein and Köhler tried to create a hybrid cell by fusing a myeloma cell with a normal spleen cell taken from immunized mice. This they hoped would generate an immortal cell line capable of secreting antibodies with known specificity. As Milstein explained, "We would be applying the well-established cell-fusion technique to a new purpose, namely to fix in a permanent cell line a function that is normally expressed only in a 'terminal' cell: the plasma cell derived from a B lymphocyte stimulated by an antigen."[60]

The antigen they decided to target was sheep red blood cells (SRBC) because the mouse's immune system was known to react vigorously against them. Antibodies against SRBCs could also be easily detected by Jerne and Nordin's plaque essay test, a procedure that Köhler had learned from Herman Waldmann at Cambridge University. With the skilled technical assistance of Shirley Howe, by December 1974 various experiments were being conducted in earnest. Initially three different myeloma cell lines (P3, 289, and P1) were selected as fusion partners for the spleen cells.

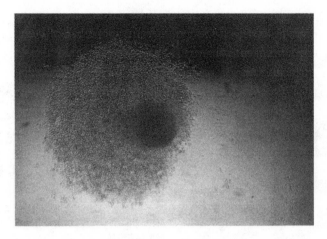

FIGURE 1.3. Microscope photo of a hybridoma cell secreting
monoclonal antibodies (Geoff Hale)

Eventually, however, Köhler determined that the most successful myeloma
fusion partner was X63, his variant of a subclone of the P3 myeloma cell
line originally prepared by David Secher, then a postdoctoral student at
LMB. It originated from Horibata and Harris's adaptation of Potter's
myeloma cell lines in Cohn's laboratory at the Salk Institute. The advantage of X63 was that it was resistant to azaguanine, a reagent used to
promote fusion. Köhler grew the cells in a HAT medium and added inactivated Sendai virus to promote fusion.[61]

Next, Köhler adapted Jerne and Nordin's plaque test to determine
whether any of the hybrid cells he produced would bind to SRBCs, by link-
ing SRBCs with a fluorescein dye that glows green when put under an
ultraviolet light. Should any of the antibodies produced in the experiment
lock on to the surface of the SRBCs, he would be able to detect a bright
green halo.[62]

By the end of December Köhler could see a number of cells growing
in the HAT medium, but was unsure whether any had generated hybrid
cells secreting antibodies with specificity for the SRBCs. Furthermore,
by the time he could analyze the cells, some fungi had contaminated the
culture so he was forced to go back to square one. Finally, on January 24,
1975, he was ready to try out his plaque test on some cells he had created
by fusing X63 with the spleen cells taken from a mouse immunized
against SRBCs. Expecting the process to take several hours, Köhler started

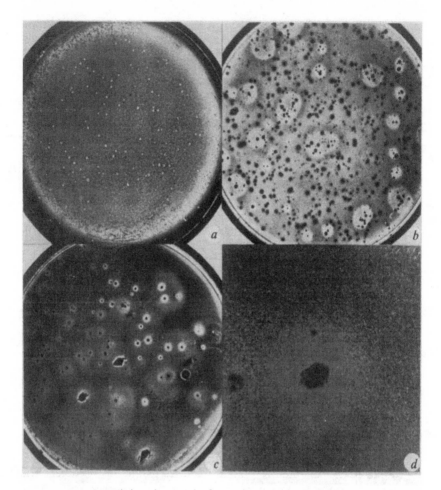

FIGURE 1.4. Petri dishes showing the first Mabs grown by César Milstein and Georges Köhler (G. Köhler and C. Milstein, "Continuous Cultures of Fused Cells Secreting Antibody of Predefined Specificity," *Nature* 256, no. 5517 [1975]: 495–97, fig. 2)

the test at 5 p.m., then went home. He returned some hours later with his wife as company because he expected boring results. He recalled, "I looked down at the first two plates. I saw these halos. That was fantastic. I shouted, I kissed my wife. I was all happy. The other results were positive as well. It was the best result I could think of." Not only had he created hybrid cells that secreted antibodies that bound to SRBCs, but the number of antibodies they had generated was also far greater than anticipated.[63]

Following this success, Köhler and Milstein repeated their experiment twice more to see if the technique was reproducible. When these experi-

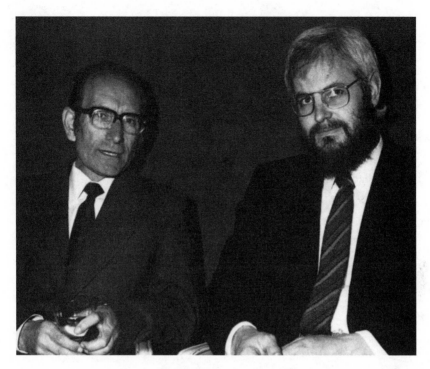

FIGURE 1.5. César Milstein (*left*) and Georges Köhler in 1984, around the time of their Nobel Prize (Celia Milstein/MRC Laboratory of Molecular Biology)

ments proved positive, they excitedly realized that they possessed a tool that scientists had been striving to make for many years: an immortal cell line capable of producing endless quantities of identical antibodies with known specificity. Their method would later be dubbed "hybridoma technology" and the antibodies it produced "monoclonal antibodies," to signify that they were derived from a single hybrid cell (Figure 1.3). In May 1975, the two scientists submitted a paper announcing their experiment to *Nature*, one of the most prestigious scientific journals in the world, in which they declared their technique to be a promising development for both medicine and industry. Yet the significance of their achievement eluded the journal's editors, who asked Köhler and Milstein to shorten their article and did not include it in the section reserved for findings of major importance. The article was published in August 1975.[64]

The hybridoma technology marked the culmination of years of research into fighting infectious disease and understanding the immunological mechanism by which living organisms defended themselves from foreign invaders. In 1984, Milstein and Köhler were awarded the Nobel Prize jointly with Jerne "for theories concerning the specificity in development and control of the immune system and the discovery of the principle for production of monoclonal antibodies" (Figures 1.4, 1.5). Their discovery was achieved despite many blind alleys and fierce theoretical battles. Now, at last, it seemed possible that scientists had found the powerful "magic bullet" against infectious disease that Paul Ehrlich had envisaged many decades earlier. But exactly how monoclonal antibodies could be applied in this way remained unknown.

CHAPTER TWO

A Hesitant Start

PATENTS, POLITICS, AND PROCESS

IT IS EASY TO IMAGINE that monoclonal antibodies, which are now recognized as one of the major advances of biotechnology since the early 1970s, were adopted overnight. But their dissemination necessitated complex negotiations among actors in numerous scientific laboratories across the world, negotiations that also played out on the political stage. Central questions arose over who possessed rights to the technology, and whether those rights should be protected. Much of the debate about rights was shaped by whether scientists believed the technique was revolutionary or merely part of a long chain of scientific discoveries. Mabs were not particularly new either theoretically or conceptually in 1975, because similar antibodies had been produced before. The difference was essentially one of scale.[1]

Milstein recognized the technology's potential early. One letter he wrote in July 1975, a month before publishing the technique in *Nature*, underlines the practical utility that he and Köhler ascribed to it: "We believe the technique described, for the derivation of tissue-cultured lines synthesizing antibodies against red cells, could be of more general application for the production of permanent cultures of cells synthesising other antibodies. . . . The great advantage of cell cultures is that one can not only standardize the product but also obtain antibodies of the

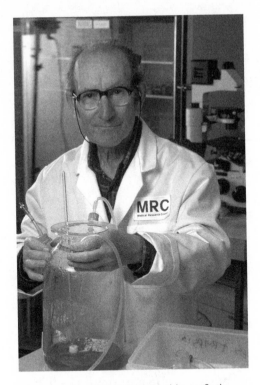

FIGURE 2.1. César Milstein holding a flask
containing Mabs growing in a fluid (MRC
Laboratory of Molecular Biology)

mono-clonal type, i.e. of a uniquely defined specificity. We are at the
moment rather excited about these possibilities" (Figure 2.1).[2]

John Newell, a scientific correspondent for the British Broadcasting
Corporation's World Service, was one of the first outside Milstein's circle
to grasp the technique's possibilities, and he immediately publicized the
promise that Mabs held out for new diagnostics and drugs. Alerting radio listeners to what sounded like "science fiction," he asserted that the
technology could have "big applications, both in clinical medicine and
in the drug industry." Huge numbers of antibodies could now be manufactured outside the human body, opening new vistas for research and
for medical applications.[3]

Niels Jerne, the BII director, also quickly understood the enormous
potential of Mabs. Upon reading the *Nature* article, he immediately invited Alfred Pletscher, head of Global Research Roche, to his office, and

explained the great potential of this novel technology for diagnostics. He urged Pletscher to initiate a "Project of Applied Immunology" (PAI) at Roche. Following this, Roche created twenty-two new scientific positions for the development of Mab diagnostics.[4]

Another champion of the technique was Tony Vickers, a Medical Research Council (MRC) administrator with scientific training. After hearing Milstein present his work to an MRC internal meeting on the safety of genetic engineering, and reading proofs of the *Nature* article, Vickers wrote to Milstein in mid-July 1975: "Your paper confirms my feeling that this approach to antibody synthesis has great commercial implications. It is most important that action is taken as soon as any exploitable idea gets to the stage where patent protection can be applied for. I have therefore taken the step—and I do hope that you will forgive me for acting without consulting you first—of drawing the attention of the National Research and Development Corporation (NRDC) to your preprint." His intervention was designed to prompt action from the NRDC, the body responsible for patenting MRC innovations.[5]

NRDC officials, however, were slow to react. In October 1976 they finally replied, claiming that they could not "identify any immediate practical applications which could be pursued as a commercial venture" and concluded, "Unless further work indicates a diagnostic application or industrial end product which we can protect . . . , we would not suggest taking any further action ourselves." Overall, Milstein was given to understand that patents of his technique were "out of the question."[6]

In part, the NRDC's response reflected the initial difficulty that many had in understanding how the technique could be used. James Gowan, for example, who headed an MRC unit that heard Milstein's presentation at the same meeting as Vickers, remembered being "mightily intrigued" by the science, but did not imagine "there was a vast catalogue of diagnostic reagents just waiting on the horizon, or perhaps even [therapeutics]."[7]

The NRDC's inaction was to become highly controversial in the late 1970s when the British economy was in decline and unemployment soaring. One solution was thought to lie in harnessing the power of biotechnology, which was then spawning an exciting new industry in America. The NRDC's failure to patent Mabs rallied those concerned about the country's economic future, who depicted it as yet another example, alongside penicillin, of Britain's failure to exploit its scientific discoveries commercially. As a *Nature* reporter asked: "Has Britain lost large potential royalties through a failure to recognise the commercial potential of antibodies?"[8]

Margaret Thatcher took the nonpatenting issue up particularly forcefully after she became the British prime minister in 1979. At an impromptu conference on the matter at 10 Downing Street, she was heard to remark that the days of the NRDC were "numbered." Thatcher was a trained chemist so had a keen understanding of the technology, and she wanted private capital to back its development. Another strong critic of the NRDC was Keith Joseph, secretary of state for industry, who was looking for an excuse to privatize nationalized industries. He had no understanding of Mabs or what they could do. Strong criticism was also published in a report from a working party then investigating how to advance biotechnology in Britain. This group largely laid the blame on the scientists themselves. Milstein was to feel the brunt of this attack for many years.[9]

The British government's bitterness was heightened by the fact that in October 1979 and April 1980 Hilary Koprowski (Figure 2.2), director of the Wistar Institute in Philadelphia, and his colleagues, were granted two U.S. patents for Mabs using myeloma cells originally supplied by Milstein in September 1976.[10] These patents covered Mabs produced against influenza and tumor antigens. The broad claims made by the patents were especially troubling. In an article in the widely circulated journal *Science* in 1980, a scientific journalist, Nicholas Wade, referred to Milstein's unhappiness about the Wistar Institute's extensive claims—as Milstein apparently put it, "they are essentially patenting our procedure." Many other scientists shared this view. Wade claimed that Koprowski had broken an agreement with Milstein not to patent any product based on his cells.[11]

Incensed by Wade's implication of theft, Koprowski and his colleague Carlo Croce quickly drafted a response that the editors at *Science* eventually agreed to publish after being legally threatened. Koprowski and Croce disputed having contravened any agreement, claiming the patent subject had never arisen in the Koprowski-Milstein correspondence about the cells. Milstein's papers, however, reveal a more complex picture. By early 1977, it was standard practice for recipients of cells to agree in advance not to patent any products. In May 1977 Milstein gave Koprowski permission to transfer the Cambridge cells to another colleague, on the condi-

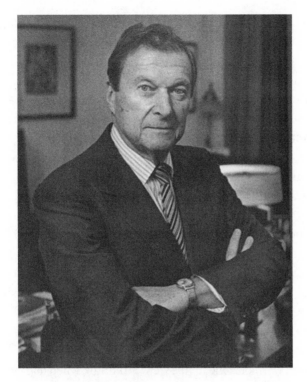

FIGURE 2.2. Hilary Koprowski, first scientist awarded a patent for Mabs and co-founder of Centocor (Wistar Institute, Wistar Archive Collections, Philadelphia, PA)

tion that "the products will not be made subject of any patent rights." Poignantly, Milstein later penned on this letter, "Yet Koprowski took up a patent in June 1977!" Similarly, in February 1978, an American colleague wrote to Koprowski emphasizing Milstein's request that no products made from his cells should be patented. Despite this, the first Wistar patent application was officially filed in April 1978, the second in June 1978.[12]

Milstein's correspondence makes it clear that he was totally unaware of Koprowski's patent intentions. In November 1976 Koprowski wrote to Milstein stating: "Croce's and my studies with your line progress satisfactorily," adding, "If we get any positive results in producing monoclonal antiviral antibodies we will let you know immediately." After this Koprowski and Croce successfully generated hybrid cells by fusing Milstein's myeloma cells with spleen cells from mice that his colleague

Walter Gerhard had immunized with influenza cells. These hybrid cells secreted Mabs specific to the influenza-A virus. Gerhard then replicated this work. Milstein, however, heard nothing about this. On the letter Milstein received from Koprowski dated November 1976—in which he promised to inform Milstein if they produced antiviral Mabs— Milstein subsequently noted that "he never did! Instead . . . he took [out] a patent without ever letting me know." Although Milstein and Koprowski met face-to-face in London in July 1978, soon after Wistar filed its patent applications, the topic was never discussed.[13]

Milstein first learned of Wistar's filing from Eric Tridgell, an NRDC official, in March 1979. The news took Milstein completely by surprise. He was shocked to see that the Wistar application requested "a blanket patent for deriving *any* clone directed against *any* virus and using myeloma cells from *any* origin." Incredulously, Milstein wrote: "It is obvious that animals immunised with an immunogen (and viruses are immunogens) will give rise to plasma cells which can be hybridized. Nothing is new therefore in the patent except the *specific* lines they [the Wistar scientists] have derived."[14]

Milstein was not alone in this view. Strikingly, when questioned about Koprowski's application for a patent, Robert Gallo, a colleague of Koprowski's at the U.S. National Cancer Institute, admitted, "I wouldn't have done it for fear of reprimand." "But," he continued, "on the other hand, science needs catalysts to speed up the process. In those days, it might have taken five years if everyone had sat back and waited for Milstein/Köhler and the British to take the next step."[15]

The confusion over the dealings with Koprowski highlights the casual way that the Cambridge cells were initially supplied. The only conditions imposed on recipients in the very early days were that they acknowledge the source of the cells in publications and that they seek Milstein's permission when passing them to others. This type of flexibility was common at the time. Indeed, the MRC encouraged its scientists to share materials. As Michael Clark, one of Milstein's doctoral students in 1978, recalled, LMB researchers regularly exchanged cells and reagents, with the LMB acting as a "swap shop." Such sharing was necessary when scientific materials could not be purchased. LMB scientists often opened their freezers to other researchers knowing that this was usually reciprocated. A note to Milstein in 1982 illustrates the informality of these years:

"May I give you a little reminder about the way we have traditionally treated requests for mouse cell lines. When we first started sending these (P3) lines out we created a note giving the conditions that recipients were asked to comply with. This was sent with the cells and we never did ask people to sign and return it—although some did so spontaneously."[16]

A more formal procedure was established only in 1978 at the instigation of the NRDC after Milstein developed a new line of Mabs based on rats. From this time on, all recipients were expected to sign a form waiving the right to any patents before cells were sent. Nonetheless, as an MRC official admitted to Milstein in 1979, how far this could be enforced was debatable. He advised omitting the restriction.[17]

Whatever the legalities, an important consideration in the patent saga is the way that Koprowski and his team regarded the Cambridge technique. Papers they published in the early years, and interviews conducted with them later on, indicate that while they viewed Köhler's and Milstein's myeloma cell line to have "excellent properties," they did not regard the hybridoma technology as anything particularly different from the cellular hybridization process deployed by the Wistar Institute and elsewhere since the 1960s. They also did not consider Köhler and Milstein's Mabs as particularly original because they had already produced antibodies using the Klinman method outlined in Chapter 1. The only difference was that Köhler and Milstein's technique facilitated the reproduction and survival of the antibodies. From Koprowski's perspective the Cambridge myeloma cell was merely a useful agent for the institute's ongoing experiments to develop antibodies against viral antigens and cancer, and in any case, he pointed out, their fusion procedure originated from John Littlefield. Koprowski was equally dismissive of the Cambridge Mabs because they targeted sheep red blood cells. This he regarded as only of curiosity value with no clinical significance.[18]

The views of the Wistar scientists were not universal. Massimo Trucco, a scientist who moved from the BII to the Wistar Institute, wrote to Milstein shortly after reading Wade's article, commenting: "To be honest I feel—let's say—guilty to be here at the Wistar, ie in the only place in the world were [sic] some of your work not only is, by purpose, under evaluated but also, and what is worst somehow stolen [spelling and grammar as in the original]." In acceding to Milstein's request not to patent any product derived from use of the cells supplied, another researcher wrote, "I appreciate the frustration and effort involved in developing the strain and the fusion technology, and your concern for reasonable use of the strain by other laboratories." Similarly, another colleague, upon reading Wade's article, commented, "Frankly, I think your attitude of sending the hybridomas to scientists who need them for their work is exemplary. I, for one, sure as hell did not go into science to make money."[19]

Koprowski's decision to patent partly reflected the very different context of scientific work in the United States where, starting in the late 1960s, the National Institutes of Health (NIH) allowed institutions to petition for patents for research covered by their grants. From 1968 Koprowski and the Wistar Institute had been successfully filing patent applications for techniques and discoveries related to rabies and rubella vaccines. When commercial organizations sought to develop these vaccines, these patents brought in lucrative royalty income.[20]

The Wistar's strong patenting culture was unusual for the time. Furthermore patent law governing genetic engineering, the domain with which Mabs are often associated, was still in its infancy. In their letter of October 1976, NRDC officials argued that it would be difficult to patent the hybridoma technology because "the general field of genetic engineering is a particularly difficult area from the patent point of view." The patent application for recombinant DNA, or genetic splicing, another biotechnological landmark, was filed in November 1974. Devised by Stanley Cohen and Herbert Boyer at Stanford University and the University of California in 1973–1974, the technique was patented in December 1980, just days before the application was due to expire and after prolonged deliberations in academic and government circles. The U.S. Supreme Court's ruling on *Diamond v. Chakrabarty*, which allowed the patenting of life forms for the first time, also occurred only in June 1980.[21]

The NRDC's decision not to patent was not completely misjudged: the British patent office later turned down the Wistar patent application on the basis that the invention was "trite" and "devoid of inventive substance," since "all antibodies are immunoglobulins and the specificity of a particular antibody depends simply on the antigen which has given rise to it." Overall, it claimed, the process that Koprowski and his colleagues were trying to patent "did not go beyond prior art" because the development of Mabs against viral and tumor antigens was "an 'obvious' application of Milstein's technique," having already been suggested in a *Lancet* editorial.[22]

The fact that Köhler and Milstein published their method before the NRDC could consider patenting further complicated issues. In contrast to U.S. patent law, which permits the granting of patents if an application is filed within one year of the discovery's initial publication, British law allows no room for public disclosure of any kind. One of the reasons that NRDC officials gave in October 1976 for not patenting was because Köhler and Milstein had already published their work. This reason, however, was given a full thirteen months after Vickers had informally contacted the NRDC. At that time, the *Nature* article was still pending publication so could theoretically have been delayed while a patent was considered. Why the NRDC did not take any action following Vicker's letter has generated much speculation. The NRDC's response came only after the MRC made an inquiry after a visit from Sydney Brenner, divisional head of molecular genetics and cell biology in the LMB, to find out what had happened. Claiming they had no record of receiving the original *Nature* manuscript, NRDC officials requested a copy—which Milstein duly supplied. But by then it was too late for a patent to be filed.[23]

Some have asked why Milstein himself was not more proactive. Years later when asked whether he was unhappy not to have patented the technique, he was heard to remark, "I was not unhappy, Margaret Thatcher was." In general, he viewed patents as slightly distasteful and best left to lawyers and kept separate from scientific discovery and invention. Years later, Milstein reflected that the NRDC's refusal to patent his technique was a blessing because it allowed him greater freedom to publish and share his results, and to get on with his research. Had he received a patent, he would have been forced to be more secretive.[24]

Over the years many doubted whether the missed patent resulted in any long-term loss. Royalties would probably have been negligible, since the Köhler-Milstein Mab had limited applications and required considerable refinement to be clinically useful. In 1993, David Secher, one of Milstein's former postdoctoral researchers and later an MRC industrial liaison officer, argued: "It is doubtful, within the system operating in 1975, whether the commercial exploitation of the technology would have been more successful if patent protection had been applied for."[25]

Overall, Milstein's inaction should be viewed alongside the more general dislike of commercialization in the LMB in the 1970s. According to Secher, while the MRC's policy favored patenting to protect "its inventions," the culture at the LMB did not. As John Finch, a contemporary of Milstein's at the LMB, wrote, "The general feeling in the LMB at that time was that patenting was acceptable for machines that would be built by outside firms, but research results and techniques should be openly published and available, and so there was no strong pressure by César to chase things further." Milstein also had misgivings about the NRDC, having had a bad experience with its staff in the past. The reluctance to push for patents due to a lack of incentives was true of most government-funded British biomedical laboratories at the time. Nobody, for example, considered filing a patent on the protein and DNA sequencing techniques developed by Fred Sanger between the 1950s and 1970s at Cambridge University's Department of Biochemistry and the LMB. Until 1980, any royalties from patents arising out MRC unit discoveries were automatically assigned to the NRDC. The atmosphere changed only in 1986 when the MRC allowed for the sharing of royalties among inventors, individual units, and the central organization.[26]

The patenting question has to be considered also in terms of the initial expectations that Milstein and Köhler had for their technology. Milstein's informal transfer of cells to Koprowski shows not only how far the patent issue was from his mind in 1976, but also that the technique's exact application was still not determined. Milstein later admitted that he himself had originally been reluctant to draw attention to the technology's medical and industrial possibilities in the *Nature* article lest it seemed that "we were blowing our own trumpet too much." His most important consideration at the time was to publish ahead of his competitor, Matthew Scharff at the Albert Einstein College of Medicine, New York, who was adapting mouse myeloma cells for cell culture in order to understand antibody diversity.[27]

What is often forgotten in the history of the patent saga is how fragile and untested the technique was at the time. As Secher commented, "With hindsight one can focus back on a shattering invention, but there was doubt as to how easy it would be to reproduce, how easy it would be to translate into an industrial process . . . there was even doubt as to how easily it could translate to another laboratory or to another month."[28]

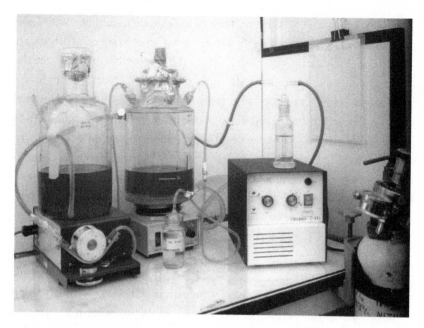

FIGURE 2.3. Equipment for the continuous growth of myeloma cells used in generating Mabs (MRC Laboratory of Molecular Biology)

Just as Köhler and Milstein's paper was accepted by *Nature,* the scientists faced a major crisis. Suddenly they were unable to achieve any fusions, despite the technique working on seven previous occasions. As subsequent attempts failed, Milstein considered withdrawing his and Köhler's paper. With the validity of their results threatened, the two scientists faced six stressful months trying to fathom what had gone wrong. Their very basic and hazardous working conditions, and the multiple steps and ingredients that their technique required, added to their woes. Finding out what had gone wrong was further hampered because by then Köhler had returned to Basel. Eventually Giovanni Galfré, a newly recruited LMB postdoctoral researcher, identified the problem—an incorrectly prepared stock solution of HAT medium, which "instead of selecting cells" was "killing them." Later, they discovered that other variables were also contributing to the erratic results (Figure 2.3).[29]

Milstein and Köhler were also concerned that others might not be able to replicate their technique. This fear was not unfounded, as the experience of G. Wilkinson, a junior pathology researcher based at Guy's

Hospital, London, shows. He was one of the first to be supplied with LMB myeloma cells, in January 1976. While he was able to successfully establish the cell line in his laboratory, he found it impossible to reproduce the technique despite numerous attempts over nine months. When he inquired whether he had been sent the wrong cell line, Milstein informed him that his team had faced similar problems and that various factors could be at fault: "In one case we strongly suspected the serum batch, in another the Sendai virus preparation, and in one case we could demonstrate a toxic effect from a (probably incorrectly prepared) HAT concentrate. The Sendai virus problem was so acute that . . . [we have recently] moved on to polyethylene glycol fusion. Likewise we are now using foetal calf instead of horse serum for fusion experiments." After more unsuccessful attempts, Wilkinson was finally invited to visit Milstein's laboratory in March 1977.[30]

Wilkinson's difficulties were not unique. In October 1977, Joan Macnab, a Glasgow scientist, wrote thanking Milstein for his cells, but added: "I hesitated to write earlier in the hope that I might have succeeded in propagating the cells successfully. However, we have had some trouble with our tissue culture. . . . I hesitate very much to trouble you further but would appreciate if you could send me some more cells . . . together with exact instructions on how you grow these cells with regard to medium, number of splits, etc." It was only when the Cologne-based immunologist Klaus Rajewsky successfully replicated the technique in 1977 that Köhler felt confident it could be reproduced and could think their method was "of some importance."[31]

Researchers continued to struggle even after improvements to the process and the cell lines. Many of the problems mirrored more general difficulties inherent in tissue culture, such as contamination and cell instability. Much depended on how the cells were sent. Some felt that cells were easier to propagate if they were sent frozen and accompanied by tested fetal calf serum rather than in medium. Sending serum was important, given the difficulty of establishing in advance which serum was best. No uniform cell samples were sent. Some received myeloma cells or serum containing antibodies taken from immunized mice. Others were sent whole hybridomas (hybrid cells) that produced Mabs. Alternatively a sample of the medium in which Mabs were growing could be sent, from which Mabs could be isolated.[32]

Hybridomas were the easiest to send out as they were constantly being grown in culture in flasks, but their survival was dependent on quick transportation in cold, but not freezing, conditions. This optimum temperature was often not available in the freezing baggage compartment of an airplane. Other samples required more preparation: they had to be taken out of liquid nitrogen and placed on dry ice before they could travel safely by air in polystyrene containers. Serum samples were the easiest to transport because they survived at room temperature.[33]

How samples moved from one place to another varied enormously. Those that could be carried in a cell suspension in a test tube were often collected in person. Others were sent in parcels via postal services, which employed trains or airplanes for transport. The logistics of transportation, however, could easily break down, and securing permits from relevant governmental authorities to get packages cleared through customs could take time. On occasion industrial disputes at airports held up shipping, and sometimes transport networks were disrupted by military coups. Any delay or changes in temperature could damage the cells. To avoid some of the logistical distribution problems, Milstein and his staff advised those requesting cells that, where possible, they try to obtain them from previous recipients located closer to hand.[34]

In addition to transport logistics, laboratories did not always have ideal conditions for nurturing the cells after their arrival. On more than one occasion laboratories reported trouble storing the cells because of problems with their own liquid nitrogen systems. Recipient laboratories also frequently reported contamination.[35]

Unstable materials, delivery complications, and contamination were not the only difficulties. Scientists needed various levels of knowledge and skill to replicate the Cambridge technique. The immunization of animals, for example, required expertise in immunology, the fusion procedure necessitated experience in cellular biology and genetics, and immunochemistry and biochemistry were important for determining which hybrid cells to select after fusion and for their characterization.

Scientists had to know not only how to create hybrid cells, but also how to maintain them. While the cells grow automatically, the medium that they grow in requires regular replenishing. Much of this can be done easily, though knowing what to look for is important. The vital sign is the color of the liquid in the flask containing the medium and the Mabs. If it turns from its original orange to purple or yellow, the Mab-producing cells have used up all the medium's nutrients. Maintaining the right level of carbon dioxide is also important. Training is needed even for an apparently simple procedure like putting the mature cells in storage, because it involves using a centrifuge to spin the medium that contains the Mab-producing cells in order to make pellets that are then suspended in polyethylene glycol (PEG). Should the correct grade of PEG with the right consistency and no excess water not be used, the cells can be damaged. The pellets are then frozen in liquid nitrogen, a well-established procedure in tissue culture. The aim of freezing is to temporarily interrupt cell division and metabolism. The process needs careful watching to ensure that no ice crystals form because they can burst cells. It is equally important to thaw the sample slowly when the pellets are taken out of storage to be grown again in a medium, so as to prevent damage to the cells. Defrosting and nutrient requirements vary between cell lines, raising further complications. This is a general problem for tissue culture, and can be even worse when growing cells in a recently established laboratory, where slight variations of each particular new piece of equipment and reagents are yet unknown.[36]

Some of the difficulties that scientists experienced in the early years were articulated by Roger Wilsnack, who after failing to make myeloma cells for some time described the process as "art." Much of the knowledge and skill involved in producing Mabs was tacit and unwritten, and could not be easily picked up from a written protocol. This meant that scientists depended on experimental learning and knowledge acquired informally. As Heddy Zola and Robert Knox pointed out in 1982: "The newcomer to hybridization is well advised to learn the technique in a laboratory which is already practicing fusion. . . . newcomers to the technique are relatively unsuccessful initially and obtain many hybrids after some practice, although [even] an experienced observer cannot see any differences between the technique used on the first day and in subsequent, successful experiments. The best approach is to learn from an experienced laboratory and practice until hybrids are obtained."[37]

Milstein's papers show that many scientists needed guidance. Their questions ranged from the type of equipment to be used to what growing cells looked like. One scientist, for example, was concerned that his cells, while growing well, tended to bunch together. Milstein's research assistant responded that this was normal if the cells were grown in flasks or spinner cultures, and that the clumps would disperse once the cells reached the fusion stage. He further suggested that, if possible, the cells should be grown in roller bottles.[38]

It was difficult to determine the right conditions for success. A manual put together in 1980 by Köhler and colleagues from the BII and Roche's PAI summed up the technique's fickle nature: "The fusion does not invariably work. Often a repeat of the fusion process without obvious change results in successful hybridisation." Capturing the frustration of the early years, Milstein recalled, "There were all sorts of rumours: you should use this or the other reagent, from this make or the other make, and this is better than the other, . . . no one really had any magic formula."[39]

Echoing this sentiment, another scientist observed wryly, "I consider that the actual fusion has a lot of voodoo. There [are] a lot of things people do, they don't know why. I don't know why but I just copy what they do and they say: 'If you do it differently, it will not work.' They told me I had to spin the fusion cells with the top open. Why the top open? It doesn't make any difference, this is a small, desk top centrifuge, it doesn't matter whether the top is open or closed. I think the history of it is [laughter] that you can't regulate the speed that well, so initially when people used to do it, they would open the top and see how fast it would spin. Now people know how to regulate the speed and they don't really have to look at it any more, but they leave the top open. I am supposed to be a scientist. I don't believe the top has to be open. But I am not going to put it down, because if the fusion did not work, they would tell me it's because I left the top down." Over time, each laboratory developed its own methods. These could be very simple, such as fusing the cells in a Petri dish on a flat surface or in a centrifuge tube. In part the variety of methods reflected the fact that each of the cell lines behaved differently.[40]

Nor did finding the right method guarantee continued success. As Köhler and Milstein had found, highly successful researchers could suddenly fail. There were also individual differences among members of the same research group. It was crucial to learn how to interpret visual clues, such as the color of the culture liquid or the formation of cells under the microscope, and to acquire the motor skills for handling cells. When asked to comment on why not everyone was successful, a cell biologist who had managed to achieve the technique quickly replied, "Because there were small tricks. For example, when you add polyethylene glycol to the cells they become very fragile. People who work for years with the cells . . . are used to vigorous shaking. So if you pipet [sic] those cells strongly, you disrupt them and you lose your experiment. Things like that."[41]

What might seem like small issues could make a big difference to results. This was most noticeable in terms of maintaining sterility, which was greatly dependent on how scientists controlled and coordinated their movements. One major difficulty in solving the problem was that by the time contamination is visible it is usually too late to determine its cause. Without immediate feedback about which action had undermined sterility, it was tricky to know what changes to make.[42]

The difficulties that novices had in preventing contamination led Milstein to divide tissue culture work between two separate laboratories. The first, known as the "dirty laboratory," located in the LMB basement, was where newcomers who had little experience of tissue culture and producing Mabs started their work. Only once they had proven themselves were they allowed into the "clean laboratory" normally reserved for experienced staff. Milstein's establishment of a two-tier system of laboratories was particularly important given the many visitors who wanted to learn how to produce Mabs.[43]

Given the complexity of growing Mabs, it is not surprising that many different protocols emerged over the years (Figure 2.4). These protocols, could not, however, alter the fact that success was heavily reliant on knowledge and skills that could not be learned from a textbook. Not surprisingly, laboratories that were already highly experienced in cellular fusion, such as those at the Wistar Institute, were among the first to adopt it.[44]

Reflecting the obstacles producing Mabs, Milstein initially received very few requests for his cells. As he noted in 1993, "The derivation of the first hybrid myeloma cell line (or hybridoma, as we now know it) against a predefined antigen was not received with wild enthusiasm by the scientific community at large—nor even by immunologists." Again in 1999 he commented, "People now think that everybody was asking me for cell lines as soon as the thing was published. There were very few, very, very few requests in the beginning."[45]

This lack of interest is borne out by the testimony from Melvin Cohn who was at the forefront of cellular hybridization in the 1970s. In 1990, he recalled that after reading the Nature article, "We didn't even attempt

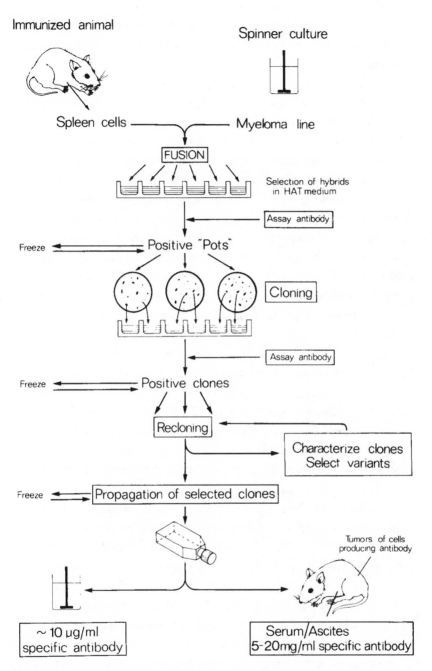

Immunized animal

Spinner culture

Spleen cells ———————— Myeloma line

FUSION

Selection of hybrids
in HAT medium

Assay antibody

Freeze ◄———— Positive "Pots"

Cloning

Assay antibody

Freeze ◄————► Positive clones

Recloning

Characterize clones
Select variants

Freeze ◄———— Propagation of selected clones

Tumors of cells
producing antibody

~ 10 µg/ml
specific antibody

Serum/Ascites
5-20mg/ml specific antibody

FIGURE 2.4. Basic protocol developed by Georges Köhler and César Milstein for
making Mabs (G. Galfré and C. Milstein, "Preparation of Monoclonal Antibodies:
Strategies and Procedures," Methods in Enzymology 73 [1981]: 15)

to reproduce the first Milstein P3/Sendai experiment. We knew that it wouldn't work with our line." Moreover, he was not particularly impressed with the method, because of its low frequency of fusion. As he argued, "If we had gotten it, we would have published it in the way that he did, but we would have considered it marginal." Only after Cohn learned that others had used it successfully did he request samples from Milstein's cell line. Ironically, this cell line was a derivative of one that Cohn and his team at the Salk Institute had developed some years earlier.[46]

Milstein's notebook shows that in 1976 cells were sent to only eight scientists. All had close ties with Milstein or his colleagues. One of the factors limiting uptake of the technology was ignorance about its usefulness. As Gerhard pointed out, when the Nature article appeared in 1975 "many people may have said, 'It's nice but so what, what can we do with it?'" He had no such hesitation, having already had some expertise in using Klinman's method to produce antibodies against the influenza virus. He therefore quickly grasped the utility of Köhler and Milstein's technique.[47]

Gerhard, however, was unusual. For most scientists, the practical utility of the technology was not obvious. It took Milstein himself time to understand its practical possibilities. Like most people, he admitted, he "had a very restricted view of the use of the monoclonal antibody in the very early days." This was also true of many others who were skilled in cellular cloning, and could have adopted the technique with relative ease. Even by the end of 1976 questions remained about its applicability.[48]

The number of cells dispatched from Milstein's laboratory continued to be small into the first half of 1977. From September 1977, however, demands began to increase: seven people were sent samples in that month alone. This interest was awakened in part by an article that Milstein had published with Galfré and others in Nature the previous April, which demonstrated the practical applications of Mabs for the first time.[49] Critically, it illustrated the possibility of synthesizing Mabs against antigens of clinical interest: rat major histocompatibility complex antigens.[50] Such antigens helped identify the "unique identity of a given organism's tissues." This opened up new avenues for human tissue typing, which was important for successful organ transplantation. It also allowed for the exploration of the distinction between self and nonself, a concept fundamental to immunology. In addition, Milstein and Galfré indicated that Mabs could be produced for a specific antigen even if nonpurified immunogens (foreign particles that trigger immune responses in the body) were used. They pointed out that scientists therefore now had a "powerful tool in the study of complex antigenic structures," and an established cell line that offered an "unlimited permanent supply of material." All of this made possible "worldwide standardisation."[51]

Some of the excitement the article aroused can be seen from the accompanying news and views section of *Nature* written by Ken Welsh, an immunologist based at East Grinstead Hospital. In the wake of his fury that the NRDC had not patented the technology, Welsh argued that it represented "a major step forward" for many of "the clinical and biological problems then confounding tissue-typing associated with human transplants."[52] As he pointed out, "Tissue matching for skin, cornea, bone marrow and kidney transplants depends to a large extent on stocks of reasonable titre monospecific typing antibodies against the major histocompatibility antigens. These precious sera, obtained from immunised volunteers, multiparous women, transplant recipients or primates take months or even years of laborious work to produce, test and become accepted as standard agents." Commercially, Welsh believed that the new technique promised to convert "antibody production from a biological science with all its inherent variability and non-reproducibility into the realms of synthetic chemistry where any desired reagent is available off the shelf and can be assumed with reasonable confidence to be identical to the same reagent in any other laboratory."[53]

Similar enthusiasm was expressed in a *Lancet* editorial in June 1977, which claimed that this latest research could have "profound implications for medical practice." Apart from its potential use in transplants, the technique, according to the editorial, could be important for diagnostics—helping, for example, to diagnose rare blood groups, hepatitis, and tumors, as well as prevent Rhesus disease in the newborn. The editorial also pointed to its possible use in cases of drug overdose, snakebites, and life-threatening infections.[54]

A paper that Milstein published with his colleague, Alan Williams, and others in November 1977 generated even more excitement. It showed how Mabs could be used to differentiate cell surface markers. Crucially, the paper "jumped the boundaries of immunology into the world of general biology," prompting a flood of requests for Milstein's cells. In later years Milstein admitted that the research had been a turning point in his own understanding of what could be achieved with hybridoma technology.[55]

The 1977 publications helped popularize Mabs' potential in the wider scientific and medical community for the first time, but a small number of scientists had already begun to consider the utility of antibodies. In late 1975 an Anglo-American symposium held in New York and sponsored by the Royal Society of Medicine and Royal Society of Medicine Foundation brought a number of scientists together to think through the diagnostic and therapeutic implications of recent advances in antibody research. At this forum, potential medical applications of antibodies were recognized. In addition to discussing those mentioned in the *Lancet*'s editorial, forum attendees raised the possibility that antibodies could be used for fertility control and to detect damaged tissue in heart attacks. Some idea of the mood at the symposium can be gleaned from Edgar Haber's introduction to the published collection of papers it generated. "The wanderings of a fertile imagination can readily speculate upon many more applications of the powerful drug or reagent which antibody represents," he wrote, "particularly when a specified and uniform product can be produced in indefinite supply. It is certainly a worthy goal for the expenditure of considerable effort."[56]

Milstein and Köhler's technique was discussed at this meeting, but it was seen merely as one prospect among others for the production of antibodies using cellular culture and chemical synthesis. Haber stressed that while "elements of *in vitro* antibody production" appeared to be at hand, experiments were still needed to choose "the best and most efficient approach" for the production of "optimal quantities."[57]

By 1977, however, Milstein had begun to be inundated with requests for his cells. Answering these requests meant not only growing, packaging, and labeling the cells, but also sending numerous telexes and phone calls to arrange for their transport as well as letters to ensure the cells had arrived safely.[58] Recovering the costs of shipping the cells, given the bureaucracy involved, was often not worth the hassle. As Milstein's secretary wrote to one researcher in 1981,

Thank you for your letter . . . concerning payment of shipping costs for Dr Milstein's cell line. We quite appreciate that it is

difficult for some laboratories to arrange for payment to be
made (especially abroad) without a formal invoice. . . . as all
our accounting is done by the Medical Research Council head
office in London, we have to deal with a rather cumbersome
machinery to arrange for invoices to be sent. In the circumstances, and as the sum involved is relatively small, it really
would be best if you were not to worry about . . . payment. It is
kind of you to be concerned about . . . this matter, but in fact
we have not received payment from many . . . recipients.[59]

By 1983, however, as the requests increased, and the financial burden of
covering the various costs became excessive, recipients had to send payment in advance.[60]

Milstein's laboratory struggled to manage the distribution alone. Rescue came in February 1977 when David Murray, founder of Sera-Lab, a
company producing and marketing antisera as a research reagent for scientists, knocked on Milstein's laboratory door. He was visiting on the off
chance of selling fetal calf serum, and initially had no idea whose door
he was knocking on. But Murray was familiar with Milstein's work, having been alerted to it by Ken Welsh, who had contacted him and other
company executives in his effort to find a commercial solution to the
NRDC's failure to patent.[61]

Having wrestled with standardizing antisera reagents for many years,
Milstein's technique offered Murray a way forward. As he put it, "Here
was, for the first time, a method of raising extremely . . . high titre and
absolutely pure antiserum with each batch identical to the previous one
in every respect." Excited by the prospects Murray quickly wrote to Milstein, at the beginning of 1977, to see if he could use his cell lines to prepare a range of antisera to be marketed by Sera-Lab.[62]

When Murray launched into his sales pitch for fetal serum, Milstein
quickly interrupted him to say how impressed he had been with his other
proposal, for the cell lines. It was only when Milstein started hunting for
Murray's letter that the penny dropped for Murray. Soon the conversation turned to Milstein's frustration at having to meet all the requests for
his cells; for the past few months he had been involved in "running down-
stairs to the refrigerator, thawing a vial, pouring out an aliquot [a frac-
tion], packing it up in dry ice and posting the parcels all over the world."

Murray quickly proposed Sera-Lab's help in distributing Milstein's cells. It was to take at least another year before the agreement was formalized by the MRC, but by early 1978 Sera-Lab was promoting the sale of Milstein's cell lines in its catalogs. For Milstein the arrangement rid him of his "distribution problems," which, as he pointed out, "if not done by Sera-Lab, would fall on our already overstrained administrative services."[63]

Under the arrangement, Milstein initially supplied Sera-Lab with different cell lines. Later his lab supplied incubators and other equipment for the company to establish a tissue culture laboratory to reproduce the cells. By April 1979 Sera-Lab had its own facilities and had established a research program to develop its own cell lines. Through the years Milstein's laboratory continued to liaise with the company, ensuring the quality of production and transferring new cell lines as they developed. In return, the LMB received a percentage of the income generated from Sera-Lab's distribution of the cells. The NRDC retained the rights to the cell lines. By July 1980 Sera-Lab had invested £250,000 in Mab technology and was the leading provider of Mabs in the world, with a network of twenty-eight distributors across the globe. It had paid over £3,000 in royalties to the MRC.[64]

The collaboration between Sera-Lab and Milstein's laboratory provided the first commercial channel for the global dissemination of Mabs, and established an important foundation for future research in the field. Crucially, Sera-Lab took out much of the "donkey work" involved in the production of Mabs. This proved of vital importance in efforts to determine new applications for Mabs in the world beyond Milstein's laboratory.

CHAPTER THREE

Breakthroughs at the Bench

RESEARCHERS WERE QUICK to capitalize on Mabs for their laboratory work in fields ranging from immunology to neuroscience, oncology to cardiology, perhaps because they were unprotected by a patent and somewhat easy to make. By 1981, between 25 and 50 percent of articles in immunology journals showed that Mabs were an intrinsic part of the research and a large number of projects might never have started without them. As Alan Rabson, deputy director of the U.S. National Cancer Institute, reported in 1982, Mabs were "a rapidly escalating phenomenon . . . it is such a powerful technology that I think it will dominate much of immunology." Out of the new grants granted by his division at that time, 70 percent involved Mabs.[1]

Conceived of as a tool to analyze the genetic origin of antibody diversity and specificity, Mabs soon opened new frontiers in research well beyond immunology and transformed the way that scientists investigated and analyzed biological phenomena more generally. Reflecting this dynamism, between 1981 and 1983 U.S. National Institutes of Health funding for Mabs rose from $78 million for 768 projects to $206 million for 1,940 projects. Critically, the technology enabled the detection of unknown molecules and established their function for the first time. Spearheading the movement were scientists who quickly applied Mabs to the tasks of unraveling the mechanisms underlying disease, and improving diagnosis and treatment. This work attracted the interest of the commercial world as well. In 1980 the British biotechnology company Celltech predicted that the world market for research Mabs would soon be £6 million. Similarly, in 1984, the U.S. Office of Technology Assessment estimated that the U.S. market for monoclonals was worth between $5 and $6 million and predicted that by 1990 its value would increase to between $300 and $500 million.[2]

Yet the rise of Mabs was not inevitable or straightforward. As Alan Williams, an early collaborator of Milstein's, pointedly observed in 1986, "It does irritate me that nowadays the Mab story is written as though everyone saw all the possibilities from the start." Milstein himself reflected, "I have often been asked if we were aware of the future revolutionary impact that the hybridoma technology would make when we developed the first monoclonal [anti] sheep red cells antibody. . . . The answer is that although we realised that the methodology could have an important application in medicine and industry its true impact ranging from basic research in all branches of biology to the stock market escaped us in 1975. It also escaped others, I hasten to say, as shown by the fact that *Nature* refused to publish the paper as a full article because it was not considered of sufficient general interest."[3]

Early on Milstein realized that he would have to devote time and energy to demonstrating the application of his and Köhler's technique, even if this meant temporarily leaving his long-term endeavor to understand antibody diversity. His efforts to spread the word about Mabs were not only fundamental to the rapid adoption of Mabs, but also highly unusual among scientists at the time.[4]

Critically, Milstein needed to prove the value of Mabs over conventional, or polyclonal, antibodies. This was not easy because the specificity of antibodies, that is, the ability of antibodies to target and bind to particular antigens, was still being debated. As Milstein recalled, "Among many unknowns, the specificity of antibodies was a matter of controversy. The possibility that the specificity of antisera [polyclonal antibodies] was more the result of heterogeneity of the polyclonal response than of specific molecular recognition was discussed many times. . . . So the possibility that monoclonal antibodies were in fact never going to be highly specific was open. It remained quite possible that although we could make antibodies to a specific antigen, the antibody itself may be too cross-reactive to be of any practical application."[5]

The precise specificity of Mabs came to be compared favorably with the specificity of polyclonal antibodies. This is particularly striking because until 1975 conventional antibodies were considered very specific tools. Later, however, scientists regarded them as inferior to Mabs in discerning targets. In his quest to determine the utility of Mabs, Milstein sought collaborators from a variety of disciplines. Soon after the *Nature* publication, Milstein approached experts trying to resolve problems in other fields and suggested they use Mabs.[6]

One of Milstein's first collaborators was Claudio Cuello, a fellow Argentinian attached to the MRC's Neurochemical Pharmacology Unit in Cambridge between 1975 and 1978 and then, starting in 1978, the departments of pharmacology and human anatomy at Oxford University (Figure 3.1). Their partnership, begun soon after publication of the 1975 *Nature* article, was a natural extension of their deep friendship and mutual interests. At the time Cuello was struggling to characterize Substance P (SP), a kind of neuropeptide that since the 1930s had been known to be involved in pain and neurotransmission. Cuello wanted to determine whether SP was a peptide transmitter, and to map its pathway in the body, then a hot topic in neuroscience. He was also keen to understand the relationship between SP and disease. Milstein brought to the project his skills in tissue culture, while Cuello contributed his expertise in immunohistochemistry and anatomy.[7]

The two scientists saw their venture as a way both to advance Cuello's research and to demonstrate the application of Mabs more generally. They hoped specifically to prove the utility of Mabs for immunohistochemistry. Sometimes known as immunocytochemistry, immunohistochemistry is a common laboratory technique that exploits the binding mechanism of antibodies to specific components of cells to analyze and identify different cell types. The antibodies act as markers to locate and measure cells in biological samples. By the 1970s scientists had successfully attached various fluorescent dyes, radioisotopes, and enzymes (especially horseradish peroxidase, a yellowish-brown pigment) to antibodies as a means of staining tissue and identifying various cells in biological samples. Tests using antibodies conjugated with radioisotopes are known as radioimmunoassays (RIA). Immunofluorescence is the test that employs fluorescent labels. And those tests that use enzymes are known as enzyme-linked immunosorbent assays (ELISA).[8]

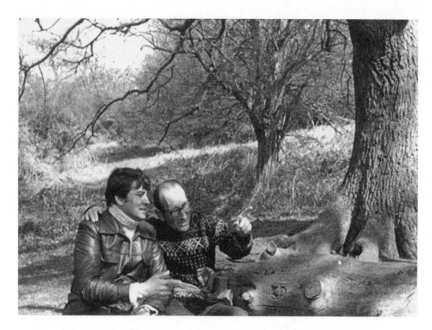

FIGURE 3.1. César Milstein (*right*) and Claudio Cuello, ca. 1975, in earnest discussion during one of their many walks together (Claudio Cuello)

A major advantage of the immunobased tests was that they could be used in conjunction with an electron microscope. But they relied on conventional antibodies, which were difficult to standardize. Jonathan Howard, one of Milstein's colleagues, explained,

> When an animal is immunized with an antigen, no matter how simple, the antibody response is phenomenally complicated. Hundreds, even thousands, of different antibodies are produced, each of which recognises the antigen in a slightly different way. The mixture is called an antiserum, and it is with these antisera that immunologists and those who use immunological tools have been obliged to work. No two antisera are identical: repeated immunization of one single inbred animal with a pure antigen yields a complex response which evolves slowly over time. One tube of antiserum may be good for some purpose, the next, from the same animal, bad. Eventually the good tube is emptied and the unfortunate scientist must wait until a thousand different antibodies fall

again into that happy conjunction which is called a good antiserum. And it will not be the same as the last one, only similar.[9]

Overall, conventional antibodies involved extensive preparation and purification and had a limited shelf life. This made it difficult for scientists
to reproduce their results or compare them with others.[10]

Despite these limitations, immunobased tests were routinely used as
diagnostics in fields such as parasitology, virology, immunology, and cancer. Few scientists, however, had explored their use for neuroscience.
Cuello was already familiar with immunobased tests, having partially
worked out the structure of SP using guinea-pig serum that contained
antibodies raised against SP. He and his team had also successfully vi-
sualized the peptide in the spinal cord of rats using immunofluorescence,
thereby becoming the second laboratory in the world to reveal the cellular location of SP. (Until then its location had been theoretical.) Yet this
work had proved time-consuming and unreliable. Among the problems
they confronted was that guinea-pig serum provided only a limited supply of antibodies and because they were not specific to SP, they cross-
reacted with other substances. This made it difficult for Cuello and his
colleagues to reproduce their results and those of other scientists.[11]

Hybridoma technology offered a way of generating unlimited standardized antibodies highly specific to SP. Not everyone was convinced that
it would work. One scientist commented scathingly, "Claudio, whatever
you do with monoclonals can be done by a rabbit!" Nevertheless, by 1979
Cuello and Milstein had successfully generated a Mab highly specific to
SP that proved extremely versatile for characterizing the peptide. Cuello
and his Oxford colleagues, Rejean Couture and Eric Pioro, went on to use
Mabs to unravel many neurotransmitter pathways in different neurological specimens. Their work was helped by access to postmortem material
specimens collected by Trevor Hughes and from the Brain Research Institute in Düsseldorf. The institute's collection included samples from the
German physician and neurologist Oskar Vogt, who had started gathering
human brain specimens in the 1930s. Over time, the results by Cuello and
his colleagues provided a major reference point for neuroscience.[12]

Cuello and Milstein's work on SP represented the first of many Mab
applications in neuroscience. Together with others, these scientists also
developed Mabs to detect and map other neural proteins, including

serotonin and enkephalin. By showing the power of Mabs as tools for neuroscientific dissection, Cuello and Milstein opened up investigation into the brain and the central nervous system on an unprecedented scale, which in turn led to better understandings of the causes of neurological disease and the means for neuropharmacological intervention. By the early 1980s, for example, Mabs were being used to dissect unknown components of the synapses and for the pathological investigation of diseases like Alzheimer's and Parkinson's. Mabs proved particularly useful for demonstrating the relationship between loss of memory and cholinergic function (that is, the function of nerve fibers that release the neurotransmitter acetycholine), as well as the part played by cortical lesions in Alzheimer's disease.[13]

In addition to extending the boundaries of neuroscience, the two scientists transformed immunobased tests, prompting the revival of many techniques neglected because of inadequate supplies of pure antibodies. Critically, they demonstrated the feasibility of conjugating Mabs with radioisotopes and various enzymes, which enabled them to be slotted into preexisting RIA and ELISA techniques commonly deployed for laboratory work and diagnosis. Mabs' major advantages were that they offered not only an abundant, standardized reagent, but also high sensitivity and specificity, which minimized unwanted cross-reactions and improved signal detection. Mabs also reduced the number of procedural steps necessary for developing such tests.[14]

In 1984, Cuello and Milstein also developed bispecific antibodies, which recognized two different antigen epitopes, the portion of an antigen that binds to antibodies. Compatible with ELISA and RIA tests, bispecific antibodies enabled the construction of single-step assay systems, thus eliminating the need for second antibodies. By helping to improve the sensitivity of immunochemistry and signal detection, and by simplifying the staining procedure, bispecific antibodies permitted a much more refined and detailed structural analysis than was heretofore possible.[15]

With Mabs, scientists could now run hundreds of replicable tests and compare their results with others on an unprecedented scale. The excitement that Milstein and Cuello's work generated is illustrated by the comments of one neuroscience professor at Washington University in Missouri who in 1981 wrote to Milstein: "I am sure [your discovery] will excite a great deal of interest and because it is so simple (perhaps dangerously so), I am sure it will become widely used." Similarly, the pathologist Elaine Jaffe remembered that in the 1970s "immunohistochemistry with monoclonal antibodies exponentially increased the different views one could have of the same tissue, and was the source of endless wonder and excitement."[16]

Not everyone was ready to embrace Mabs, however. A Swedish correspondent to the *Lancet,* for example, doubted whether a Mab targeting serotonin could replace existing techniques for the diagnosis of carcinoid tumors, one of the most common forms of neuroendocrine tumor. In dispute was the degree of accuracy that Mabs offered over older methods. Such skepticism was not uncommon. An executive of Cytogen, a small biotechnology startup, commented in 1982, "I don't see monoclonal antibodies as improving on conventional antiserum tests already in existence. Both would detect the same compound in the same way. What's the advantage of another system?" Even those who had some experience with Mabs were cautious. As Yelton and Scharff pointed out,

Hybridomas are attractive reagents since, once generated, they provide a perpetual source of a well-defined antibody. In many ways a monoclonal antibody can be used like a conventional antiserum, but because of the fundamental differences between the two reagents it is unsafe to assume one can automatically be substituted for the other. . . . Although a great boon, hybridomas are not a panacea for all serological woes. In view of the quality, reproducibility, and relative cost effectiveness of monoclonal antibodies, it seems inevitable that they will replace polyclonal antibodies in most large-scale routine serology. But in the basic science laboratory, where smaller amounts of antibody are required, conventional antisera may still be preferable for many purposes. It usually takes four to six months to generate a stable hybridoma, if all goes well, whereas producing small amounts of antisera requires less time, energy, and expense.[17]

Despite these reservations, Milstein was soon inundated with visitors eager to learn how to produce Mabs. Many were keen to join forces with him to see how Mabs could be exploited. One of these visitors was

Leonard Herzenberg, an American geneticist who joined the LMB for a few months' sabbatical in late 1975 to improve his skills in molecular biology. Herzenberg had been developing an instrument to automate the separation of cells so as to determine the function of cell subsets that co-exist in the blood and various organs. Working together with his wife, Leonore, and colleagues at Stanford Medical School, he aimed to improve the traditional immunofluorescence techniques used to observe and count cells. This was part of a wider effort to automate clinical diagnostic practices, such as the diagnosis of cancer and the counting of white blood cells, and to automate biological equipment for unmanned space flights.[18]

By the time Herzenberg arrived in Cambridge, he and his colleagues had devised an automatic fluorescence-activated cell sorter (FACS), which could sort five thousand live, functional cells per second. Its sorting mechanism relied on conventional antibodies coupled with fluorescent tags. These antibodies acted as probes that would attach to proteins found in certain cell types; these were then picked up with the help of a laser that could detect fluorescence. Commercialized by the medical device company Becton, Dickinson, the instrument was already in use by a number of European and American laboratories. Yet the FACS was having some teething problems because conventional antibodies were in limited supply and tended to cross-react. Conjugating the antibodies with staining agents was also laborious and slow.[19]

Fruitless attempts had been made to improve the FACS's performance by calibrating the amount of fluorescein attached to antibodies. Once in Cambridge, Herzenberg realized that Mabs offered a better solution because they provided a standardized reagent. Initially unaware of what the FACS could achieve, Milstein was hesitant to partner with Herzenberg. Nevertheless, by late 1977 the two scientists, helped by Leonore and Vernon Oi, a Stanford University graduate student, had generated the first Mabs in mice suitable for use in the FACS to screen antibodies according to cell surface determinants.[20]

The development of Mabs for the FACS significantly enhanced the instrument's reliability and popularity. The number of FACS being used increased from half a dozen in the 1970s to more than five hundred in the early 1980s. They were deployed for a range of purposes. In biological research, for example, FACS proved critical for investigating cellular structures and functions, measuring metabolic processes in cells, and determining how viruses infect cells. On the medical front, they became instrumental for counting white blood cells (leukocytes), a routine test for assessing the efficacy of chemotherapy for diseases like leukemia.[21]

FACS were found to be particularly powerful for identifying and characterizing protein molecules found on cell surfaces. Known as differentiation antigens, these molecules appear on the membranes of living cells during sequential stages of maturation and differentiation. Today, analysis of differentiation antigens is instrumental for the investigation of cellular development during normal and abnormal growth and for cell classification. The antigenic structure of a cell's surface allows scientists to determine a cell's lineage and to define subsets of cells. Differentiation antigens enable a distinction to be drawn, for example, between B and T lymphocytes, types of white blood cells that each perform different functions in the immune system. T lymphocytes, for example, can be determined by a Thy-1 antigen marker on their cell surfaces. Not all subsets of cells have specific markers, however. Most are characterized instead by the collective presence of particular distinctive "differentiation" antigens.[22]

By the mid-1970s, a handful of scientists were already developing and testing various cell-surface marker reagents. Much of their work was dedicated to investigating T and B cells to better understand leukemia, cancer of the blood or bone marrow, at the cell's morphological level—with the object of improving its diagnosis and treatment. By this time leukemia was divided into four categories: acute, chronic, myeloid, and lymphatic. These categories were important indicators for a patient's overall prognosis and were determined by staining cells.[23]

Until the 1970s, research into T and B cells for leukemia was slow, hampered by the inability to secure standardized antibodies for use as cell-surface marker reagents in immunobased tests. Securing enough antisera against acute lymphatic leukemia could take three months of highly skilled, yet repetitive, laboratory work. The work was further hindered by a more general ignorance about the significance of differentiation antigens.[24]

Research into differentiation antigens was to gain much greater momentum with the emergence of Mabs in tandem with the introduction of the FACS. Spearheading this work was Milstein in partnership with Alan Williams, an Australian immunochemist at Oxford University. Keen to understand the structure and biochemistry of immunological reactions, Williams had been attempting since the early 1970s to purify antigens and antibodies to develop quantitative methods for analyzing cell surface antigens. Antigens and antibodies provided a way of distinguishing lymphocytes with different functions and identifying cell surface molecules involved in the mediation of lymphocyte functions. By 1975, Williams and his colleagues had successfully purified a Thy-1 antigen for use as a marker for locating T lymphocytes in mice. They had also identified a leukocyte-common antigen using antibodies taken from the serum of rabbits immunized against rat lymphocytes. This work, however, had been slow due to inadequate supplies of antibodies with the right strength and specificity. Anti-lymphocyte serum had multiple specificities.[25]

In June 1976, a chance conversation between Williams and Milstein at a conference in Cold Spring Harbor, New York, prompted them to explore whether Mabs could offer a solution. The task, which was to be carried out with the assistance of Milstein's postdoctoral researcher Giovanni Galfé, was daunting. They did not know whether they could produce a Mab efficient enough to detect a cell-surface antigen, and they had no idea if Williams's RIA technique was sufficiently sensitive.[26]

Overall, the tissue culturing was to be done in Cambridge and the serological work in Oxford. With eighty-five miles separating the two teams, the project posed major logistical challenges. According to Milstein,

> The basic protocol of the collaboration was as follows. We produced the cultures and clones and sent the supernatants by urgent mail. As soon as he got them, Alan proceeded to do the binding assays, . . . usually within 24 hours. He would phone (no faxes in those days) the results (perhaps 100 assays per round) for us to proceed with clonal selection. Speed turned out to be essential. We discovered that contaminating clones or chain-loss mutants all too often conspired against us. Indeed, literally hundreds and hundreds of failed attempts taught us a lot about the technical problems involved and how to tackle them.[27]

An invaluable partner in this effort was the automated FACS that Williams had in his laboratory, which was used to isolate and characterize the function of the different Mabs produced. Crucially, it facilitated the sorting out of the large cell population on the basis of their size and surface-antigen pattern.[28]

Initially, the team worked out their approach by using the Mabs generated against SBRCs developed by Köhler and Milstein. This provided what Milstein called "fantastic" results, prompting Williams to predict that Mabs would allow them to "detect as many as 10,000 surface molecules per cell." Thereafter the collaborators created a mouse Mab that targeted rat T cells. This provided a major breakthrough. Milstein recalled, "In that one attempt we defined three new antigenic specificities, a task that might have required years of sophisticated immunology by conventional methods." They produced three Mabs with specificities for distinct subsets of T cells in rats; the most exciting one was code-named W3/25. This later turned out to be the rat equivalent of the human antigen CD4, which in the mid-1980s was identified as the receptor for the AIDS virus.[29]

Importantly, the partnership proved that Mabs could be produced to unknown cell surface antigens and deployed to understand the function of the unknown cell surfaces. Publishing their results in 1977, Milstein and Williams excitedly claimed that Mabs might not only be used for investigating immune cells, but also "for the analysis of cell surface molecules of any sort." They could potentially be produced to "recognise an individual chemical structure in any complicated mixture of molecules."[30]

Developing Mabs against antigens found on human cell surfaces initially proved difficult. As a clearly frustrated Milstein explained, "If we did not get what we wanted, we had to learn to love what we got!" In the spring of 1977, however, Milstein launched a project with Andrew McMichael in the Nuffield Department of Surgery, Oxford, that moved things forward. McMichael had been a doctoral student in Brigitte Askonas's laboratory, which had developed single antibodies with B cloning, and had some expertise in the area. He was also versed in typing human leukocyte antigens, having worked with Hugh McDevitt and Rose Payne at Stanford University.[31]

Milstein and McMichael began their joint venture following a chance conversation at a joint conference of ICN Pharmaceuticals and the University of California, Los Angeles, held in Utah in March 1977. They saw their new partnership as an extension of Milstein's collaboration with Williams, work that McMichael was already familiar with because he and Williams were friends. The aim was to raise Mabs to antigens in humans similar to those developed to rat T cells so as to increase knowledge about the immune response in humans.[32]

McMichael's team was tasked with immunizing mice with human thymocytes (precursors to T cells) to generate Mabs against human leukocytes. Mabs, in the form of supernatants, were then sent by mail to Milstein for fusion with myeloma cells in his laboratory. Once fused, the cells were posted back to Oxford for RIA analysis. The work was not easy. Initially, the scientists battled to perfect fusion with the cells. Having finally achieved this, a fungus then contaminated the cellular culture. The project was rescued only because some earlier cells had been fortuitously stored in a freezer.[33]

By late 1978, the partners had produced a Mab that proved highly specific for human thymocytes. This was the first Mab produced to detect a human leukocyte differentiation. Despite this achievement, editors from the *Journal of Experimental Medicine* rejected their article on the subject, asserting that it was of "little scientific interest" and did not describe anything new. Finally published in 1979 in the *European Journal of Immunology*, the article went on to become a citation classic.[34]

The initial rejection partly reflected a more general ignorance of the significance of differentiation antigens and of what hybridoma technology could do in the early years. With many still struggling to produce stable Mabs, skeptics doubted whether hybridoma technology could truly produce Mabs against different antigens, let alone against T cells. Even Stuart Schlossman at Harvard's Dana-Farber Cancer Center, who successfully isolated the first human T-cell subclass in 1976 using conventional antibodies, was reluctant to use hybridoma technology despite his shortage of antibodies to reproduce his earlier result. He was using purified polyclonal antibodies from rabbits immunized against human T cells taken from a patient with T-cell leukemia. Schlossman had been present at the same ICN-UCLA conference in Utah as McMichael. During this conference Milstein and others had showed how Mabs generated against T-cell antigens could be "useful sources for biochemical and physiological studies of specific T cell subpopulations." Schlossman, however, decided to continue using purified polyclonal antibodies because of problems reported in securing stable Mabs.[35]

It was Patrick Kung, a young Taiwanese immunologist who learned about hybridoma technology as a postdoctoral researcher at MIT, who converted Schlossman to using Mabs. In 1978, Kung joined the immunologist Gideon Goldstein at Ortho Diagnostic Systems (a subsidiary of Johnson & Johnson), on a project designed to understand the regulatory role of thymopoietin, a hormone produced in the thymus, in the immune system. Lacking a standard test to detect the effects of thymopoietin, Kung set out to devise one. Rather than using conventional antibodies, which was the norm, he developed a Mab against T cells for the test, seeing it as a way of differentiating cell subsets.[36]

By 1978 Kung had generated promising Mabs, but they needed testing and classification. To do this, he turned to Schlossman, one of Ortho's consultants, who possessed a bank of twenty thousand leukemic cell samples from patients. Established in the early 1970s as part of his research into T and B cells, Schlossman's bank contained well-defined human T cells that could be used to test Mabs. Schlossman also had cellular immunoassay techniques for characterizing Kung's Mabs. Soon Kung and Schlossman, and their colleagues, began mapping Kung's Mabs against human T-cell antigens that had already been identified using conventional antibodies. In 1979, they published the first of their papers outlining their development of a series of Mabs for targeting various T cells, which they coded OKT (for Ortho, Kung, T cell).[37]

Kung struggled to persuade his Ortho colleagues of the value of the new Mabs. Goldstein saw the OKTs as only ancillary to his thymopoietin research. His view was not unique. A company survey indicated no prospective market for the OKTs. Only eleven people showed an interest in buying them—and they happened to be Kung's friends. It took months of wrangling before Kung could coax Ortho into commercializing the OKTs.[38]

This early reluctance began to disappear once scientists became more familiar with the hybridoma technique and better able to generate stable Mabs. Soon the technology had opened up a "goldmine" for studying and understanding human differentiation antigens and their relationship to health and disease. By 1981, no fewer than 150 Mabs had been identified for research into differentiation antigens on human leukocytes. Within five years this number had risen to 850.[39]

With an unlimited supply of Mabs, scientists could experiment with the same reagents and compare results on an unprecedented scale. Yet challenges remained. The key difficulty was ensuring that a Mab produced in one laboratory had the same qualities as one made elsewhere, and so provided comparable data in tests. This issue became increasingly pressing as more laboratories began producing Mabs. By 1983, fifty thousand Mabs had been produced and ten thousand new ones were being generated each year. With so many Mabs in existence, the potential for chaos was great—a problem compounded by the fact that no classification system existed for coding them. In an effort to cope, registries and bulletins began to be set up to monitor and list Mabs as they became available. Repositories were also established. These not only stored cells, but also compiled information on them based on data gathered from both published papers and unpublished sources.[40]

One of the earliest repositories was that set up at Sera-Lab by Murray, who soon after gaining access to Milstein and Köhler's Mabs in 1978 persuaded other scientists to follow suit. In exchange for free donations, scientists were offered royalties on any Mabs that were sold. Sera-Lab promised to store the cells in triplicate to ensure their safety, and to check their quality and the antigens they recognized. The company also created data sheets outlining the unique quality and specificity of each Mab. Having little information apart from what could be gleaned from publications, the process was labor-intensive.[41]

With scientists still battling to produce Mabs of their own, Sera-Lab rapidly became an essential resource for researchers new to the field, because it not only provided access to its own cells, but also helped researchers find sources for Mabs that it did not have in its repository. As Robert Tindle, Sera-Lab's head of research from 1984, recalls, it acted as a clearing house or like a newsagent that stocked all available newspapers. By 1979, Sera-Lab was receiving daily requests for the Mabs generated by Milstein and his colleagues and its catalog listed twenty-two Mabs, mostly from MRC researchers. This number grew substantially in the following years (Table 3.1). By 1986 Sera-Lab's repository represented one of the most extensive collections of Mabs then in existence. Many of the cells collected had no commercial value but were vital for research. They could be purchased either in purified form, or as ascites or supernatants. Production adhered to U.S. good manufacturing practice.[42]

Table 3.1

Number of Mabs listed in Sera-Lab catalogs

DATE	NUMBER OF MABS
1979	22
1983	68
1986	221

Source: Sera-Lab, *Catalogue* (1979), 11–14; Sera-Lab, *Catalogue* (1983), 8–13; Sera-Lab, *Catalogue* (1986), 35–53. Catalogs kept by Jenny Murray.

Across the Atlantic, another repository was set up by Melvin Cohn at the Salk Institute in San Diego. This was an extension of a cell bank of immune-related culture and tumor cell lines from mice that he had created in the early 1970s with funding from the National Cancer Institute (NCI). Cohn initiated the Mab collection after being inundated with requests for the P3X63Ag8 cell line he had received from Milstein in 1977. Applying to the NCI for extra finance to cope with the administrative demands of his ever-expanding collection of Mabs, in October 1980 he claimed his bank was fast "becoming the unofficial standard reference center for hybridoma cell lines." Indicating a number of scientific investigations worldwide directly or indirectly dependent on his bank, he depicted it as the primary repository for the new hybridoma products then "revolutionizing many facets of biological research." Scientists could apply to the repository in the event they accidentally lost their own cells.[43]

Both the Sera-Lab and Cohn's enterprises represented the informal and decentralized nature of Mab storage, distribution, and cataloging in the early years. A more centralized approach began to emerge in the early 1980s. By 1983, an international Hybridoma Data Bank (HDB) had been established under the auspices of the Committee on Data for Science and Technology of the International Council of Scientific Unions and the International Union of Immunological Societies. Its headquarters were in Rockville, Maryland, at the American Tissue Culture Collection (ATCC), which had been set up in 1925 to serve as a worldwide repository and distribution center for cultures of micro-organisms. It had established its own cell bank for Mabs, in 1980, and had become responsible for Cohn's collection in 1981. In addition to its headquarters at the ATCC, the HDB had databank branches in France, Japan, Canada, the United Kingdom, and India.[44]

The HDB provided a locator service to prevent scientists from duplicating their efforts. It offered comprehensive information on each cell line and product, including information on the reactivity patterns of the Mabs, their fusion partners' histories, who had developed them, their availability, their distributors, applications, assay procedures, and the class of antibody to which they belonged. The HDB depended on donations of Mabs from individual scientists, who were expected to complete data-reporting forms. This information was supplemented with data from published papers, commercial catalogs, and patent applications.[45]

By the early 1980s some large commercial companies were also actively distributing Mabs. This included Becton, Dickinson, which became engaged in the enterprise through its commercialization of Herzenberg's FACS. Unable to supply Mab reagents from his own laboratory for the FACS, Herzenberg persuaded the company to take it on in exchange for his training its staff in the procedures for standardizing the Mabs and for quality control. Certified to a specified standard, these Mabs were supplied with data sheets outlining the Mabs' known reactivities. Starting in 1980, Ortho Diagnostics also began distributing Kung's OKT Mabs, which were soon identified as important markers for tissue typing.[46]

The establishment of repositories and the commercial distribution of Mabs were vital not only for helping to standardize and disseminate information about emerging Mabs, but also for circulating them to researchers. This assistance became especially important after the Wistar patent of 1978, which made scientists more wary of giving out their Mabs. As Milstein commented in 1979, "I myself feel that monoclonal reagents are not being made as easily and generally available as I had hoped." Such possessiveness was linked not only to patent concerns, but also to researchers' desire to retain them for their publications. From the late 1970s, access was increasingly dependent on whom one knew. As Leonore Herzenberg put it, "This created a situation of haves and have-nots. It wasn't a question of whether people wanted to use the antibodies. It was a question of whether they could. For the most part everybody was playing very close to the bat. They gave their friends some antibodies, but they. . . . were generally not going to make them publicly available."[47]

Some scientists were outraged by their difficulties in accessing Mabs. A particularly stinging attack came from the director of the Max-Planck-Institut für Biologie at Tübingen, Germany, Jan Klein. Klein, a Czech-American immunologist, complained:

> Not so long ago, I urgently needed large quantities of monoclonal Lyt antibodies and so I wrote letters to several investigators asking them for the antibody-producing hybridomas. The replies surprised me. One said . . . that he had handed over (translate "sold") the rights to distribute the antibody to a commercial company and that I could buy it from them. Two answered that their respective universities were working out policies on how to distribute the antibody and that they could not help me until these policies were decided. The fourth promised me the hybridomas but . . . , despite repeated urging, I have not received them.

Klein drew analogies with Jacob and Esau and Shakespeare's Jewish merchant, Shylock, arguing,

> The new Merchants of Monoclonal Antibodies are smart fellows too. First they spend public money on centrifuges, hoods, media, glassware, mice, and technicians, and then they sell back to the public what they have produced using this equipment and manpower. Some even try to protect their merchandise by patenting it! There is nothing legally wrong with this practice (or is there?) but it is trickery and in keeping with that of the young Jacob and Shylock.

He hypothesized,

> Perhaps we should use Old Testament ethics to combat the new Shylocks in science: an eye for an eye, a tooth for a tooth. . . . If you refuse to share your cell lines you will not get any cell or mouse lines from me. This measure might be the only way to make the Shylocks realize that Jacob's morals are not good for science.[48]

Klein would later regret his Shylock analogy because of the offense he unwittingly caused.[49] Nonetheless, his concern reflected that of many contemporaries. The Herzenbergs, for example, while highly critical of Klein's use of Shylock because of its anti-Semitic undertone, pointed out that they and many Jewish and non-Jewish colleagues shared Klein's "irritation with investigators who have allowed business to dictate their scientific ethics." While they had aimed to ensure maximum availability of their own mouse Mab reagents when drawing up a commercial contract with Becton, Dickinson, others had not followed their example. They were indignant about the restrictive covenants that some of their colleagues had entered into with commercial bodies, agreements that they believed interfered with the open exchange of reagents. As they put it, "We see no a priori reason for this state of affairs save the naivete of scientists who accept the argument that this is the only way business can operate and the equal naivete of business school graduates who think that owning clones (which are easily reproduced) will guarantee their profits. Greed may be a motivating factor." They pointed out, however, that Mabs not only generated "piddling amounts of money," but the money was usually returned to the laboratory and the university. They continued,

> Perhaps we should look to the habits of investigators who in
> the past refused to distribute their research "products" for
> academic reasons and now find commercial rights a more
> convenient excuse. . . . Whatever the underlying causes, how-
> ever, the problem of how reagents are distributed needs to be
> addressed if immunological research is to survive and flourish.
> Students cannot be trained in an environment of secrecy
> and cupidity. Data lose their value if experiments cannot be
> repeated elsewhere because the reagents are under lock and
> key. Science, by its very nature, progresses through cross-
> checking and combining of information from many sources.
> There is certainly ample grounds for criticizing the kinds of
> behavior we have witnessed recently.[50]

Mab distribution was tied up with not only concerns about ownership rights, but also the extent to which their release sowed further confusion. A vigorous debate arose, for example, during Ortho Diagnostics' investigation into selling OKT Mabs. On the one side were the industrial executives who were keen to distribute the Mabs to qualified investigators to build up the generality of such tools, and on the other were the academics who preferred to limit circulation initially to a few private hands "in order to clean up the field."[51]

Attitudes shifted considerably after a series of international workshops on differentiation antigens of human leukocytes initiated by the French scientists Laurence Boumsell and Alain Bernard at Hôpital Saint-Louis in Paris, a major center for leukemia research and treatment. The workshops aimed to bring some coherence to the rapidly expanding number of Mabs then appearing in both the public and private domains. Known as the HLDA workshops (with HLDA standing for human leukocyte differentiation antigens), they originated from a meeting held on leukemic markers in Vienna in 1981. While those at the meeting were excited by the abundance of data being generated for characterizing normal and malignant leukocyte populations, they feared that the sheer number of Mabs being created, and the lack of organized understanding about them, could become an obstacle. As they put it, "The lack of an exact correspondence between the specificities of the various Mabs in use might act as a break on this major technological advance." In the worst-case scenario, "The elaboration of a plethora of individual systems of nomenclature would create complete confusion, render impossible any coherent dialog between those concerned, discourage others from joining in this work, or simply prevent people from being able to understand it."[52]

In October 1981, Boumsell and Bernard brought together a number of scientists, including Milstein, Schlossman, and McMichael, to design the HLDA workshop protocol. Also present was Jean Dausset, a hematologist and immunogeneticist similarly based at Hôpital Saint-Louis who had recently won a Nobel Prize for discovering the importance of leukocyte antigens for tissue typing in organ transplants. Dausset had helped set up of a series of international workshops directed toward the systematization of human leukocyte antigens (HLA) used in tissue typing. Launched in 1964, these workshops brought together investigators to compare their reagents, techniques, and results, and to publish their findings. The first three workshops included "wet" sessions where scientists could experiment together in the same laboratory using the same panel of cells. They were designed to determine whether the specificities of antigens defined in one laboratory matched those similarly defined in other laboratories. By 1980 eight workshops had been held. These provided a valuable set of reliable data for research into HLA antigens and understanding their disease associations. Critically, the workshops also showed how scientists could come together and share information in an open and friendly international environment.[53]

Like the HLA workshops, the HLDA meetings were intended to be "as open as possible" and had no limit to the number of participating groups or Mabs studied." Undertaken in the spirit of "intensive and unselfish international cooperation," the workshops were designed to find answers to questions that laboratories could not answer alone or that required "unduly long and painstaking efforts." Their overall objective was to provide a multi-laboratory, blind, comparative analysis of antibodies.[54]

The first workshop was held in Paris in 1982. Sponsored by the Institut National de la Santé et de la Recherche Médical (INSERM) and the World Health Organization, it focused on analyzing antibodies in terms of their reactions with leukocyte populations. It included fifty-four research groups from fourteen countries, who tested 137 Mabs. Using immunofluorescence, they demonstrated that a number of the cell types had "clusters of differentiation," thereby laying the foundation for a new classification system. Antibodies detecting the same antigen were allotted a specific CD number (for "cluster of differentiation"). Initially, the CD code implied a distinct molecular entity, but it was later used to designate the antigen. Scientists now had a common nomenclature, so results could be communicated in a universal language. This advance also helped to standardize the many different Mabs.[55]

The workshops became a regular four-year event. Table 3.2 lists the various workshops and illustrates the increasing number of laboratories and Mabs that were involved. Each of the workshops followed a similar pattern. Workshop organizers would code the Mabs submitted for review and then send them to multiple participating laboratories for blind analysis against an array of cell types. Data would then be collated and analyzed statistically and the Mabs and antigens assigned a CD code that was published. The workload was considerable, with "literally over 100,000 aliquots of antibodies changing hands in workshops." Tim Springer, one of Milstein's colleagues, remembered,

> The strain of organizing the workshop was enormous. After
> each workshop, it appeared that no one might be willing to
> organize the next, even bigger one. Here César's political skills

truly shone. Each time he was the force behind the scenes, cajoling or arm-twisting to ensure the next workshop. His global political vision ensured eight workshops on four different continents and the largest exchange of reagents ever organised for basic and clinical research.[56]

Many of the early Mabs submitted for review were directed toward unknown molecules that the first workshops helped define. Notably they defined the molecules CD3, CD4, CD8, and CD20, which became reference points for both basic research and diagnosis in immunology, hematology, and pathology—and were to prove particularly important in investigating HIV/AIDS. Mabs classified during the 1982 workshop, for example, helped to determine the relationship between HIV and CD4 receptors on cells. One panel of Mabs helped to reveal the way the HIV

Table 3.2

Summary of the HLDA Workshops I–VIII, 1982–2004

WORKSHOP (DATE)	CDS ASSIGNED	NUMBER OF CDS	NUMBER OF PARTICIPATING LABORATORIES	NUMBER OF MABS EXAMINED
Paris (1982)	CD1–CDw15	15	54	137
Boston (1984)	CD16–CDw26	11	N/A	N/A
Oxford (1986)	CD27–CD45	19	150	790
Vienna (1989)	CD46–CDw78	33	500	
Boston (1993)	CD79–CDw109	31	475	1,450
Kobe (1996)	CD110–CD166	55	475	1100
Harrogate (2000)	CD167–247	81	N/A	N/A
Adelaide (2004)	CD248–339	95	N/A	N/A

Source: H. Zola and B. Swart, "The Human Leucocyte Differentiation Antigens (HLDA) Workshops: The Evolving Role of Antibodies in Research, Diagnosis and Therapy," *Cell Research* 15 (2005): 691–94, table 1; F. Gotch, "Workshop Structure and Protocols," in A. J. McMichael et al., eds., *Leucocyte Typing, III: White Cell Differentiation Antigens* (Oxford, Eng., 1986), 3–14; A. L. Jackson, "Summary of the Fifth International Workshop on Human Leukocyte Differentiation Antigens," *Clinical Immunology* 15, no. 1 (1995): 1–5; P. Keating and A. Cambrosio, *Biomedical Platforms* (Cambridge, Mass., 2003), 188–89, fig. 6.5.
Note: N/A indicates data not available.

virus attaches and penetrates the CD4 receptor on susceptible cells, thereby causing infection.[57]

By providing an international framework for classifying and validating Mabs, the HLDA workshops brought most scientists together, leaving those unwilling to collaborate increasingly outsiders. Crucially, academics could submit their Mabs for characterization and classification for free, and laboratories that reviewed submissions could retain any Mabs left over from such work for their own research purposes. So important were the workshops that commercial companies such as Becton, Dickinson and Ortho Diagnostics paid to enter panels of their Mabs for review so that they could be assigned a CD classification.[58]

Aided by the classification and verifying systems established by the HLDA workshops, Mabs soon moved beyond the confines of a handful of laboratories and were applied to more and more research questions. This trend was accelerated by the growing supply of reagents provided by commercial companies. Researchers no longer had to rely on the goodwill of individual scientists to provide fundamental materials for their experiments. Soon Sera-Lab and Becton, Dickinson were joined by other companies eager to supply Mabs to researchers. Foremost among them was Serotec, established in Oxford in 1983, which rapidly became the main supplier of the workshops' Mabs.[59]

By the early 1980s, Mabs had opened up a whole new world of research. Not only did they provide more accurate pathological analyses than the older immunobased techniques; they also revealed previously hidden anatomical aspects of the body. Some of the earliest discoveries made possible by Mabs were related to the brain and the central nervous system. Yet these advances were just the tip of the iceberg as scientists began to realize the power of Mabs for exploring the vast number of human differentiation antigens, proteins located on the cell surface of immune cells. Before the arrival of Mabs, scientists had as much knowledge of the surface of immune cells as they had of the surface of the moon. Their subsequent investigations into human differentiation antigens would not only advance understandings about the network of interactions that govern the immune response, but also help identify new targets for diagnostic and therapeutic interventions that would have profound implications for human health.

CHAPTER FOUR

The First Medical Applications

AS RESEARCHERS BEGAN to use Mabs to explore the surface of cells and to probe previously hidden parts of the body, clinical applications began to open up. Writing years later Milstein reflected, "Once the exclusive specificity of monoclonal antibodies was established, the possible application of monoclonal antibodies in diagnosis and therapy became a subject of considerable importance and active research." The technology offered so many different possibilities that it was difficult to know where to start.[1] Many of Mabs' early applications appeared to have little overall pattern or logic, but their most effective uses were quickly established. In this process new relationships were forged between research scientists and industry, and Mabs' influence came to extend well beyond the confines of the small-scale laboratory. Such alliances inevitably posed challenges.

Milstein's correspondence reveals the wide range of applications that researchers sought for Mabs, including in the areas of immunology, parasitology, virology, bacteriology, oncology, endocrinology, hematology, pharmacology, and embryology. Many researchers hoped, too, that Mabs would improve the sensitivity and specificity of diagnostic techniques already in use. As the Canadian-based scientist Jacqueline Lecomte told Milstein, "My intentions are to use this cell line for producing monoclonal antibodies against Herpes, polio, rubella, IVC etc . . . with the hope of producing better viral diagnostic reagents."[2]

Optimism was not confined to human health. The Brazilian scientist Helio Gelli Pereira at the National Institute for Medical Research (NIMR) in London hoped, for example, to use Mabs to control foot and mouth disease. He believed that Mabs offered distinct advantages, commenting, "Antigenic variation is one of the most striking features of these viruses, having important implications in relation to epidemiology and control of the disease. However, all the information available on this subject is based on tests performed with highly heterogeneous reagents and, not surprisingly, it has been difficult if not impossible to interpret the majority of results. . . . the use of homogeneous antibody preparations . . . obtained by the techniques you describe may be of considerable value in our studies."[3]

Mabs generated some of the greatest excitement in their potential to help purify natural substances. Milstein immediately grasped this from his work with Williams. As Milstein put it, "The ability to derive antibodies to a [sic] single component of a 'dirty' mixture opens up a new approach to the purification of natural products." Milstein soon identified a suitable natural substance for testing his proposition: human leukocyte interferon, a group of natural proteins that cells release in response to pathogens such as bacteria, viruses, or parasites. Discovered in 1957 at the NIMR, by the 1970s interferon had been embraced as the next "wonder drug" to combat viral diseases such as cancer and the common cold. Interferon, however, remained a scarce commodity; only minute quantities are produced by the body and scientific methods for its production were limited. In 1969, a Finnish virologist, Kari Cantell, made some progress with secretions from white blood cells, leukocytes, but the preparation was crude, containing only 1 percent interferon. Interferon thus remained prohibitively expensive.[4]

By the mid-1970s, efforts to increase the yield of interferon were intensifying, inspired in part by the allocation of $1 million by the U.S. National Cancer Institute for research in this area and its launch of clinical trials. Research laboratories, pharmaceutical companies, and small start-up biotechnology companies sought to scale up interferon production using genetic engineering. Their aim was to isolate and clone the human interferon gene so that it could be inserted into bacteria for the mass production of recombinant interferon. By 1980 millions of dollars had been poured into the effort and both alpha and beta interferon had been successfully cloned.[5]

The process, however, was far from complete. Like natural interferon, recombinant interferon required purification, and although several methods for purifying interferon had been deployed from the late 1950s, these could not deliver the several-thousand-fold purification needed for enabling its use in the clinic. One of the most promising techniques for purification was immunoadsorbent chromatography, which worked by isolating and selecting a protein based on the binding properties of antibodies and antigens. But this technique relied on conventional antibodies that were in limited supply and were difficult to standardize. Part of the problem was that the animals used to make the conventional antibodies were often immunized with impure interferon, which meant that contaminants, rather than interferon, could be the actual targets of the antibodies.[6]

Early on Milstein and David Secher, one of his postdoctoral researchers, wondered whether Mabs might provide the key to improving immunoadsorbent methods for purifying interferon (Figure 4.1). A chance conversation in 1976 between Secher and Derek Burke—an expert in interferon who had worked with Alick Isaacs, a co-discoverer of interferon—led to their collaboration, with Milstein offering encouragement from the sidelines. Secher and Burke's project provided an ideal opportunity to demonstrate the practical and commercial utility of Mabs. As a consultant for Burroughs Wellcome, a pharmaceutical company, Burke had access to the human interferon it produced for clinical trials. Although it was only partially purified, it could be used to immunize mice so as to produce antibodies. These could then be fused with myeloma cells to develop hybridomas to secrete Mabs for use in purifying interferon.[7]

The work was painstaking. Three years were to pass before the team managed to develop a Mab suitable for use in immunoadsorbent chromatography. By March 1980, they had found a way of creating, in a single step, a much purer form of interferon than anything achieved before. And because they now had an infinite supply of standardized antibodies for immunoadsorbent chromatography, scientists no longer needed to generate antibodies by immunizing mice with interferon, which was also a scarce commodity.[8]

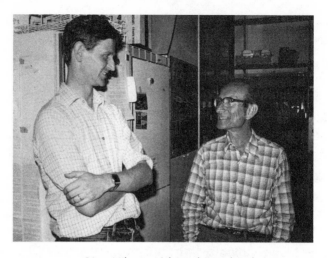

FIGURE 4.1. César Milstein (*right*) with David Secher, ca. 1980
(Photographer unknown; MRC Laboratory of Molecular Biology)

The new Mab also paved the way for improving process and quality control in the production of interferon. Even scientists in the best laboratories had an error rate of plus or minus 50 percent when creating interferon. Mabs not only offered greater accuracy but also made automation possible, allowing a single person to assay hundreds of samples in a single day. Because Mabs could be used to test for interferon in biological fluids, they also provided a way of monitoring the progress of patients taking the substance.[9]

Excited by the commercial potential of his and Burke's innovation, Secher quickly informed the MRC and the NRDC, the body responsible for patenting MRC inventions. His haste was due in part to the current political furor in Britain over the lack of a patent for Milstein and Köhler's technique. As mentioned earlier, any application for a British patent needed to be submitted ahead of publication for it to be valid. The MRC and the NRDC, however, declined to file for a patent, claiming that Secher and Burke's technique had no obvious application. Fearful that a patent application would delay publication of their research, Secher and Burke were initially relieved by this news. Secher, however, changed his mind days before submitting an article to *Nature* that outlined the broad applications of their purification technique and covered the main points required for patenting it. He asked MRC and NRDC officials to reconsider their decision. They, however, would not do so.[10]

The refusal posed a major dilemma for Secher, who was acutely aware of how Milstein had been pilloried for the failure of the MRC and NRDC to patent his and Köhler's innovation. Under the Patent Act of 1977, however, for a small fee he was free to file the drafted article for *Nature* with the Patent Office without a patent agent. Doing so would not comprise a full application, but would allow a full application to be submitted within a year. Sydney Brenner, then director of the LMB, discouraged Secher from patenting the technique, reminding him that he risked being fired if he went against MRC advice. With the support of Milstein, Secher nevertheless decided to file his and Burke's paper with the Patent Office at the same time as they submitted it to *Nature*.[11]

Once filed, Secher thought no more of the patent. Little did he realize that just about a year later the MRC's attitude would change with the establishment of the government-supported British technology company Celltech in November 1980. Shortly before the twelve-month patent deadline, and now encouraged by Brenner who sat on Celltech's Science Council, Secher disclosed his initial patent application to Celltech. Its executives understood the implications of this revelation and agreed to take responsibility for the final legal work and costs required for the full patent application. This was fortunate, since it was an expensive procedure that would have been difficult for Secher and Burke to finance on their own. Any thought the MRC may have had of disciplining Secher vanished once Celltech was interested in the patent.[12]

Owning the rights to the interferon patent was an attractive proposition for Celltech. Unable to compete with companies that were already ahead in the race to clone interferon, Celltech hoped to build a lucrative business by contracting to purify it for them.[13] Despite this, Celltech did not launch the interferon project with the urgency that Milstein and Secher expected. After attending a meeting of Celltech's Science Council in April 1981, Milstein reported with disappointment that the group felt "that immunoadsorbent chromatography with monoclonal antibodies was not going to be an economic proposition in [the] manufacturing industry." With many industrial executives now having "no great difficulty [accepting] the idea of mass-production using bacteria," Milstein could not understand why Celltech viewed the "mass growth of cultured cells" in "a completely different light." As Milstein put it,

> Tissue culture methods are still in their infancy and even now we can grow hybridomas in serum free media. With a certain amount of ingenuity and industrial development it ought to be possible to make continuous cultures of cells giving supernatant spent medium consisting perhaps of monoclonal antibody at a concentration of 100 mg per ml and 60% pure. That is, one gram per 10 litres of spent medium. At present the *laboratory* cost of 10 litres of tissue culture medium is under £20. And 1/2 of that cost is to sterilize it! A suitable immunoadsorbent column can easily be used ten times and, with proper development, probably many more times.[14]

Milstein was so angered by Celltech's lack of engagement that he wanted to cancel the contract when it came up for renewal. His dissatisfaction was shared by other LMB staff, who feared that Celltech's disinterest would lead to their inventions being commercialized in the United States and Europe rather than in Britain. They concluded that it might be better to collaborate with established companies like the Wellcome, ICI, and Unilever. Milstein felt Celltech's only "redeeming factor" was its "aggressive attitude" toward patenting. The company filed the official interferon patent application in April 1981, and it was granted in 1983. Tensions between the LMB and Celltech eventually eased in 1986 when Secher moved to Celltech to direct its research and development program dealing with therapeutic Mabs.[15]

Much of the strain between LMB scientists and Celltech arose because scientists elsewhere were gaining ground in the application of Mabs for the purification and biological testing of interferon, particularly recombinant interferon. At the forefront of this research was Sidney Pestka, who joined the Roche Institute of Molecular Biology in New Jersey in 1969. He had been investigating interferon since 1966 and from 1975 had spearheaded efforts to clone and purify it. In 1978, unaware of Secher and Burke's efforts, Pestka telephoned Theophil Staehelin in Basel to see if he could generate Mabs for use in immunoadsorbent chromatography to purify the recombinant interferon he was then developing. Staehelin had just moved from the BII to F. Hoffmann–La Roche to head up its efforts to commercialize monoclonal antibodies.[16]

Initially, Staehelin was cautious in his response to Pestka. In part, this was because he was still establishing his base in Roche and he and the colleagues who had come with him from the BII were unfamiliar with hybridoma technology. He was also unsure about the cost-effectiveness of using Mabs to purify interferon. Much would depend on how many times an immunoadsorbent chromatographic column coated with Mabs could be reused in the purification process. Staehelin, however, had two advantages. He had strong ties with Köhler, established when they were both at the BII, and he could call on the BII for the technical knowledge and most up-to-date reagents for generating Mabs.[17]

In 1979 Staehelin started working on the development of Mabs against interferon, using some fractions of interferon sent by Pestka. Containing between 2 and 10 percent interferon, these were used to immunize mice, creating what Staehelin later called the "million-dollar mouse." The mice were then sacrificed and their spleen lymphocyte cells harvested for fusion with myeloma cells. Fusion, however, proved difficult. Like other researchers, Staehelin's team struggled to prevent the mammalian cells from becoming contaminated with mycoplasms, a form of bacteria that feed off live mammalian cell culture. This problem was difficult to re- solve because mycoplasms are hard to detect with a conventional micro- scope. Some progress was made by adding the antibiotic chlortetracycline to the myeloma cell line, but the mycoplasms reappeared five to seven days later. Many of the fused cells also shriveled and died within ten days. Eventually the research team overcame the problem by injecting the sur- viving fused cells into the peritoneum of mice, which enabled the ani- mal's immune system to both destroy the mycoplasms and accelerate the growth of the Mabs, reducing production from a matter of weeks to just days.[18]

By the end of May 1980, Staehelin's group had sufficient quantities of Mabs to build a purification platform. This involved the attachment of two Mabs to beads on a solid support that acted as a column over which Pestka's interferon could be passed for purification. These Mabs bound to interferon simultaneously but without interfering with each other. The result was a "sandwich-type" dual antibody radioimmunoassay. This technique proved highly effective at measuring interferon concentrations in a single one- to two-hour incubation step.[19]

By October 1980, Pestka had one kilogram of crude recombinant interferon with which to begin testing the new platform, which he obtained in partnership with scientists at Genentech. The same month Staehelin flew to New Jersey to begin the purification process. He carried with him an immunoadsorbent column of about 18 milliliters, as well as reagents for a radioimmunoassay to monitor interferon concentration in all fractions of the purification process. Upon his arrival, he began to purify the interferon using the antibody column, which took four days and five nights of work. The end product was twenty milligrams of more than 99 percent pure interferon in thirty milliliters of buffer.[20]

With Staehelin's team's purification system, Pestka was able to achieve recombinant interferon that was a thousand times purer than that obtained through tissue culture and biochemical methods. Natural interferon used in clinical trials at this time was, by contrast, only 1 to 2 percent pure. A key advantage of Staehelin's technique, like that of Secher and Burke's, was that recombinant interferon could be purified in one step and the Mab column used repeatedly without losing efficiency.[21]

The platform created by Staehelin and his colleagues put Roche in the lead in the race to develop recombinant interferon for clinical use, ahead of the Hungarian-Swiss scientist Charles Weissmann, who had cloned interferon alpha for a newly formed biotechnology company, Biogen, seven months ahead of Pestka and Genentech. At one stage Weissmann had attempted to establish a collaboration with Staehelin to develop Mabs for purification. He, however, had not pursued the matter any further because he did not want to partner with Roche. Instead he used biochemical methods for purification, which took much longer. In any event, Roche lost its early advantage during the clinical testing, which put it neck and neck with Biogen when it came to the final marketing of the drug for leukemia in 1986.[22]

During the commercialization and patenting of interferon as a drug, the Mab purification of interferon became a major matter of contention between Celltech and Roche. At stake was which group of researchers— those in Britain, or those in Switzerland and the United States—had originally conceived of using Mabs to purify interferon. The matter was settled in Britain in the early 1990s, when the U.K. Patent Office ruled that the innovation rested with Secher and Burke. In the United States, however, Roche was able to assert its rights to a patent because Pestka and Genentech's research had been carried out there. The matter was finally settled out of court in the United States. Beyond the realm of patents, the successful use of Mabs to purify interferon clearly demonstrated the utility of Mabs for purification purposes. Interferon proved to be the first of many genetically engineered drugs purified with the help of Mabs.[23]

While the adoption of Mabs for the purification of interferon was part of a deliberate research program, Mabs came to be used for a completely different application—blood typing and grouping—by chance, as a by-product of research to produce Mabs against cancer cells. Physicians had been carrying out blood transfusions since the seventeenth century. While this procedure had long been risky, often resulting in the death of patients, its safety improved greatly as a result of Karl Landsteiner's work in the early twentieth century. When mixing blood from different individuals, Landsteiner discovered that red blood cells agglutinated, that is, clumped together, when different types of blood were combined. From this he deduced that humans do not all have the same type of blood. Exploring this further, he classified human red blood cells into four main groups, A, B, AB, and O.[24]

Exploiting the binding mechanism between antibodies and the antigenic material found on the surface of red blood cells (erythrocytes), which manifests itself in the agglutination of the cells, physicians could now mix the blood of a donor with that of a recipient to check for clumping before proceeding with transfusion. This idea was first suggested in 1907 by Ludvig Hektoen, a pathologist at Chicago's Institute for Infectious Diseases, though he did not perform the test himself. A year later, however, Reuben Ottenberg, an American physician at Mount Sinai Hospital in New York City, mixed the blood of a wife (donor) with that of her husband (recipient) prior to a transfusion. The blood did not clump, and he was able to proceed with a successful transfusion. Based on this result, Ottenberg argued that a serological clinical test could be devised for cross-matching blood before transfusions. The test would require only a pipette and a test tube.[25]

Serological testing of blood took time to become established, but by the 1940s it had become a common procedure to test for ABO incompatibilities before transfusions. In 1945 such testing was improved as a result of the work of Robin Coombs, an English pathologist at Cambridge University investigating hemolytic disease among newborns. This condition results from Rhesus incompatibility and occurs when antibodies in a mother's blood destroy her unborn baby's blood. Importantly, Coombs devised a test to identify antibodies reactive with erythrocytes that fell outside of the main ABO blood grouping system. This was critical because even though more than four blood groups had now been identified, severe transfusion reactions were still common. The Coombs test enabled the management of rhesus incompatibility and reduced transfusion complications.[26]

By the late 1970s, two techniques existed for grouping blood. Both provided results that the naked eye could detect. The first, which was quick and routinely used in emergency medicine, involved mixing the blood sample to be typed with antiserum on a blood-grouping glass tile and checking for any signs of agglutination. The second method, most commonly undertaken in hospitals, involved mixing a blood sample in a test tube with a saline solution and then checking after two hours for any sedimentation (which indicated agglutination). A centrifuge could be used to expedite the process in emergencies.[27]

Milstein himself was one of the first to recognize the utility of Mabs for blood typing, which until the late 1970s was dependent on conventional antibodies sourced from human antiserum. In Britain, most human antiserum was obtained by screening blood donated by volunteers to the National Health Service (NHS). By contrast, in Europe and the United States, it was supplied commercially from blood donated by hyperimmunized donors, that is, people specifically immunized with samples of purified blood group substances different to their own. This was potentially hazardous: not only was there the risk of adverse reactions to the procedure, but also any plasma used for immunization could be contaminated with diseases like hepatitis. Yet hyperimmunized serum was of a higher potency than that obtained from the blood donated to the NHS, and met the high standards required by the FDA. Hyperimmunized serum was also considered to be the most reliable reagent for use in the rapid tests done on glass tiles. By contrast, NHS antiserum reacted more slowly than hyperimmune-based reagents, so was unsuitable for emergency typing of certain groups of blood. The NHS reagents, however, were sufficiently reliable for use in the test-tube-based method.[28]

Efforts had been made to improve the potency of the NHS antibody reagents by immunizing some donors. Hyperimmunized serum, however, was expensive, reflecting the labor and time involved in its production. First there was the lengthy process of immunizing donors. Then extensive assaying had to be carried out on samples taken from the donors before they could be used, a process that had to be repeated for each sample obtained. The resulting reagents cost between £250 and £600 a liter—a high figure in 1970s Britain.[29]

Even antiserum obtained from the screening of blood donated to the NHS was expensive at an average of £250 per liter. This price was due, in part, to the complexity of the blood typing process. Britain's Blood Group Reference Laboratory, for example, required 1,200 liters of human serum generated from six thousand blood donations every year to carry out blood typing. Collecting the blood was also wasteful: at least 30 percent of all sera collected from a large number of small individual donations had to be discarded because it failed to meet the required standard. In addition, only 7 percent of the British population screened had the B category blood group, which was an important source for anti-A serum. This meant that supplies of potent anti-A serum were limited, and hospitals had to buy it from commercial outlets. If obtained from hyperimmune donors, this serum could cost £450 per liter.[30]

Over the years other sources had been evaluated for securing antibodies for blood typing, including sera drawn from trouts' eggs and snails. These efforts had not worked, however, and the supply of appropriate antiserum remained limited. A surge in blood typing to meet the increasing frequency of major surgery and the critical importance of human blood serum for other medical purposes also put an enormous pressure on supplies. The problem was compounded by the fact that no two human sera are alike, and it is difficult to secure a sufficient amount of antiserum with adequate antibody potency to provide reliable results.[31]

As early as 1975, Milstein and Köhler attempted to produce Mabs against the Rhesus (Rh) blood group, but had little success. They made more progress in generating a Mab against another group of blood cells known as type A. This was developed by chance with those Mabs that Milstein had produced with Williams in order to differentiate antigens on the surface of immune cells found in rats. Based on this, Milstein launched a collaboration to develop Mabs for blood typing with Douglas

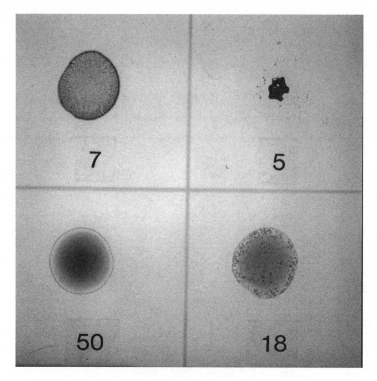

FIGURE 4.2. Slide 5, prepared by Steven Sacks, shows the distinctive clumping of blood group A with an anti-A Mab. (Steven Sacks)

Voak, a pathologist based in the Regional Transfusion and Immuno-Haematology Centre, Addenbrooke's Hospital, across the road from his laboratory. While the first Mab reagent they created had some problems, they soon had in hand one that proved effective for typing blood group A.[32]

Shortly after they started their venture, Milstein and Voak were joined by Steven Sacks, a medical graduate who joined the LMB in 1978. Sacks wanted to understand a strange phenomenon he had observed among some Mabs he had generated against cancer antigens for Ed Lennox in order to investigate immune responses to tumors. He had noticed an unusual clumping in a disc-like formation when the Mabs were placed on a small plastic plate with cancer cells (Figure 4.2). In addition to binding tumor cells, these Mabs appeared to be targeting other cells. With Voak and Milstein's help, Sacks found to his surprise that he had produced a Mab that targeted antigens on the surface of human-blood-group type A cells. Further investigation revealed that this had happened because he had immunized a mouse with human bowel cancer cells originating from a patient with the blood group type A. The resulting Mab only seemed to target group A and left group B or O cells alone. They subsequently found that mice most commonly produce anti-A antibodies.[33]

To the team's disappointment, the anti-A Mab proved a weak reagent for blood typing compared with human serum, but a month later, they managed to develop another anti-A Mab. Made on purpose, this Mab was a more potent blood-typing reagent than conventional serum. As Sacks wrote:

> Monoclonal anti-A produces a clearly visible reaction with red cells, improving the recognition of A and AB cells. The clearest benefit is seen with the weaker blood types of A poorly detected by conventional grouping serum. . . . Our present reagent is about three times as potent as conventional serum. Additional improvement in the speed and strength of red cell clumping can be achieved by concentrating the monoclonal antibody four times so that it equals the potency of hyperimmune commercial serum.[34]

Sacks reported that the Mab was particularly well suited for use in the blood-grouping machine that had begun to be introduced from 1963 onward. These machines facilitated the automated pipetting of samples and reagents into sample wells. Within this context the red cells were mixed with antibody in one of several channels, then the mixture's degree of agglutination was assessed either by passage through a light beam or by inspecting the ejected sample of cells on blotting paper. By the mid-1970s the automation of blood typing had been advanced through the introduction of plastic micro-liter plates that used solid-phase and gel technologies—technologies that decreased the volume of reagent required. Nonetheless, the process still required considerable work by technicians, who continued to have to manually prepare the reagents, identify the patient sample, and interpret and record the results. By the time the Cambridge team began their work, the introduction of laser scanners and computers had made it possible to identify and record labeled samples automatically—especially when Mab reagents were used. Sack reported, "Machine operatives greatly favoured the monoclonal reagent since the tighter pattern of red cell clumping enabled detection of weak A_2B bloods that are missed by conventional anti-A. In a recent run of 31 AB blood samples all were correctly identified by monoclonal anti-A whereas human anti-A failed to recognise seven of them."[35]

Following their development of the anti-A Mab, the team turned their attention to developing an anti-B Mab. This proved more difficult than anticipated, in part because most mice produce anti-A Mabs when immunized. But the goal was eventually achieved, after many different strains of mice were immunized with a group B blood group substance.[36]

By 1982 the collaborators had developed a number of different anti-A and anti-B Mabs and had studied them as blood-typing reagents for more than three years. From this they had determined one anti-A and one anti-B Mab that were good for routine use in ABO blood typing. The two Mabs had been evaluated using thousands of blood samples done both manually and by machine (the anti-A Mab was tested against 91,000 samples, and the anti-B Mab was tested against 65,000 samples). Importantly, the Mabs offered greater sensitivity than other Mabs for detecting different subtypes of each blood group and did not give false positives.[37]

The Cambridge scientists saw the adoption of these Mabs as a major opportunity to reduce costs in blood typing. While the average cost of hyperimmune serum at the time was £250 per liter, the team estimated that Mab reagents would cost only about £150 per liter, a difference that would save £100,000 on a typical yearly production of thousand liters. They argued further that "the financial saving from using monoclonals includes the benefit of saving the 6,000 donations at present used annually to make NHS reagents. This is less than 1% of all the plasma used to prepare blood products, but it . . . represent[s] over £31,000 of blood products. . . . Also it may save most of the unknown cost of commercial ABO reagents sold to hospitals at between £290 and £600/[liter]." Overall, they believed,

> The main cost benefit of monoclonals stems from their being
> produced in large batches, which reduces the expensive testing
> workload by more than 90%. At present tests are on batches of
> 2.5 [liter] antiserum pools, requiring initial screening tests
> and 13 detailed studies on 12 individual serum donations.
> Tissue culture-produced [Mab] reagents need only a few tests
> to monitor potency during culture and one detailed set of tests

on the final batch of perhaps 100 or more litres of culture medium.

The significant advantage of Mabs, then, was that they could be standardized and what was learned about one batch could be reused for the next.[38]

Armed with these positive results and MRC backing, in 1981 Lennox and Sacks filed for patents, which were subsequently granted in Europe, Japan, and the United States. These patents provided the basis for producing Mabs as reagents for ABO blood testing. Leading the commercialization of the reagents was Celltech. The company estimated the world market for these products at £7.5 million for hospital sales and £3 million for other sales. In contrast to the delays surrounding Mabs-related advances in interferon production, Celltech rapidly developed Mabs for blood reagents, probably in part because of the influence of Lennox, who was hired as Celltech's director of research in 1983. That year Celltech began to develop Mabs as blood reagents in earnest, having tested them at thirty-four British hospitals and transfusion centers.[39]

The commercialization of Mabs as blood reagents was uncharted territory. Until then, only small quantities of Mabs had been required as a tool for research or diagnosis, or even for purifying interferon. These small amounts had been supplied by either growing hybridomas in cell culture, or inserting these hybridomas into the peritoneal cavity of rats or mice and harvesting the fluid that gathered there, known as ascites. While ascites provided the greatest concentration of Mabs, this method was not a viable commercial option for creating the many kilograms of purified Mab needed for blood grouping. At least twenty thousand mice would be needed to produce just one kilogram of purified Mab. Executives at Celltech considered this approach not only impractical, but also unethical.[40]

Celltech's foray into the commercialization of Mab-based blood reagents catapulted it to the forefront of improving Mab manufacturing methods. What it needed was to find a way of producing Mabs that would provide blood reagents that were comparable in cost or even less expensive than those already on the market. Its executives decided the way forward was to optimize cell-culture production. This could be achieved by scaling up and reengineering the vessels in which the Mabs were grown. Celltech could draw on industrial techniques developed in the 1950s for scaling up the production of the polio vaccine, which was the first commercial product generated using mammalian cell cultures (in that case, monkey kidney cells).[41]

One of the most important sources of expertise for Celltech came from Burroughs Wellcome, a major established British pharmaceutical company that during the 1970s had devised a system for the commercial production of human interferon for clinical trials by using Namalwa cells, a cell line derived from a child with Burkitt's lymphoma. Able to grow mammalian cell cultures in eight-thousand-liter batches, Burroughs Wellcome had found a way of avoiding many of the difficulties encountered earlier in scaling up cell culture, thereby becoming a world leader in cell-culture production. Its system provided the foundation for the production of many other protein-based drugs, including those made through genetic engineering.[42]

Until the 1970s, most Mabs were generated on a small scale, using either static flasks or roller bottles. Celltech scientists realized that they could scale up production by taking advantage of the fact that hybridoma cells could be grown in suspension. This meant they could use deep-tank fermenters, large vessels commonly used in the industry to grow microorganisms such as bacteria for antibiotics. Celltech's goal was to adapt the airlift fermenting reactor, first used by Burroughs Wellcome for producing human interferon, which would provide the simplest means for monitoring and controlling the environment around the cells. Celltech also improved the culture medium used for growing hybridomas. As a result of these advances, within a short time Celltech was successfully producing Mabs on an industrial scale. While the productivity of hybridoma cell lines varied greatly, by 1986 Celltech had achieved a yield that represented a "four- to fivefold increase over those obtained in simple laboratory culture systems such as roller bottles." In 1989 its chief executive officer, Gerard Fairtlough, reported that Celltech had two thousand-liter and one two-thousand-liter airlift fermenters in operation as well as many smaller-sized vessels. Overall the company had managed to produce a hundred different cell lines in quantities of over a hundred grams, for a total of about six kilograms of Mabs. This put the company ahead of many of its competitors.[43]

By 1989, over half of the world's blood-typing reagents were based on Mabs produced by Celltech. The company's success reflected the growing acceptance of Mabs as blood reagents. Hybridoma technology offered many advantages: the uniform batch-to-batch control and the quality of the Mabs often exceeded that of conventional U.S. FDA licensed reagents; and unlike conventional blood serum, Mab reagents were free of contaminants and could be produced on a large scale. In just eighteen days, the company could produce a thousand liters of Mab supernatant, the equivalent of two thousand individual human donations—donations that had to be evaluated one by one and that involved the risky practice of immunizing volunteers to secure conventional reagents.[44]

The demand for Mab-based ABO blood reagents was reinforced by the outbreak of AIDS, which raised concerns about the safety of blood banks and transfusion. Nowhere was this concern more apparent than in France, where it was discovered in the mid-1980s that hemophiliacs and other recipients of transfusion had been given HIV-infected blood. Although the French uptake of Mabs as substitutes for human plasma-derived products was initially slow, it increased rapidly in the late 1980s. Between 1985 and 1987 the use of Mabs as reagents for blood typing of ABO blood groups before transfusion grew from 18.8 to 35.7 percent. Thereafter, the percentages grew to 48.7 percent in 1989, 56 percent in 1993, and 82.2 percent in 1995.[45]

Despite the rapid success of Mabs for ABO blood typing, the ability to create Mabs for other blood groups took longer to materialize. This was particularly noticeable in the case of anti-Rh Mabs, which Köhler and Milstein had failed to produce in 1975.[46] Such a Mab was highly sought after, because the Rh blood group is one of the most clinically important, especially given the increasing scarcity of plasma rich in anti-Rh antibodies. From the early 1970s mothers known to be rhesus negative who were carrying infants with rhesus-positive blood were routinely injected during their pregnancies with antibodies collected from the plasma of immunized volunteers. While this technique was highly effective at preventing hemolytic disease among newborns as well as complications among mothers, it dramatically reduced the number of women naturally sensitized during pregnancy.[47] The success of the treatment, then, not only reduced the stocks of plasma available, but also increased demands on the source. Alternative sources of the plasma could only be secured from donors following a mismatched blood transfusion, or by the deliberate immunization of volunteers. Immunization, however, required donors to have booster injections of red blood cells if they were to produce plasma with adequate potency of antibodies, which in itself carried risks.[48]

One of the problems scientists faced was that mice do not produce antibodies to Rh blood antigens. Some headway was made in 1983 by researchers at University College London and the North East Thames Regional Blood Transfusion Centre, who used the Epstein-Barr virus to modify B lymphocytes taken from donors with hyperimmune anti-D antibodies. Disappointingly, however, these first few Mabs proved less effective than conventional human antiserum. The final breakthrough was achieved in 1986 by scientists at Cambridge and Oxford universities. The reagents they developed proved useful both for rapid emergency slide tests and for the saline-based test-tube technique. Despite their utility, however, countries varied in their readiness to use the new Mabs. Adoption was faster, for example, in France than in the United States, reflecting the scarcity in the United States of plasma that was rich with anti-Rh antibodies.[49]

Despite the early difficulties, scientists soon began to produce Mabs to match many other blood groups. By 1989, for instance, Mab reagents had virtually displaced conventional serum for typing the M and N blood groups. Overall, Mab reagents transformed blood typing, obliging producers to improve their quality and standardization procedures for all the blood reagents they produced. Mabs also proved to be powerful tools for learning about the structure of antigens found on the surface of red blood cells, thus advancing work in the field.[50]

In addition to more efficient and effective blood typing, Mabs helped improve tissue typing for transplant surgery, a procedure that had been routine since the early 1960s. Traditionally, serological methods had been used to match the HLA antigens found on the surface of white blood cells in both donors and recipients to prevent incompatible or sensitized transplants (and so minimize organ rejection). First developed in 1964, the test for tissue typing was known as the micro-lymphocytotoxicity assay. Like blood-typing tests, this technique relied on antisera. The most effective source was serum drawn from women who had experienced several pregnancies and therefore had been exposed repeatedly to non-self paternal HLA antigens expressed by the fetus. Patients who had undergone transfusions or a previous transplant were also a useful source of antisera, albeit to a lesser extent.[51]

Tissue typing with Mabs uses the same basic principles of the lock and key mechanism between antibodies and antigens used in blood-typing tests, but instead of testing for antigens on red blood cells, tissue typing looks for antigens on the surface of white blood cells. The number of Mabs developed against HLA antigens increased exponentially from the late 1970s. By 1989, no fewer than 181 HLA Mabs had been evaluated for use in tissue typing, and several had proved useful. Although during the 1990s DNA probes also began to be used for tissue typing, Mabs continue to be important for this task.[52]

By showing the utility of Mabs in purifying interferon and for blood and tissue typing, the scientists discussed in this chapter not only demonstrated the clinical effectiveness of hybridoma technology, but also proved its commercial potential. By helping to bridge the gap between the academic world and industry, they developed the mechanisms needed for the bulk production of Mabs. Because of their efforts, those seeking to use and improve Mabs were no longer reliant on a few university-based researchers or limited to the small quantities they could produce. Armed with the expertise to generate Mabs on a large scale, scientists in both the academy and industry now had the capacity to explore the use of Mabs for a wide range of diagnostic and therapeutic purposes.

CHAPTER FIVE

Joy, Disappointment, Determination

EARLY CLINICAL TESTS

AS SCIENTISTS began to find practical applications for Mabs, clinicians were exploring their use for improving patient care. Indeed, many believed that Mabs were medicine's long-sought-after magic bullet. When, for example, a large group of scientists was asked by the U.S. Food and Drug Administration to appraise and rank 150 emerging technologies, they rated Mabs "the most useful medical discovery for the rest of the century."[1]

Many were optimistic that Mabs would defeat cancer. In 1982, John Minna of the U.S. National Cancer Institute (NCI) predicted that Mabs would revolutionize cancer diagnosis within five years. The adoption of Mabs as probes for targeting and identifying the multitude of antigens on different cell types seemed to herald their use in detecting and classifying tumors on a hitherto unthinkable scale. Mabs also promised to deliver more precisely powerful tumor-cell-killing agents, such as chemotherapeutic drugs, radioactive isotopes, or toxins, and to provide a way of harnessing a patient's immune system to attack tumors.[2]

Work in the cancer field, however, proved less straightforward than anticipated. In part this was because much of the initial endeavor was undertaken by researchers in academic laboratories and clinics with limited resources. Funded by government and charitable sources, their work had only minimal support from industry. In addition, new cancer drugs faced stiff regulatory and ethical tests.[3]

The idea of using antibodies to fight cancer had a long history. As early as the 1860s, clinicians, encouraged by successes in fighting infectious diseases, began to investigate the use of vaccines to stimulate an immune response against cancer. Based on observations that tumors shrank in patients with a skin infection called erysipelas, clinicians attempted to cure cancer patients by inoculating them with streptococcus, which caused erysipelas. In 1899, William Bradley Coley, a New York surgeon, together with the pharmaceutical company Parke, Davis & Co., developed a vaccine for the treatment of sarcoma. It contained a combination of the heat-killed bacteria streptococcus and *Serratia marcescens*. Clinicians also explored serum therapy for treating cancer. In 1895, for example, the French physicians Jules Héricourt and Charles Richet injected cancer patients with serum taken from an ass and two dogs immunized with an extract of a human osteosarcoma (a kind of bone tumor). The use of vaccines and serum therapy, however, failed to make any significant headway against cancer.[4]

In 1929 Ernest Witebsky, the German immunologist who described the antigen characteristics of tumors for the first time, laid the foundation for the use of antibodies in the diagnosis and treatment of cancer. The search for cancer diagnostics and therapeutics gathered momentum after 1948 when David Pressman and Geoffrey Keighley at the California Institute of Technology were able to localize in an intended target (in this case, a rat's kidney) antibodies conjugated with radioactive isotopes. Soon after, they showed that radioactively labeled antibodies in rats, dogs, and humans could detect tumors and could deliver low-dose radiation to kill them.[5]

By the early 1970s radioimmunoassay and immunofluorescence tests had identified a number of tumor antigens, and many scientists believed that it would be only a matter of time before clinicians could detect minute amounts of tumor antigens in the blood, allowing for cancer to be diagnosed and managed on a large scale. The advent of the hybridoma technology, which introduced virtually unlimited quantities of purified antibodies with known specificity to particular tumor antigens, represented significant progress toward this goal.[6]

Some of those most active in this area were scientists based at the Wistar Institute in Philadelphia, which in 1972 was nominated one of the first seven NCI-designated Cancer Centers in the United States. Much of the Wistar's cancer research was driven by its director, Hilary Koprowski, whose mother had suffered ovarian, breast, and throat cancer. Others involved in the work were Zenon Steplewski, a Polish cancer biologist with expertise in cellular fusion and cancer-cell preservation techniques; the German veterinarians Dorothee and Meenhard Herlyn, who were skilled laboratory investigators; and Barbara Knowles, an American immunologist studying cell differentiation and the immune response of mice to cancer.[7]

From early on, the Wistar group investigated the development of antibodies from fibroblast cell lines in order to devise a tool for detecting and defining tumor antigens. Their progress, however, was limited—at least until Koprowski secured Milstein's myeloma cells in September 1976. These cells, when fused with antibodies from the spleens of mice that had been immunized with tumor cells taken from patients suffering melanoma and colorectal cancer, helped generate a panel of Mabs that the Wistar team then slotted into radioimmunoassays. The resulting technique meant that by 1979 they could detect human melanoma and colorectal carcinoma cells.[8]

Yet the transformation of the Wistar team's laboratory achievements was not easy to translate into clinical applications. Early on the Wistar team discovered that their hybrid cell secreted a random assortment of Mabs that targeted multiple antigens. They wrestled for two years to find a Mab that targeted an antigen on only a single type of tumor so that it could be used as a diagnostic tool. Speaking to the First Annual Congress for Hybridoma Research held in Los Angeles in 1982, Steplewski summed up the challenge: "Up to now, there is not a single antigen that you could call tumor-specific—found on tumor cells but nowhere else. If you look long enough you will find it somewhere else."[9]

Finding a suitable Mab for diagnostic purposes involved arduous labor. In 1981, for example, researchers at the NCI reported having to screen between fifteen thousand and twenty thousand Mabs to find one specific for small-cell carcinoma of the lung. After combing through thousands of Mabs produced against different antigens, scientists began to realize that identifying a single Mab that bound to a specific antigen found on a particular tumor could be impossible. The best they could hope for was finding Mabs that targeted "tumor-associated" as opposed to "tumor-specific" antigens.[10]

Overall, the Wistar scientists found that Mabs generated against colorectal cancer were less reactive with other human cells than those developed against melanoma antigens. This was painstaking work. In 1979, they reported that of the 104 hybridomas generated using antibodies taken from the mice immunized against five colorectal carcinoma cell lines, only twenty-five bound to human cells when tested in radioimmunoassays, and of these only two proved specific for colorectal carcinoma cells. Nonetheless, they concluded, Mabs would one day be of "value in the classification of colorectal carcinomas by their antigenic determinants and may be applicable to immunodiagnosis and eventually to immunotherapy of one of the most common among the malignant tumors in man."[11]

Joining the Wistar group in their efforts was Henry Sears, an American oncologist based at Fox Chase Medical Center in Philadelphia. Sears first learned of Wistar's research by attending one of its meetings in the late 1970s. Excited by what he heard, Sears offered to help the Wistar team test their panel of Mabs to identify those with the greatest specificity for gastrointestinal tumor antigens. One they isolated from Mabs produced from serum taken from seventy-seven patients with a range of gastrointestinal cancers and thirty-nine healthy volunteers proved effective at identifying a specific antigen circulating in the blood of three-quarters of patients with colorectal cancer. Another analysis of serum taken from 108 healthy volunteers and 374 patients with colorectal, gastric, or pancreatic carcinomas indicated that Mabs could distinguish between antigens in cancer patients and those in healthy individuals. In another investigation of eighty-five patients with primary colorectal carcinoma, the researchers identified two anti-colorectal-cancer Mabs as "valuable prognostic aids for making clinical therapeutic decisions and appropriately stratifying patients for clinical trials." Following this, the Wistar group scrutinized the thousands of hybridomas they had produced against human gastrointestinal cancers for a Mab that could both act as a diagnostic tool and block tumor growth. By 1979 they had found a suitable candidate. Labeled 17–1A, it was produced from the spleen of mice immunized with colon cancer cells from an eighty-three-year-old Texan.[12]

After preliminary tests in mice indicated that 17–1A could help control colon cancer, the team launched a pilot study of patients with terminal gastrointestinal cancer in December 1980. The scientists were anxious
about this trial, fearing that patients would develop allergic reactions to
the mouse component of 17–1A or, even worse, suffer an anaphylactic
shock or cardiac arrest. All patients were therefore given a skin test prior
to treatment to check for possible sensitivities to the 17–1A. With emergency equipment kept on hand during the trial, each patient's respira-
tion, temperature, and physical condition were monitored during the
drug's infusion and over the next twenty-four hours. Blood samples were
also taken before and immediately after treatment, and at regular intervals thereafter for three months, to monitor liver and kidney functions,
measure the circulation of 17–1A, and detect any antibodies produced in
response to it that could trigger an adverse reaction.[13]

Jeffrey Mattis recalled the apprehension in the air: "Around 1981–82
I was involved in the process of developing and purifying an anti-cancer
antibody, 17–1A, which was to be given to a cancer patient at the Fox Chase
Cancer Center who was terminally ill and in the end stages of cancer.
This was one of my scariest experiences." To the team's relief, the reactions of the first four patients treated indicated that it was safe to administer a mouse Mab targeting a human tumor antigen directly to an affected
organ, and that the Mab circulated in the body for lengthy periods. Nevertheless, the patients experienced negative immunoreactions when 17–1A
was infused too fast, and although this problem was remedied by slower
infusions, it ruled out repeated doses of the drug. Thereafter, leukophoresis was explored for administering 17–1A to see if this made the Mab
more effective. Leukophoresis involved isolating a patient's white blood
cells (leukocytes) and incubating them with the Mab so that they would
be programmed to attack tumors before being infused back into the patient. It was a time-consuming and laborious process.[14]

By January 1983 a further sixteen patients had been tested. None experienced any immediate allergic or other adverse side-effects to 17–1A
either during or after the trial. Encouragingly, three appeared tumor free
when followed up ten, thirteen, and twenty-two months after treatment.
Hoping to engage more collaborators, Koprowski publicized the results
to a hybridoma research meeting in Los Angeles in February 1983. This,
however, sparked a "verbal shoot-out" between himself and U.S. Food and

Drug Administration officials attending the presentation. The dispute was over "whether mouse-derived monoclonal antibodies, in any dose, form, or combination, were ready for human use at all." Koprowski left the meeting determined to "prove the skeptics wrong." Undertaking trials on a large scale posed significant risks. As Marshall Goldberg, one of Koprowski's colleagues, put it, "The National Cancer Institute conducts such 'therapeutic trials' all the time and when they fail, as many understandably do, little is said. But for an independent institute, lacking its own treatment facility, to undertake such an extensive study represents a steep gamble for all involved."[15]

With each treatment costing approximately $7,000, further trials would also be prohibitively expensive. Regulations for clinical testing posed another hurdle. American regulations specified that patients could be tested with novel drugs only after all other therapeutic avenues had been exhausted. This left Koprowski with what he called "essentially hopeless cases to work on." These were "people who were in the last stages of cancer whose immune systems were reeling from all the other drugs and procedures that had been tried on them." Koprowski solved the conundrum by partnering with clinicians in Europe where the rules were more permissive and so would allow 17–1A to be tested in patients with less advanced cancer. The European patients were also likely to have less compromised immune systems than their American counterparts, because chemotherapy following surgery was less common in Europe than in America. One of Koprowski's key European partners was Gert Reithmüller, a German immunologist based at Ludwig Maxmilian University, Munich, who had developed a Mab with similar properties to those of 17–1A.[16]

By 1986 eight groups were testing 17–1A across the world and a meeting was convened in April to assess their results. Overall, 376 patients had been treated, of whom 105 had received the drug to test its toxicity, and 271 had taken it as therapy. The data revealed that 26 patients had been disease-free for two years and 69 were stable. These results were not particularly spectacular, however; instead they were equal to results for other forms of therapy. In addition, patients had been drawn from a mixed population and varying doses of the drug had been given, so it was unclear what dose was sufficient to destroy cancer. It was also unclear whether leukophoresis enhanced the effectiveness of 17–1A, which had implications for whether the procedure could become routine beyond a hospital setting.[17]

Encouragingly, however, the trials did indicate that 17–1A could stimulate a patient's immune system to attack tumors. The theory was that the Mab either prompted an attack by the immune system's T and B cells, or activated a series of proteins known as "complement" that, as mentioned earlier, helps fight off bacterial and viral infections. Alternatively, the Mab was thought to be stimulating macrophages, a type of white blood cell that surrounds and destroys foreign substances. This theory was backed by microscopic investigations by the Wistar team, which showed that macrophages primed with Mabs were capable of destroying cancer cells.[18]

The idea that an antibody could destroy cancer by prompting an internal immune response was not new. Research in the early 1970s by the British immunologist husband-and-wife team Freda and George Stevenson at the Tenovus Research Laboratory, Southampton University, had revealed that antibodies could kill tumor cells by activating complement and other immune defense cells known as natural killer or NK cells. They had demonstrated this with antisera raised in sheep immunized with cells taken from leukemic guinea pigs.[19]

In addition to identifying the power of antibodies to stimulate an immune response, the Stevensons discovered that malignant B lymphocyte cells involved in leukemia, lymphoma, and multiple myeloma secrete unique "marker" proteins on their surface that include a particular marker known as an "idiotype." Because it is present only on cancer cells and not on normal cells of the body, the idiotype offers a very precise tool for diagnosing and treating such cancers. The Stevensons capitalized on this discovery by developing anti-idiotype antibodies, which proved highly selective in targeting leukemic cells in guinea pigs, and so offered a very promising way to reach and target these cancer cells in humans as well.[20]

By 1976, with the help of colleagues, the Stevensons had successfully created anti-idiotype antibodies targeting human chronic lymphocytic leukemia (CLL), one of the most common forms of leukemia, by injecting sheep with CLL cells taken from patients. These anti-idiotype antibodies, which were shown to be capable of slowing down and even eradicating the growth of lymphocytic leukemic cells in guinea pigs and mice, were infused into a seventy-three-year-old man with CLL in 1980. The antibodies, administered by leukophoresis, destroyed the patient's leukemic cells by activating his complement.[21]

Despite these promising findings, manufacturing anti-idiotype antibodies proved cumbersome and time-consuming. By 1980 the team had secured only enough antibodies to treat one patient. Moreover, the antibodies had prompted only a modest response in the patient, because the antibodies had been internalized in the patient's body within minutes of being infused. To resolve this problem, the Stevensons' group tried purifying large quantities of rabbit and sheep antibodies and modifying them with enzymes. While this reduced the rate of internalization of the antibodies and increased their potency to kill tumors, it failed to produce enough antibodies for treating patients. This led George Stevenson to approach Milstein to see if hybridoma technology could offer a way forward, but Milstein felt the technique was still in its infancy and had not yet produced sufficiently robust Mabs for therapy. He also believed that creating tailor-made Mabs for individual patients as the Stevensons had done with conventional anti-idiotype antibodies would prove impractical and logistically difficult. The Stevensons team therefore decided to persevere with their enzyme modification method.[22]

Little did the Stevensons realize that across the Atlantic, Ronald Levy, an American oncologist at Stanford University, was beginning to generate anti-idiotype Mabs for diagnosing and treating leukemia and lymphoma. He saw this work as an extension of the Stevensons' research and that of Jean-Paul Mach, who had demonstrated that conventional antibodies, labeled with radioisotopes, could target tumor-associated antigens in humans. Initially Levy had used Klinman's splenic fragment technique, but this had generated only minuscule quantities of antibodies, which died quickly. While good for analytical work, they were unsuitable for diagnostic and therapeutic purposes. The publication of Köhler and Milstein's hybridoma technique in August 1975 marked a turning point for Levy. Accessing Köhler and Milstein's cell lines from Leonard Herzenberg, a Stanford colleague who had just returned from a sabbatical in Cambridge, Levy mastered the new method easily and soon had Mabs "growing as weeds."[23]

Within a short time, Levy had generated Mabs able to determine and categorize leukemia and lymphoma cell subtypes. Importantly, they could distinguish between malignant cells associated with leukemia that originated from myeloid cells made in the bone marrow and those linked with lymphoma produced by the lymphatic system. This enabled him to identify which type of disease individual patients had and their ideal course of treatment. By 1979 Levy and his colleagues had produced a series of mouse hybridomas that secreted Mabs against human acute lymphocytic leukemia (ALL), of which two had proven useful for subtyping ALL cells in lymphoid tissues. A year later they reported on the development of an anti-idiotype Mab derived from cells of a patient with nodular lymphoma. This Mab, which could recognize the surface of lymphoma cells in the patient's serum, provided a means to track the progress of lymphoma and monitor its treatment. It also opened an avenue for mounting an attack on tumors by stimulating a patient's immune system.[24]

Levy's first patient was Philip Karr, a sixty-seven-year-old industrial engineer who had received treatment at Stanford's Clinical Cancer Research Center over a number of years and whose lymphoma no longer responded to that treatment. After agonizing over what to do, in 1981 Levy decided to try a customized Mab that had been produced from Karr's own lymphoma cells and stored in Levy's freezer for a year. In accordance with some preliminary experiments in mice, Karr was given seventeen infusions of the Mab at steadily increased doses over ten weeks. Within two weeks of his first dose Karr had improved significantly and continued to make progress with each infusion. Nor did he suffer immunoreactions. By August 1981 his disease had gone into remission, and the following month he resumed hiking and gardening, something he had not been able to do before treatment. In 2004, now aged ninety, Karr recalled that before receiving the Mab he had been unable to swim even the width of a pool, but within a few days of treatment he was able to swim a width, and soon thereafter its length.[25]

While Karr's experience was encouraging, Levy was apprehensive about trying it on others. His anxiety was not helped by Henry Kaplan, one of his mentors and a successful pioneer of radiotherapy for non-Hodgkin's lymphoma, who had warned Levy when he began Karr's treatment, "The experiment better work the first time!" Following Levy's positive results, Kaplan demanded another trial, only to be flabbergasted when its results proved positive once again. Levy received more support from Milstein, whom he encountered at a conference in France. Thrilled

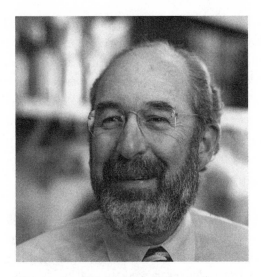

FIGURE 5.1. Ron Levy helped pioneer the development of rituximab. (Ron Levy)

to hear of Karr's improvement, Milstein urged Levy to continue developing the treatment (Figure 5.1).[26]

While it seemed to be effective and have few side effects, Levy's Mab
had a major downside: it had to be tailored to individual patients because
it targeted surface antigens of the lymphoma tumors unique to each patient. Customizing a Mab was inevitably time-consuming, taking up to
six months, and so was also prohibitively expensive. Treatment of just one
patient was estimated to cost $50,000. Because Levy's sole source of fi-
nancial support came from government and charitable bodies, progress
was inevitably slow. By 1983, he had treated seven more lymphoma patients, five of whom experienced some improvement. Yet other researchers struggled to replicate his results. Not only did they find it difficult to
produce Mabs with the right tumor specificity, but patients also developed immune responses to the mouse component of the Mabs, which
neutralized the therapeutic efficacy of treatment.[27]

With the jury still out on Levy's approach, reports began to surface
about the use of Mabs for bone marrow transplants (BMT), a procedure
that by the 1970s was becoming routine in the treatment of leukemia,
lymphoma, and multiple myeloma. A spongy material found in the
cavities of most major bones of the body, bone marrow is responsible for

the production of millions of stem cells that are converted into the red and white blood cells necessary for carrying oxygen around the body, fighting infections, and clotting. Any bone marrow damaged or destroyed by a disease like cancer, or by chemotherapy or radiation, can result in life-threatening shortages of blood cells. The BMT procedure involves injecting a cancer patient with healthy bone marrow so as to replenish his or her own bone marrow and boost the production of blood cells. The bone marrow is either harvested from the patient prior to treatment or from a matching donor.

BMTs were first pioneered in the early 1950s not for the treatment of cancer, but as a biological tool for investigating the effects of lethal radiation released by atomic bombs and accidents at nuclear reactors. By the 1960s BMTs were regularly performed for the treatment of blood disorders (marrow aplasia, leukemia, and anemia) and for organ transplants. The procedure is not risk free. As is the case for any tissue grafting, any incompatibility can mean a BMT will set off unwanted, and at times severe, immune reactions that can lead the recipient's immune system to reject the donated bone marrow and attack it as foreign. By the 1970s, improvements in matching techniques, which allowed for better screening of the immunological compatibility between donors and recipients, and the introduction of immunosuppressive drugs such as methotrexate and cyclosporine, meant that the incidence of graft rejection among patients had greatly diminished. Nonetheless, BMTs could still cause graft-versus-host disease (GVHD). First identified in 1959, GVHD is caused when the transplanted bone marrow (graft) attacks the recipient's body's organs and tissue cells, which it regards as foreign. Sufferers experience severe damage to their skin, liver, and gut, and have a high risk of chronic disability or even death. The incidence of GVHD remained so high during the 1970s that BMTs were not widely performed.[28]

Given its risks, particularly the high incidence of GVHD, the use of BMT for cancer treatment looked to be of limited use for the foreseeable future. The arrival of Mabs, however, provided a new way of conquering GVHD. One of the researchers quick to seize the opportunity opened up by Mabs was Herman Waldmann, an immunologist and clinician who had been appointed to the department of pathology at Cambridge University in 1973 after completing a doctorate on the process of immune-system regulation. Waldmann had first been alerted to Mabs when he was asked to teach Köhler the plaque assay necessary for launching his and Milstein's first Mab experiments. His interest in Mabs was further aroused when he was invited to hear Milstein and Köhler discuss their technique at one of the LMB's weekly meetings held just before the team published their August 1975 article in *Nature*. One comment made during this meeting by Sydney Brenner proved particularly thought-provoking for Waldmann. Brenner asked whether it would now be possible to make Mabs against anything, including, as he put it, "against my mother-in-law."[29]

Interested in developing Mabs for studying immune tolerance, Waldmann took a sabbatical with Milstein at the LMB between 1978 and 1979. He believed that Mabs could help him understand why the immune system could respond so quickly to pathogens and yet ignore self-antigens, molecules that exist in a person's own body. In particular, he wanted to test the prevailing theory that immune tolerance signified a lack of cooperation among lymphocytes in the immune system. One way of assessing the validity of the theory, he speculated, would be to reduce the number of lymphocytes in an experimental animal and then expose it to a new antigen. If immune tolerance was linked to a lack of cooperation among lymphocytes, then the animal's immune system should become tolerant to the antigen. An anti-lymphocyte Mab provided the ideal means to reduce the number of lymphocytes in an experimental animal (Figure 5.2).[30]

Soon after starting his work on developing an anti-lymphocyte Mab for use in animals, Waldmann shifted his attention to its development for use as a clinical tool to prevent GVHD. This was a natural extension of his research, since animal experiments conducted in the early 1970s had shown that mature T-lymphocyte cells were responsible for GVHD. He believed that such a Mab could help remove these T cells in human marrow and thereby eliminate the risk of GVHD. Purging T-cells from human marrow to improve BMTs was not a new concept. Various researchers around the world were investigating this route. In 1980 a team of researchers based at the Memorial Sloan-Kettering Cancer Center in New York reported some success in separating T cells from human marrow using the plant called lectin soybean agglutinin and sheep red blood cells. The technique was, however, time-consuming, so its use was limited.[31]

Elsewhere researchers were also investigating the utility of Mabs for such a purpose. This included the OKT series of Mabs described in

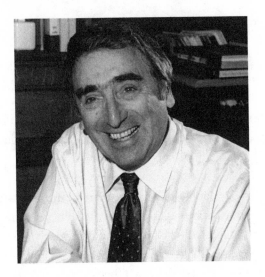

FIGURE 5.2. Herman Waldmann, ca. 1970.
Waldmann and his team were responsible for the
development of the first humanized Mab, which is
still used for combating leukemia and transplant
rejection and has proven effective in controlling
autoimmune disorders like multiple sclerosis.
(Herman Waldmann and Geoff Hale)

Chapter 3, which Kung and Schlossman had developed specifically to
target T cells. Initially these Mabs were deployed to classify leukemias
and lymphomas of T-cell origin, but scientists soon realized that they
could help coat T-cell receptors and thereby prevent their attack on transplanted tissue. One Mab in particular, labeled OKT3, was considered
particularly effective, because it was thought to inhibit T-cell functions
in the same way as an anti-idiotype antibody. Much of the attention was
focused on its use as a therapeutic agent for immunosuppression to prevent organ rejection, but it was also explored for BMT, in a technique
whereby the Mabs were incubated first with donor marrow or spleen
cells so as to coat the T cells before they were infused into patients. The
aim of the treatment was to stimulate the recipient's immune system to
remove and destroy the T cells. While OKT3 went some way toward preventing GVHD, it did not completely eliminate the disease. This was partly
because OKT3 did not work in tandem with cells made by the patient's immune system to cause the removal of the T cells infused with the bone

marrow. Although it was designed to seek out and bind to a particular target on the T cell, OKT3 was not intended to function as a killer cell and could not activate the human immune system to destroy the T cells.[32]

In fact, although most Mabs developed against T cells in the late 1970s and early 1980s targeted T cells effectively, they could not kill the cells by themselves. They only did so if combined with a second reagent that killed or at least separated out the unwanted T cells. Some researchers tried to overcome the problem by tagging Mabs with the plant toxin ricin. Others tried combining them with human complement, a small protein made by the immune system to help antibodies and phagocytic cells clear pathogens from the body. Unfortunately, the only source of complement known at the time to bind with Mabs was from heterologous serum taken from rabbits, which was hard to procure in a reliable, standardized form. Some batches of rabbit complement had also proven toxic to stem cells. Screening for such toxicity added not only complexity to the process, but also time and expense.[33]

In view of these problems, Waldmann aimed to generate a Mab that could both activate the human complement and bind to T cells while simultaneously sparing stem cells. His goal of developing a functional Mab with "operational" specificity was highly novel. Most researchers at the time were focusing their energies on producing Mabs against certain binding sites on cells, with the goal of investigating the antigens on their surface, rather than developing one with a particular function, and many of his colleagues were highly skeptical that he could generate a single Mab that would activate human complement. Up to this point, as Waldmann recalled, "Only polyclonal anti-lymphocyte antisera, which contained many antibody specificities, were expected to coat lymphocytes with sufficient antibody so as to activate C_1, the first component of complement." To achieve his objective, Waldmann began exploring the possibility of developing an anti-T Mab that would facilitate the controlled lysis (dissolving) of the T cells in a donor's bone marrow in a test tube before that marrow was infused into a patient.[34]

Waldmann was joined in his work by a number of other young researchers from various fields eager to participate in cutting-edge immunological research. They included his doctoral student, Stephen Cobbold, a biochemist by training; Geoffrey Hale, a postdoctoral protein chemist; and two postdoctoral cellular biologists with expertise in culture systems,

Sue Watt and Trang Hoang. He was also helped by Alan Munro, his former doctoral supervisor based in the Pathology Department, and Don Metcalfe, an expert in stem cells who had come to Cambridge on a sabbatical from the Walter and Eliza Hall Institute of Medical Research in Melbourne. An additional team member was Michael Clark, a biochemist who joined after completing a doctorate with Milstein.[35]

In 1979, Waldmann's team, funded by the Medical Research Council, started the ball rolling by immunizing a rat with a human lymphocyte. The rat's spleen cells were then fused with a rat myeloma cell line, known as Y3/Ag1.2.3, which had been developed recently by Giovanni Galfré and Bruce Wright at the LMB. The choice of developing a Mab using rats, rather than the more traditional mice, offered technical advantages, notably more efficient fusions and the ability to attain greater quantities of Mabs than had been possible previously. It also provided an easier means of producing Mabs to human cell antigens.[36]

By 1980 Waldmann and his colleagues had successfully generated a diverse range of antibodies to human cells, of which one set appeared to have the ability he had sought: to lyse T cells with human complement. This set of antibodies came to be referred to as the Campath-1 (for "Cambridge Pathology") family of antibodies. Further experiments in animals proved Campath-1 to be particularly efficient at activating complement and virtually eliminating T cells while sparing the bone marrow's stem cells. Subsequent collaboration with colleagues at Addenbrooke's Blood Transfusion Centre revealed that the set of Mabs recognized the same antigen, a GPI-anchored dodecapeptide now known as CD52, that, while present on nearly all human lymphocytes, was absent on human red blood cells.[37]

One Mab, labeled Campath-1M, was found to be most efficient at lysing lymphocytes with human complement. After some laboratory testing and some safety studies with Campath-1M in primates, the first pilot study was launched in humans in 1982 to check for the antibody's safety before beginning larger studies to investigate its use for preventing GHVD in BMTs. The first patient treated was FB, a man suffering from end-stage non-Hodgkin's lymphoma, a type of blood cancer. He was a patient in the Hematology Department next door to Waldmann's laboratory. Disappointingly, the Mab cleared FB's tumor cells only temporarily.[38]

Although FB died shortly after completing treatment as a result of his underlying disease, he had tolerated the treatment well and had

experienced no toxic effects with repeated doses. This encouraged Waldmann and his team to test Campath-1M in other patients. The second
person treated was a man called AP. Again, while he responded well to
the treatment initially, he died when it ended as a result of his underlying disease. Following AP, Campath-1M was given to a woman suffering
from leukemia. While it had little impact on her leukemia, it proved effective in removing her T cells and activating complement. She also tolerated the drug well. From the pilot tests, Waldmann's group concluded
that Campath-1M merited clinical investigation for BMT. Not everyone
was so convinced. Reviewers for the *Journal of Experimental Medicine and
Blood,* for example, refused to publish their work and editors at *Blood* were
initially reluctant to publish it.[39]

The challenge the team faced was how to find an appropriate patient
for testing the value of Campath-1M for BMTs. They were anxious about
conducting such a trial, in case their Mab killed patients' stem cells along
with their T cells. The first person chosen for testing was a woman at
Hammersmith Hospital suffering from severe aplastic anemia, a condition that occurs when the bone marrow produces insufficient new cells
to replenish blood cells. The woman faced a strong possibility of dying if
not given a BMT. Unable to find a suitable matching sibling donor, she
was slated to receive bone marrow from an unrelated but genetically
matched donor. Receiving bone marrow from an unrelated donor, however, was still highly experimental and carried a high risk of GVHD.[40]

In 1982, Waldmann, working with Jill Hows and Ted Gordon Smith
during a clinical training stint at the Hammersmith Hospital, gave the
woman Campath 1-M. To their delight her marrow appeared to recover.
Subsequent analysis of her marrow, however, suggested that her own stem
cells rather than those of her donor were responsible for reconstituting
her blood system. This was unexpected because prior to receiving Cam-
path-1M she had been unable to make any of her own bone marrow cells.
While the result was good news for the patient, it made the Hammersmith clinicians afraid that the Mab was affecting stem cells, so they called
a halt to the work.[41]

After the experiment at Hammersmith was abandoned, the team collaborated with Shimon Slavin, a clinician based at Jerusalem's Hadassah
Medical Center, whom Cobbold had met by chance at a transplant conference in California. Already performing experimental BMTs in leukemic

patients, Slavin was eager to try Campath-1M, seeing its power to deplete T cells as a promising method for preventing GVHD. Together with Waldmann's team, Slavin launched a trial of Campath-1M in a small cohort of eleven leukemia patients whose prognosis was poor. All patients received bone marrow taken from matched donors mixed with Campath-1M prior to infusion. Campath-1M was found to reduce the incidence of GVHD from 40 to 10 percent in the patients, even without any posttransplant prophylaxis. Some of the patients continue to be alive and well today, more than thirty years on.[42]

Despite reducing the incidence of GVHD, however, the bone marrow grafts in two out of the eleven patients treated at Hadassah Medical Center were rejected during treatment and could not be rescued with a second or third graft. Waldmann and his team hypothesized that the rejection could have been due to residual cells from the conventional treatment that the patients had received, which tried to destroy a patient's own T cells so as to condition their body to accept tissue from a donor. Based on this reasoning, they wondered whether they could resolve the problem by administering Campath-1M directly into patients rather than mixing it with their bone marrow prior to infusion. Because this method posed a significant risk, however, they decided to take a break from clinical testing and return to the laboratory to investigate further. It was important to establish first which T-cell subsets were responsible for rejecting marrow and then determine if a Mab could be developed for combating the problem.[43]

Until then, Waldmann's group had been testing an IgM antibody, a kind of antibody that is produced by the immune system immediately after exposure to a foreign invader. Such antibodies exist only temporarily and usually disappear from the body within two to three weeks. They are then replaced by IgG antibodies, which last a lifetime and thus provide long-term immunity against a disease. Based on experiments conducted by Cobbold, which indicated that IgG Mabs helped prevent both graft rejection and GVHD in mice given BMTs, the team focused their efforts on developing an IgG antibody for use in humans. This necessitated studying the genetic structure of Mabs and screening 20 million different monoclonal antibody clones, a time-consuming and painstaking task undertaken by Hale. In 1985, a suitable IgG Mab was eventually identified for clinical testing. This was labeled Campath-1G.[44]

The first patient chosen for testing was a man suffering from chronic lymphocytic leukemia (CLL) who was being treated in the Hematology Department. His leukemia was rapidly getting worse and had failed to respond to chemotherapy, though his tumor cells appeared sensitive to Campath-1H when tested in a test tube. He was given his first dose of Campath-1G in 1987. His response to the Mab went well beyond what Waldmann and Hale described as their "most optimistic expectations." Ten days after treatment he had gone into what seemed to be complete remission, and his tumor cells had been completely cleared from his blood and bone marrow. The result was astonishing. Waldmann and Hale recalled, "Many sincere prayers had been offered for this man and it did cross our minds that divine intervention might have overruled our efforts!" Just a few days later, however, the team discovered large tumor cells in the patient's cerebrospinal fluid. In a bid to save him, the team infused Campath-1G directly into his cerebrospinal fluid. While well tolerated by the patient, unfortunately the infusion had no effect on his tumor cells. He died a few weeks later, having failed to respond to other therapies. His death was attributed to his underlying disease.[45]

Although Campath-1G had failed to rescue the patient, his initial response to treatment gave Waldmann's team grounds to believe that the drug might be effective in others. To this end, they decided to treat a second patient. The candidate was a woman suffering from CLL who had been treated with two earlier versions of Campath. Helped temporarily by Campath-1M, her disease had been held in check with chemotherapy for two years, but she was now deteriorating rapidly. Campath-1G again led to a dramatic improvement in the woman's condition, helping to clear the majority of tumor cells from her blood and, to a lesser extent, from her bone marrow. A few weeks after completing treatment, however, tumor cells reappeared in her blood, albeit in a smaller number than before.[46]

Although unable to cure the CLL patients, the team now had evidence that Campath-1G had the potential to prevent GHVD. Certain challenges remained, however. Undertaking larger trials was not going to be easy given the small number of patients receiving BMTs at the time. To overcome the problem, Waldmann and his team set up the Campath Users Network for clinicians working in transplant centers around the world seeking to test the drug in different ways. The establishment of the network was supported by clinicians performing BMTs, who enjoyed participating in pilot investigations of the kind needed for testing Campath. Each of them received Campath supplies in exchange for reporting back their results from testing, so that those results could be fed into a computer in Waldmann's laboratory for analysis.[47]

While the international collaborative study undertaken by the Campath Users Network is common today, it was highly unusual in the 1980s. Clinicians involved in the study worked in transplant centers in England, Israel, Germany, the Netherlands, and South Africa. Over the next few years, the number of studies conducted with Campath for BMT continued to grow: by 2000 the Campath Users Group had collected data on 4,264 patients in a central registry. This evidence indicated that Campath-1G, and a later humanized form known as Campath-1H, were effective in preventing GVHD and graft rejection. The Mab would continue to be studied for use in BMTs over the following years. Between 2003 and 2004, for example, it was used in more than 1,500 transplants in the United States.[48]

One of the striking features of the research carried out in Cambridge, Stanford, and at the Wistar Institute is that it all was funded by government grants and supported by Mab supplies generated in-house. Overall, production was a time-consuming and fiddly process. Jenny Phillips, the chief technician involved in producing Campath, recalls that in general hybridomas produced only about two and a half micrograms of Mabs per milliliter of medium, so production involved liters and liters of medium and cells in flasks. On average a little flask of seed cells would take about a week to grow to fill up a roller bottle full and another two to three weeks to fill ten roller bottles. Each bottle contained up to a liter, and required the addition of medium on a regular basis so as to promote the growth of the cells. Approximately two hundred liters of culture medium had to be made from scratch each week. In addition to adding medium, some liquid was regularly poured out of the bottles so as to determine the quantity of Mabs produced, and three-quarters decanted to give the cells room to grow. It was easier to seed the next batch for production if some Mab cells were left stuck to the side of the roller bottles during the pouring process. Checking, feeding, and pouring had to be done repeatedly until eventually twenty to thirty liters of the mixture were collected.[49]

The time-consuming and laborious process of producing Campath in roller bottles was made somewhat easier in 1987 with the purchase of a fermenter, a hollow-fiber device that cost £1,000, a large sum for a small academic center at the time. The advantage of the machine was that it cut down on many of the manual tasks involved in production. It not only facilitated the regular feeding of medium into the culture, but also provided the steady supply of oxygen necessary for promoting cell growth. Filtration of the Mabs was also easier because the fermenter contained a bioreactor similar to kidney dialysis cartridges. The machine could operate for up to six months with little attention, providing a supply of Mabs at a higher concentration, twenty times greater than anything achieved before. The fact that the fermenter was sterile and eliminated the need to pour liquid from one container to another also decreased the risk of contamination.[50]

The last stage of production required purification of the Mabs, which could take two to three weeks. Once made, the Mabs were stored in sterilized vials and frozen until needed for clinical use. Samples were then taken from batches prepared at different times, and were regularly reanalyzed for purity and activity. This testing also ensured that the final solution was sterile and free from endotoxin, a poisonous substance produced by bacteria that could cause severe reactions in patients.[51]

Throughout production, sterility was crucial. Any form of contamination carried with it the danger of infection. Of the three research institutions discussed in this chapter, the Wistar with its well-established facilities for vaccine production was best placed. Early on, Mab production at the Wistar took place in a building away from its main research laboratories. By contrast, facilities for Mab production at Stanford and Cambridge were housed in the main laboratory, and the process was performed by staff members who had other, unrelated responsibilities. All of this made sterility a serious challenge.[52]

By 1987, the clinical demand for Campath had increased greatly as it came to be tested not only for BMTs, but also for other medical treatments. It thus became imperative to appoint additional staff and establish a separate center for production. The extra space was needed not only because the volume required for trials had increased, but also because production techniques were changing. Crucially, production was moving away from the use of animals to the use of recombinant technology and the culturing of mammalian cells in vitro. This trend increased the danger of contamination and made it necessary to move production away from the research laboratory into a separate space where tighter controls could be put into place.[53]

In 1990 the Cambridge group opened the Therapeutic Antibody Centre (TAC), funded by the MRC and a small contribution from Wellcome Biotech, a subsidiary of the pharmaceutical company of the Wellcome Foundation. Directed by Hale, the TAC was intended to be a comprehensive facility where Mabs could be created for clinical trials according to good manufacturing guidelines. (The center was not designed as a place for the routine production of drugs necessary in large-scale trials; this the team saw as the preserve of pharmaceutical companies.) Initially TAC was located in the Hematology Department next door to Waldmann's laboratory. This was an ideal location because the department already had the sterile conditions and technical expertise needed for manufacturing blood reagents. It moved to its own premises in Oxford in 1994, following Waldmann's appointment to the William Dunn School of Pathology at Oxford University.[54]

At first the TAC staff had few guidelines for large-scale production and quality control. Unlike pharmaceutical companies, which were expected to conform to manufacturing guidelines laid down under the British Medicines Act of 1968, doctors and dentists conducting clinical trials on their own patients were exempt from such rules until 2004. In the absence of government oversight, TAC developed its own guidelines based on a protocol laid down in 1985 by the Cancer Research Campaign, which it had established to protect itself against poor Mab production undertaken by its researchers. In later years TAC adopted the guidelines laid down by the European Community to control manufactured biological products.[55]

Before the TAC opened, the Cambridge team had produced fifty-six batches of different forms of Campath. Output grew substantially with the establishment of the center. Importantly, the TAC demonstrated how modest facilities afforded by an academic center could produce multigram quantities of different Mabs to a consistent quality suitable for use in early phase clinical trials. This had been achieved by using hollow-fiber fermenters and disposable plastics in a standard clean room. The use of disposable biocontainers, tubing, and similar equipment minimized the need for elaborate cleaning and changeover procedures. Trained staff were also hired to assure quality control.[56]

In addition to establishing the TAC, the Cambridge team made every effort to persuade the pharmaceutical industry to develop its Mab for applications in BMT. This proved to be an uphill struggle, however, because many companies thought the market was too small to make it worthwhile. Thus the use of Campath for BMT continued to rely on TAC production.[57]

Both Levy and Koprowski also found it difficult to gain industrial support for developing their Mabs. Levy's use of a custom-made Mab to treat lymphoma was seen as too costly and inefficient and the lymphoma market too narrow for a commercial enterprise to make a profit. Levy was able to treat only fifty patients with his personalized Mab by manufacturing it in-house with his own in-built quality control system, while the Wistar scientists had a similar battle to get 17–1A developed by the pharmaceutical industry. As we will see, both Levy and Koprowski eventually had to set up biotechnology companies to solve the problem.

While the commercialization of the different Mabs for cancer treatment remained uncertain in the late 1980s, the work of academic scientists during this period provided an important framework for the future development of Mabs in the diagnosis and treatment of cancer. Not only had they demonstrated the feasibility of developing a Mab against a particular target in the body but also, in the absence of industrial support, they had found ways of producing a product so that it could start being clinically tested. How well Mab products would fare in the cancer market would depend greatly on how far the commercial world could be persuaded to come on board and invest in their development, as well as whether these innovative products could overcome the stringent regulatory hurdles for clinical testing.

CHAPTER SIX

The Wild West of Antibody Commercialization

AS INVESTIGATORS RACED to find new clinical uses for Mabs, the technology was also being considered for more profitable ventures. This chapter discusses the pioneers who commercialized Mabs from the late 1970s. Those who did so were entering totally uncharted territory. Not only was the technique still in its infancy, but how it could be used also remained unknown. The enterprise was full of risk, because the scientists needed both to raise capital and to meet the regulatory criteria. Among these profit-seekers were both experienced entrepreneurs and novices. What united them was a sense of adventure and excitement about what the technology promised and its potential to make money.

Much of the early commercialization of Mabs occurred when most biotech entrepreneurs were focused on genetic engineering, also known as recombinant DNA (rDNA). First developed by Stanley Cohen and Herbert Boyer in 1973, this technique involved taking pieces of DNA from one organism and attaching them to another to amplify specific pieces of DNA coding for a protein of interest. News of rDNA took the world by storm, opening up the possibility of manipulating genetic material for research, medicine, agriculture, and industry. It promised a way of cheaply manufacturing clinically useful protein products on a previously inconceivable scale. Spearheading the commercialization of genetic engineering was Genentech, a small California-based startup company founded in April 1976. From then on academics, entrepreneurs, and investors were inspired by Genentech to establish their own small startup companies to exploit rDNA for the development of genetically engineered human insulin, interferon, and human growth hormone.[1]

The early commercial investment in Mabs took place with much less fanfare than rDNA and with no venture capital. David Murray (Figure 6.1) was the first to engage in the marketing of Mabs; he began to distribute Milstein's cells commercially starting in February 1977. Murray's background and means of entry into the commercialization of Mabs contrasts markedly with the experience of most entrepreneurs involved in the nascent emergence of biotechnology. Most either were from the academic departments of life sciences and medical research, where they had access to the latest scientific ideas and inventions, or were based in the world of venture capital. By contrast, Murray started his working life at age sixteen as an apprentice engineer to Ardente Acoustic Laboratories, a company that designed and installed hearing aids and intercommunication sets. During the Second World War he joined the British Royal Air Force, serving first in the special investigations branch and then as a saboteur in occupied Europe for the special operations unit.[2]

After the war Murray enrolled to study biology in America, but was called back to England to save his father's business from bankruptcy. His father, Percival Murray, owned a cabaret night club. Opened in Beak Street in Soho, London, in 1933, this club was known for its exclusive membership and its highly popular cabaret performances featuring girls in elaborate, albeit scanty, costumes. Initially the club's catering manager, David Murray soon became its general manager, helping to steer it through a major crisis in 1958 when one of its dancers, Christine Keeler, had simultaneous affairs with John Profumo, the secretary of state for war, and Yevgeny "Eugene" Ivanoc, a Soviet naval attaché in London. Prompting national security concerns, this affair not only led to Profumo's resignation and the electoral defeat of the Conservative government, but also brought the club into disrepute.[3]

Following many years of service at the Club, Murray departed in 1968, after a bitter dispute with his father. Finding himself on the street without any career prospects, Murray sold his only possession, a thirty-two-foot diesel-powered boat, for £12,000, and bought a run-down Victorian house in Crawley Down, Sussex. The house had some land and housing for animals. Helped by his life partner, Lynette, Murray launched Ranch Rabbits, a company that bred rabbits commercially. Initially they planned to supply rabbits for meat, but they quickly realized that the rabbits would be more profitable if bred for research. At that time, as many as a quarter of all rabbits purchased for research died from cross-infections each year because most were obtained from small breeders whose herds had endemic pathogens that spread easily when the rabbits were brought together in laboratories. Realizing that rabbits supplied from a single large colony could prevent cross-infection and that scientists would pay a high premium for rabbits free from pathogens, Murray and his partner set about breeding a large colony of rabbits. By 1970 they had a herd mature enough to be sold for twice the going rate for laboratory rabbits. Business, however, was not easy. Orders were frequently canceled or had to be postponed at the last minute by customers because it was difficult to predict how long a rabbit would take to produce antibodies of sufficiently high concentration.[4]

In 1971 Murray launched a new company, Sera-Lab, aimed at dealing with the bottleneck in antiserum production. Aided and encouraged by Ron Chambers, chief technician of the research division at Queen Victoria Hospital in East Grinstead, the company raised antisera in rabbits using antigens supplied by customers. This allowed customers to contract out the labor-intensive task of raising antisera, and to save the cost of maintaining an animal house. For Murray, the enterprise was also more profitable. The value of a rabbit used for antiserum production was five times greater than for one bred for general laboratory research.[5]

Sera-Lab soon established a standardized method for antiserum production. Previously, in the absence of a central mechanism for comparing best practice, each research laboratory had its own methods for raising antisera. Whenever Sera-Lab received large quantities of antigen from customers to make antiserum, its team would experiment with varying protocols, using different strains of rabbits and applying a number of antigen amplifiers. They also explored the use of range animals, including goats, sheep, and guinea pigs. Such tinkering helped improve the efficiency of antiserum production. Sera-Lab's first customer was Maidstone Health Authority in Kent, and soon after requests flooded in from others. Between 1976 and 1977 Sera-Lab produced and sold 14.7 liters of various antisera priced between £1,000 and £10,000 per liter.[6]

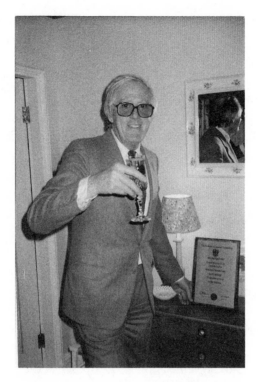

FIGURE 6.1. David Murray celebrating his
Thames TV Business Award, 1978 (Jenny Murray)

In 1976 Murray also decided to diversify his business and began producing fetal calf serum, an essential additive for tissue culturing that was
intrinsic to Mab production. Such serum was in very short supply, partly
because animal health authorities in various countries, including Britain, discouraged the importation of such serum to prevent the spread of
livestock epidemics like rinderpest and foot-and-mouth disease. Australia was one of the few countries able to supply the market with fetal calf
serum because it was not plagued by foot-and-mouth disease, but its supplies were limited.

Murray soon discovered that 10 percent of all cows sent for slaughter
in U.K. abattoirs were pregnant, contradicting a commonly held view in
the serum business that pregnant cows were never slaughtered in Britain. This gave him a ready supply of fetal calves, and after devising a new
aseptic method for collecting their serum, Murray began distributing

fresh, high-quality fetal calf serum. With tissue culturing becoming increasingly common, demand was high. At one point, the cost of a liter of the serum soared from £35 to £120.[7]

In February 1977, soon after launching fetal calf serum as a product, Murray encountered Milstein.[8] This meeting came at an opportune moment for Murray, who was then wrestling to improve anti-serum production. His key difficulty was removing the impurities in the antigens supplied by customers before he used it on the animals. As Murray noted, "Months of work may have to be spent in purifying a single microgram of a complex antigen and, even so, no matter how much care and time is taken, it is almost inevitable that very minute degrees of impurities will still remain. . . . When the antigen is injected into the host animal, the animal will react not only against the antigen but also against any impurities in it and will produce antiserum to the impurities as well as to the antigen—in addition to the antibodies it has already produced against thousands of environmental antigens, eg virus particles, bacteria, human proteins, etc." Nor was this the only factor hampering production. As Murray explained, "As any two host animals, even inbred litter mates, will react differently to the same antigen, it is possible that a percentage of host animals may react more strongly against the residual impurities than against the purified antigen. In this manner the proportion of impurities in the final antiserum will in fact be amplified in content compared to their proportion in the antigen form." All antiserum therefore required purification and this could be a lengthy and expensive process. Moreover, there was no guarantee that the final product would be 100 percent pure. Each animal also produced antisera of variable quality. According to Murray, "Some antisera have a higher titre than others, viz. are stronger, because the host animal reacted better and more fiercely to the antigen than the average. Some antisera have a greater avidity than others [avidity is the speed with which they work when used for their ultimate purpose]. Avidity is usually related to the rapidity with which the host animal reacted to the antigen."[9]

Murray quickly grasped the benefits of hybridoma technology. Importantly, it permitted duplication of any antiserum raised without purifying antigens beforehand. The end product was also fifteen times stronger in concentration than traditionally raised antisera. Already able to sell antisera at a gross profit margin of 72 percent, Murray believed that Mabs would push his profit margins even higher. The new technique gave Sera-Lab an even larger niche in the antiserum market, which was then dominated by twenty major international companies.[10]

For Murray, the market possibilities were tremendous. He pointed out, "Antisera are used in many ways both in pure research and in routine hospital diagnostics. Repeatability of results is a necessary-fundamental requirement of all research and without standard control antisera, repeatability of results is only approximate at best." He continued, "Standard antiserum where it is known that the hospital tests carried out in 1977 would relate exactly to those carried out in 1978 or 1998, or whenever, would be such a tremendous step forward that the D.H.S.S. [Department of Health and Social Security] must inevitably purchase such products. Hospitals nationwide, even worldwide, could relate to one another with total accuracy not just on the prevalence of disease in their area, but more importantly, with exact and precise percentages and degrees of gravity of such disease." He gave some idea of the market potential, pointing out, "East Birmingham Hospital Group have allocated an annual budget for Sera-Lab antisera of £12,000 and there are some twenty further such groups within D.H.S.S., all with similar purchasing power, plus, of course, an enormous potential market comprised of M.R.C. units, universities and pharmaceutical companies."[11]

Murray's desire to commercialize Mabs could not have come at a worse time for him financially. What little capital he had was being swallowed up in Sera-Lab's fetal calf business: he had had to spend £8,000 on providing equipment for abattoirs and converting a cowshed into a fully equipped laboratory. The serum was also slow to generate cash. Before buying the product, customers would take samples from three batches of serum for testing, which could take up to five weeks to complete. Much of Sera-Lab's money was therefore tied up in stock. To stem his cash burn, Murray attempted to sell batches of unfiltered serum at £10 (a major reduction given that the filtered product fetched between £30 to £40 a liter), but this did little to relieve the financial pressure. In addition, the income generated by Ranch Rabbits was being undermined by new competitors, and Murray's local bank manager refused him a loan because he believed that international companies like Seward Laboratories, a subsidiary of Unilever, would soon eliminate Sera-Lab.[12]

Just as Murray was finalizing an agreement with the MRC to distribute Milstein's Mabs, he grimly realized that he might not be able keep his business afloat, let alone find £100,000 for the purpose-built Mab unit he needed to fulfill the contract he had signed with the MRC. As he later recalled, "Times were really very desperate . . . I had re-mortgaged my house to the hilt, I had sold every personal possession of value, I had raised a small sum—I think it was £9,000—from COSIRA [the Council for Small Industries in Rural Areas], I even factored my Ranch Rabbits accounts which is a ghastly and expensive way of raising money. I remember in February 1978 sitting all night on the bank of a nearby lake, gazing over the water trying, unsuccessfully, to make myself accept the fact that Sera-Lab must be put into liquidation."[13]

In the midst of this despair, Derek Barnett, a young accountant recently hired by Sera-Lab, recommended that Murray compete for Thames Television's "Time for Business Award." This seemed like clutching at straws because the deadline for entry had already passed. Nonetheless, Murray phoned the television's organizers and cheekily asked why Sera-Lab's entry had not been acknowledged. To his surprise, they agreed to consider a proposal if submitted within twenty-four hours. This he did after working with Barnett through the night. To his astonishment, he was invited to appear on the program the following week and was then declared the winner. Only afterward did Murray realize that the prize money, £150,000, came with strings attached: Sera-Lab was expected to surrender 30 percent of its equity, which Murray believed was "an excruciatingly high interest rate." In the end, he was able to decline the prize because his bank manager finally gave him a loan as a result of the award.[14]

With funds secured, Murray erected a laboratory module built specifically to produce Mabs. This self-contained unit provided the sterile conditions and equipment necessary to prevent contamination. All staff entering were expected to wear appropriate laboratory coats, overshoes, hats, and gloves. In July 1980 Murray reported that Sera-Lab had an annual output capacity of 50,000 one-milliliter vials of serum/ascites as well as 3,000 liters of supernatants. Over the years, Sera-Lab was able to increase its output to any desired quantity, despite its shoestring budget, by adding portable cabins to the premises as production increased (Figures 6.2, 6.3).[15]

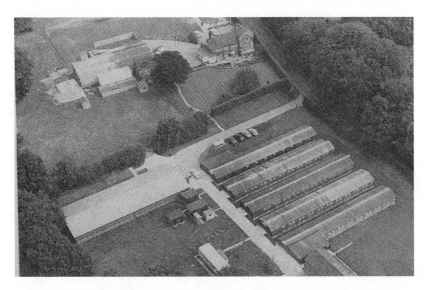

FIGURE 6.2. Aerial photo of Sera-Lab as it appeared in the company's catalog in 1986 (Jenny Murray)

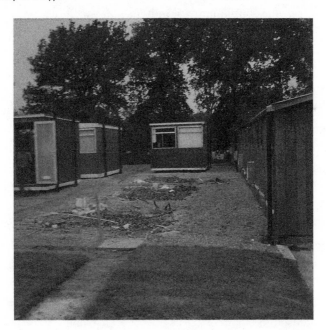

FIGURE 6.3. Sera-Lab's portable cabins in the early 1980s. Whenever business expanded, Sera-Lab increased its number of portacabins accordingly. This way the company was able to grow its business without making a major investment in new buildings. (Jenny Murray)

Murray recognized that his deal to distribute Milstein's cell lines could not last forever. As he put it, "I realised that one day soon the NRDC must wake up to the potential of what it had discarded and that my priority must therefore be to enter into similar contractual arrangements with other monoclonal research groups as soon as they appeared, to fund and collaborate with such groups and finally, of course, to carry out 'in house' research for the more commercially viable cell lines." By 1980, Sera-Lab had signed contracts with numerous scientists in the United Kingdom and internationally. While major U.S. companies quickly followed suit, in these early years Sera-Lab's listing of monoclonal antibodies remained one of the largest and most diverse.[16]

Sera-Lab had the advantage not only of being first, but also of having a marketing infrastructure in place. It could easily include Mabs in its catalog for other products. In addition, it had an established international network of distributors who were trained to deal with technical inquiries and to handle the complex process of transporting Mabs. Some distributors even set up their own in-house Mab facilities.[17]

Sera-Lab also offered researchers customized Mabs, which became a popular product because many scientists had neither the know-how nor the necessary equipment to produce their own Mabs (Figure 6.4). Sera-Lab's catalog captured the problem: "The techniques of producing monoclonal antibodies are very specialized, and the literature is large and growing. A scientist or clinician can be diverted from his own work for several costly years to produce the monoclonal antibodies he needs." Researchers would provide the immunogen and assay to Sera-Lab, and the company would then undertake the immunization and hybridization steps necessary to produce the Mab. Each Mab, supplied either as a supernatant or an ascites, would be sent to the customer for testing before clones were produced.[18]

Murray quickly realized that packaging Mabs in ready-made immunoassay kits was more profitable than growing and selling them by the gram to researchers. The kits could be sold to the in vitro diagnostics market and be used in laboratory tests on patients' blood, urine, and tissue samples. This was a lucrative market: clinical laboratories were already purchasing vast quantities of conventional antibodies in such kits, which also contained reagents, instrumentation, and similar supplies. This meant that laboratories could avoid the time-consuming and labor-

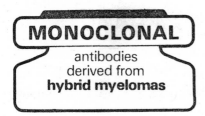

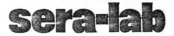

THE MONOCLONAL MESSAGE

It is accepted that antisera raised in animals by traditional methods will be subject to variables which make a product of total specificity, high titre and high avidity unobtainable; further, exact replication of any obtained level of these factors is impossible in subsequent batches. If a highly purified antigen were injected into a host animal which happened to show an immune response with great rapidity against the purified part of the antigen and a very minute and slow reaction against the antigenic impurities—then such a product would be:

1. uniquely specific
2. of very high titre
3. of maximum avidity.

The odds against such a perfect product are very great. If, however, one were willing to prepare several hundred times the amount of antigen that would be needed and use a large number of host animals and many hours of labour, then a perfect antiserum is theoretically possible—but not as an economic proposition. If, for the sake of perfection, this costly exercise were carried out, then once the "perfect" antiserum was exhausted there could be no guarantee that it could be repeated identically, even using the same techniques.

Recently it has been shown by Kohler & Milstein (Nature *256:* 495-497, 1975) that MONOCLONAL ANTIBODIES can be made from single cells grown in mass culture. *In vitro* cultures produce concentrations of about 10μg cm^{-3} of specific monoclonal antibody. Cells grown, as tumours *in vivo*, induce serum and ascites levels of about 10mg cm^{-3} of antibody. The hybrid myeloma cell can be stored for unlimited periods of time yet, when thawed and injected into an animal, or grown in tissue culture, will produce antibodies identical to those first made. Each monoclonal antibody, whether produced *in vivo* or *in vitro*, is identical in every respect with its fellows. Thus antisera need no longer be a variable mixture of antibodies which have only a small proportion of their molecules directed against the specific antigen since monoclonal antibodies ALWAYS PRODUCE AN IDENTICAL AND OVERWHELMING ACTIVITY OF IMMUNOGLOBULIN MOLECULES AGAINST THE SPECIFIC DETERMINANT. In addition, monoclonal antibodies can be synthesised with tritiated (^{3}H) or carbon (^{14}C) aminoacids incorporated. These antibodies with intrinsic labels make ideal standards for a variety of radio immuno-assay techniques.

PRODUCT PROFILES describing the original clone and its related areas of application are available upon request. A detailed bibliography of new research using these exciting products is maintained.

CONJUGATION of these products may be carried out to customer order—please enquire.

**REMEMBER THAT MONOCLONAL MEANS THE SAME ANTIBODY
AGAINST THE SAME DETERMINANT EVERY TIME**

FIGURE 6.4. This advertisement appeared in 1979 in the catalog of Sera-Lab, which first began to include Mabs in its catalogue in 1978. (Jenny Murray)

intensive process of designing and assembling their own systems. They also increased the efficiency, throughput, consistency, and control of the diagnostic process. Murray hoped to substitute the conventional antibodies in such kits with Sera-Lab's own Mabs. This change would not significantly increase the company's costs of production since only minute amounts of Mabs would be required.[19]

Developing Mabs for kits, however, required much more research and development, and more regulatory oversight, than producing customized Mabs. Sera-Lab therefore decided to partner with Bethesda Research Laboratories (BRL) in Maryland. BRL not only had the appropriate research, marketing structure, and kit production facilities, but also possessed contacts with the appropriate regulatory bodies. In 1981 Sera-Lab started promoting its first set of histology kits. These were intended for immune-histochemical staining of different pathological specimens, including tissue sections and smear preparations. Although these kits were initially marketed only for research purposes, they were soon offered for routine clinical investigations of conditions like leukemia.[20]

Within a short time, however, Sera-Lab faced serious competition. One of its first competitors was Hybritech, a small company set up in San Diego in 1978 by Ivor Royston, a newly appointed assistant professor of medicine at the University of California, San Diego (UCSD), and his assistant Howard Birndorf. Employed by a prestigious academic institution, Royston and Birndorf enjoyed circumstances very different to Murray's. And because they were based in the United States, where venture capital and the entrepreneurial culture were much more established, they could call on far greater resources than anything Murray could access in Britain in the late 1970s.[21]

Both Royston and Birndorf came from humble Jewish backgrounds. Royston, born in England, was the son of refugees from Eastern Europe who moved to the United States in 1954. His father, Polish by birth, had fought for the Polish, French, and British armies before being evacuated to England after the fall of Dunkirk in 1944. Birndorf was the American son of a shoe salesman. Of the two, Royston was the most ambitious, having entered a fast-track academic career in clinical medicine early on. By contrast, Birndorf was a laboratory technician with a master's degree in biochemistry. The two met at Stanford University in 1975 where Royston was a postdoctoral fellow and Birndorf a laboratory technician.

Royston and Birndorf were galvanised by the entrepreneurial energy then sweeping the Stanford campus following the founding of Genentech in 1976 and of the Collagen Corporation, a biotechnology company established by John Daniel, one of Royston's oncology associates. Within a short time they were exploring the promising commercial possibilities that Mabs offered, using Klinman's method to produce Mabs against cancer cells to devise a tool to investigate lymphoma. They soon shifted to the hybridoma technique, after Herzenberg supplied them with myeloma cells he had obtained from Milstein while on sabbatical in Cambridge.[22]

In July 1977, Royston moved to San Diego to head the clinical immunology department in UCSD's new cancer center and appointed Birndorf his assistant. They took with them a liquid nitrogen container that Royston had obtained when based at the National Institutes of Health between 1972 and 1975. This Royston had done without any material transfer agreement. All he had was a government document confirming that the tank was discarded property. The container was full of the cell lines and Mabs he had been working on since the mid-1970s as well as some he had collected from other researchers. Together with the expertise that Royston and Birndorf had picked up at Stanford, this tank would help lay the foundation for Hybritech.[23]

By early 1978, Royston and Birndorf had successfully generated Mabs against cells of the lymph system, but faced significant financial challenges. All they possessed was some university funding for basic equipment and a small research grant to cover Birndorf's small salary. Royston could ill afford to lose Birndorf, who was more adept than he was at producing Mabs. Moreover his laboratory was too small and his equipment inadequate for large-scale manufacturing of Mabs.[24]

Faced with these limitations, Royston began exploring potential industrial support. His efforts proved fruitless, however, in part because pharmaceutical executives were reluctant to install facilities for Mab production, which would require replacing all their existing infrastructure with another to support a largely untested technology.[25]

The solution, Royston and Birndorf soon realized, lay in the creation of Hybritech, a company designed to sell Mabs for research. Birndorf would run the company while Royston retained his university post. All they needed were some incubators, some bottles, and a fermenter. Using this experience, Royston wrote a business plan, with the help of a library book on how to start a business. He estimated he would need $178,000 in the first year, a laboratory with a thousand square feet, and a room with four hundred square feet for mouse cages.[26]

Now the hunt was on for money. Birndorf contacted some wealthy friends of his parents, as well as commodity brokers who were friends of friends. These efforts, however, came to nothing. Allegedly the business plan was so technical that no one understood it. Royston had greater success with Brook Byers, one of his wife's former boyfriends, who, unbeknownst to Royston, was not only a junior partner in Kleiner Perkins, the venture capital company that had provided seed capital for Genentech, but also had been closely involved in founding the company. When he met informally with Royston in April 1978, Byers was highly receptive and understood the similarities that Royston drew between the cloning of genes, which was the basis of Genentech's business, and the cloning of antibodies, which was to be Hybritech's platform.[27]

Encouraged by Byers, in May 1978, Royston and Birndorf rewrote their business plan and submitted it to Kleiner Perkins. In their plan, they described the range of health problems for which conventional antibodies were then being used, such as blood typing and screening, as well as various diagnostic tests and monitoring. They estimated that the price of these antibodies was between $5 and $20 per milligram, depending on their type and purity. The most popular antibodies were directed against hepatitis and other viruses (such as influenza and herpes); types A, B, and AB of human red blood cells; human blood proteins (complement, fibrin, transferrin, haptoglobulin); various human immunoglobulins; and different types of bacteria (*Salmonella, E. coli, Neisseria,* and *Shigella*).[28]

The two scientists envisaged attracting customers similar to Murray's: hospitals, blood banks, clinical medical laboratories, and academic bioscience laboratories. Knowing that they would be able to reduce the cost of antibody production and deliver antibodies of a much higher quality and specificity than those available before, they believed they could produce Mabs on an industrial scale and sell them at half the price. Like Murray, their chief competitors were the large manufacturers of antisera for medical and research purposes, whose production was still based on conventional antibody methods. Royston and Birndorf hoped that the startup would give each of them an annual income of about $100,000. They believed that the window of opportunity for exploiting the technology was small. At the time, only a handful of academic immunologists had access to the technique and cell lines, but they believed that competitors would acquire and adopt the technology within a year. They envisioned Mab laboratory reagents as no less than a launchpad for the development of Mab therapeutics.[29]

In September 1978 Royston and Birndorf were offered $300,000 by Kleiner Perkins, in return for an equity stake of 60 percent in Hybritech. This was double the equity stake that Development Capital had asked of Murray for funding Sera-Lab, but Royston and Birndorf, being new to business, agreed to the terms, which offered them far more than they had requested.[30]

In October 1978 Birndorf kickstarted Hybritech's operation in a laboratory rented from La Jolla Cancer Research Foundation, using cells derived from Milstein's cell line passed on by Herzenberg. Royston assisted him while also working as a scientific adviser. Byers was made Hybritech's part-time acting president on the recommendation of Kleiner Perkins partners so that they could retain control and maintain interests in the company. Byers, an experienced venture capitalist, quickly shifted the company toward the goal of packaging Mabs in kits for the in vitro diagnostics sector, which he believed had greater potential for growth and profit than selling Mabs to researchers. He hoped to develop a worldwide market of $100 million a year.[31]

Soon after Hybritech was founded, the team welcomed Gary David, an immunochemist. In rented laboratory space next door to Hybritech, David had established a business producing Mab immunodiagnostics, using his wife's lame horse to generate the Mabs. He was well equipped for this business, having spent six years working on the development of radioimmunoassays for the diagnosis of gastrointestinal tumors at the Scripps Clinic. But although David had hoped to build up capital to launch a larger Mab business, he soon abandoned his startup. As he recalled, "I had the option of joining Hybritech or competing with Hybritech, and since there were about five or six orders of magnitude difference in capital, there wasn't much of a choice."[32]

Soon after David came on board, Ted Greene also joined Hybritech. A Harvard Business School graduate and former McKinsey consultant, Greene was in the process of leaving Baxter-Travenol, an American medical supply company that sold blood fractions for therapeutic use and immunodiagnostics and was launching another startup called Cytex to sell customized Mabs to immunodiagnostics manufacturers for use on their existing immunoassay systems. Greene was quickly persuaded to become Hybritech's chief executive officer, because it had venture capital in hand and his Cytex team was already beginning to fracture.[33]

When Greene joined Hybritech formally in March 1979, Hybritech was being run more like an academic laboratory than a commercial organization. Most of its staff had arrived as a result of either personal contacts or word of mouth, and because they came from academic laboratories they had little experience with industry practices such as manufacturing timelines or salesmanship. Encouraged by Kleiner Perkins, Green now began to hire people with industrial expertise. Because the company could only offer modest salaries, they were incentivized with Hybritech shares.[34]

Having reshaped Hybritech into a more conventional industrial operation, Greene set about formulating a new business plan to attract more capital. He calculated that the company could break even by the end of 1980 with an equity base of $1,900,000, and set about raising $1.6 million. This was a modest sum by the standards of most venture capitalists at this time. Nonetheless, he needed a convincing plan to secure this amount, because hybridoma technology was still untested and relatively unknown. He thus portrayed Mabs as having a highly exciting commercial future as clinical diagnostic reagents, with a value that would exceed $1.1 billion in 1979. He also pitched the idea that their market would double in the next five years, and that the sales of new immunodiagnostic products—such as reagents, assay kits, and instruments—would grow even more quickly. He argued that Hybritech was in a strong position to achieve these results, highlighting the fact that he and Byers were graduates from Harvard and Stanford business schools and had attracted highly successful researchers from several prestigious scientific and medical institutions to lead its research and development.[35] This was in stark contrast to Murray's background and his Sera-Lab team.

By July 1979 Greene had secured $1.6 million by selling additional company shares to Kleiner Perkins and Sutter Hill Ventures, another venture capital company. A year later Hybritech raised more money from private and institutional investors and, in 1981 and 1982, received a further $43 million from two public offerings.[36]

As money began to flow into Hybritech's coffers, a new company was rising on the U.S. East Coast which would soon pose a serious challenge. Called Centocor, its founders, like Hybritech's, envisioned using Mabs as a means to break into the immunodiagnostics market and eventually into therapeutics. Centocor was born out of Koprowski's frustrations in persuading companies to license his Mab patents. Boehringer-Ingelheim, for example, to whom he offered a license for $500,000 annually over ten years, dragged out negotiations for six or eight months before rejecting the offer altogether, alleging that Mab products had no future.[37]

In the end Koprowski realized that the best way forward would be to establish a separate company in partnership with Michael Wall, an electrical engineer who had graduated from Massachusetts Institute of Technology (MIT). Wall had successfully founded several electronics, computer, and biological startup companies, and had been the president and chairman of Flow Laboratories, a producer of cell culture and related products, which had just been sold for $3 million. Koprowski had met Wall through Flow Laboratories. Looking for a change, Wall had various business schemes in mind, including growing orchids. His idea of founding a company based on flowers soon faded, however, when Koprowski told him that a Mab diagnostic (CA-19-9) for pancreatic cancer was imminent.[38]

Wall became the new company's chairman with scientific support from Koprowski and the Wistar Institute. After setting up an office in downtown Philadelphia in May 1979, he began to build Centocor's executive team (Figure 6.5). One of the first to join was Ted Allen, previously a marketing manager at Corning Medical. Allen had been involved in Corning's efforts to establish a strong portfolio in diagnostic immunoassays. These diagnostics were rapidly replacing the chemical-based tests that had dominated the market since the 1940s.[39]

Centocor soon attracted the interest of one of Allen's former colleagues at Corning, Hubert Schoemaker (Figure 6.6). Born to a Catholic family in

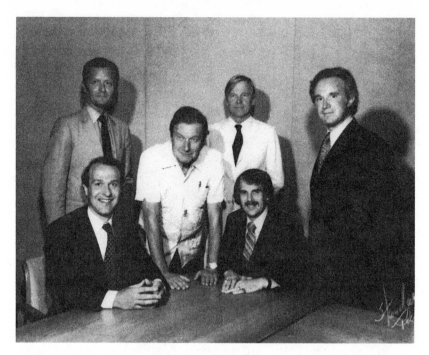

FIGURE 6.5. This photo shows the earliest founders of Centocor, ca. 1979. In the front, from left to right, are Hubert Schoemaker, Hilary Koprowski, Vincent Zurawski, and Tony Evnin. Behind Schoemaker is Ted Allen, and behind Zurawski is Michael Wall. (Tony Evnin and Anne Faulkner Schoemaker)

the Netherlands, Schoemaker came from a long tradition of risk-taking and entrepreneurship: his father had worked with the Dutch resistance movement during the Second World War and had then founded an international company manufacturing chemicals and food additives. A biochemist by training, Schoemaker had completed a doctorate at MIT in a department at the cutting edge of biotechnology research, while taking business courses at Sloan School of Management. After graduation he started working for AIM Packaging, a small company manufacturing plastic containers, but he left this position shortly after his daughter, Maureen, was born. She was diagnosed shortly after birth with lissencephaly, a rare brain malformation causing severe mental disability and motor dysfunction, and her condition made it necessary for Schoemaker both to earn a higher salary to provide for her long-term medical needs and to move to a location with appropriate medical facilities. In June

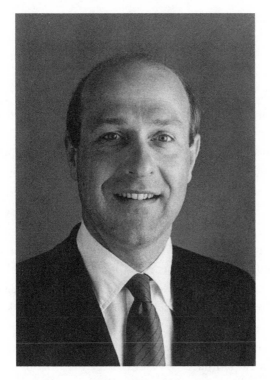

FIGURE 6.6. Hubert Schoemaker, co-founder
and chief executive of Centocor, ca. 1987
(Anne Faulkner Schoemaker)

1976, he joined Corning Medical to lead the invention and clinical testing
of several new diagnostic immunoassay tests for hyperthyroidism, hypo-
thyroidism, and cortisol, as well as to advance the firm's marketing.[40]

What drew Schoemaker to Centocor was the challenge of building a
company from scratch. Although it was a highly risky venture, Schoemaker believed that Centocor could help improve people's lives, a long-
held ambition. It was a passion reinforced by his daughter's illness.
Centocor offered him the possibility not only of developing some of the
biotechnological techniques he had learned during his years at MIT and
Corning, but also of extending his entrepreneurial skills. Initially he
worked on Centocor's research and planning in an unofficial capacity
while continuing to work for Corning. In early 1980, however, he started
to work at Centocor full-time, becoming the company's chief executive
officer in the wake of Allen's sudden departure.[41]

By August 1979 Centocor had recruited a chief scientific officer—
Vincent Zurawski, a chemist by training who had initiated Mab production at Harvard Medical School and Massachusetts General Hospital
(MGH). He had done this first as a postdoctoral researcher using Klinman's splenic fragment system, and later by deploying hybridoma technology, which he learned from researchers who had worked in Milstein's
laboratory.[42]

Like Hybritech, Centocor secured venture capital quite quickly. In late
1979, Wall, using his previous business connections, persuaded Tony
Evnin to become a director at Centocor. Evnin was a senior partner in
Venrock Associates, a venture capital firm with a strong history of investment in the diagnostics and therapeutics sector, and soon after his appointment, Venrock agreed to invest $300,000 in Centocor. Other funds
soon followed. By 1981 Centocor had raised approximately $7 million
through private placement of its stocks, and by the end of 1982 had accrued
$21 million from its initial public offering.[43]

Centocor's founders aimed to develop diagnostics and therapeutics,
targeting their products toward cancer, cardiovascular disorders, and liver
problems, which promised potentially large markets for Mab products.
In 1979, for example, it was estimated that 572 million tests were conducted annually for cancer screening, with a further 56 million tests for
monitoring drug treatment and other followup testing. Centocor's executives predicted that global sales of diagnostics for cancer detection would
total $25 million by 1980, rising thereafter to $284 million within five
years and $1.4 billion by 1995. They pointed out that the diagnostics can-
cer market was still "embryonic." Roche Diagnostics was the only company with a cancer diagnostic on the market, generating $20 million in
revenue in 1979. But this diagnostic, which was directed toward measuring the tumor marker known as a carcinoembryonic antigen (CEA), had
certain limitations. In particular, it was based on conventional antibodies, so it frequently provided false negative readings, allowing some cancers to slip through undetected.[44]

Cardiac disease was another large diagnostic market, of which myocardial infarction (heart attack) represented the largest segment. Yet no
single test for detecting heart damage existed. The best that doctors could
do was to couple two antibody tests to determine levels of lactic acid de-
hydrogenase and creatine kinase; together these were 90 percent accu-

rate for detecting myocardial infarction. These two combined tests were estimated to earn about $24.2 million in revenue in 1979; this was expected to rise to $34.1 million by 1984. Centocor's executives hoped to license a Mab from one of Zurawski's former colleagues at MGH in order to develop a single test with better sensitivity as well as specificity.[45]

Initially Centocor's founders intended to use the same Mab for developing both diagnostics and therapeutics. But as Evnin later recalled, this proved "pretty naive." Indeed, it would take many years and billions of dollars before it would be possible to use the same Mab to diagnose, monitor, and treat a disease. Like Hybritech, Centocor's team saw diagnostics as an easier area than therapeutics in which to develop products and win regulatory approval and thus lead to faster revenue growth. Their aim was to generate $17 million in revenue from diagnostics by 1984. This was an ambitious goal given the highly competitive diagnostics market, which was dominated by large healthcare companies whose own tests relied on the use of their own proprietary instruments.[46]

Unlike Hybritech, which decided to create its own diagnostics in-house and establish its own sales force and instrumentation to compete head-on in the marketplace, Centocor believed that collaboration was the way forward. The very name "Centocor," coined by Koprowski, was derived from the words "cento," which describes (in Latin) an old garment made of hundreds of patches of material or a literary or musical composition made up of parts of other works, and "cor(e)," as in the center. Its founders aimed to license diagnostic and reagent antibodies from universities, develop them for immunoassay kits, and then license the modified materials to key companies for use on their own diagnostic systems. Schoemaker recalled, "We realized it was a lot cheaper to roam academe and pay a royalty back for what we developed than start our own research facilities. Collaboration was the best way to be competitive." This strategy relied on being well connected to the academic world.[47]

Centocor's business model resembled Sera-Lab's, but its collaborative philosophy was unusual for American biotechnology companies at the time. Most, like Hybritech and Genentech, were trying to do everything internally, from discovery to development. By contrast, Centocor's founders believed that rather than depending solely on in-house research, they should also identify and fund prominent external researchers and laboratories working on antibodies that the company wanted to develop and, where appropriate, license the technology. As Wall told *Forbes* magazine in May 1985, "You can have a garage full of Ph.D.s working on a project and nine times out of ten some guy across the street is going to come up with the discovery that beats them all."[48]

The difference in Centocor's and Hybritech's approaches was most noticeable in the way they developed their first product: a test for hepatitis B. Both companies viewed their hepatitis B test as an important entry point into the diagnostics market, and hoped to take advantage of the fact that antibodies against hepatitis were among the most commonly used in medicine. They believed a Mab diagnostic would be easier to make—and thus cheaper to produce—than conventional hepatitis antibody tests.

Hepatitis B is a type of viral hepatitis with a number of different outcomes. Patients suffering from the disease may experience symptoms no more severe than a mild case of the flu or suffer far more severe complications that cause years of disability or even death. Some people can be chronic carriers of the virus without noticing any symptoms until much later, when their livers become dysfunctional and they develop fatal cirrhosis or cancer. The virus is highly infectious and can be spread in various ways: by sexual contact with an infected person, through contact with infected blood, by sharing needles for intravenous drug use, or from mother to child at birth. By the early 1970s the disease was rampant in Asia and sub-Saharan Africa. In some places, whole populations were estimated to have been infected at some point, with 15 to 20 percent of them chronic carriers of hepatitis B. Between one and two million people were estimated to die from hepatitis B each year. While the disease was less common in the West, it was still a major concern. In the United States in the early 1980s, for example, between 200,000 and 300,000 cases were reported annually and about a million people were thought to be carriers.[49]

Given this situation, many policymakers implemented measures to curb the spread of the virus, and many countries, including the United States and Britain, introduced compulsory screening of blood donations, using a serum-based antibody test, to prevent transmission. This was helped by the discovery of the hepatitis-associated antigen in 1967. By the early 1970s, every unit of blood screened for hepatitis used an antibody test kit, and the hepatitis market was one of the largest blood-testing markets in the world. In 1980 the worldwide diagnostic market for hepatitis

B was estimated to bring in $34 million in 1980, and this was expected to rise to at least $64 million by 1984.[50]

Hybritech's founders decided their best approach would be to develop a Mab internally. This was achieved within three months, although this was just the start of its development and it took the company many more months to construct a commercially viable diagnostic. Just at the point when it seemed they had a product in hand, however, Greene called a halt to the project, because he feared it would pit Hybritech directly against the diagnostics company Abbott Laboratories, which had the lion's share of the hepatitis-B testing market. Because it had put one of the first antibody tests on the market in 1972, and provided free computer equipment for reading its test results, Abbott had a considerable number of loyal customers. Abbott was fiercely competitive in the marketplace and was willing to use its large size and strong manufacturing base to compete aggressively with smaller companies on cost. In 1983 it was thought to control 95 percent of the U.S. hepatitis diagnostic market, which was worth $42.1 million. Greene was therefore wary of any confrontation. As he put it, "We didn't want to take on the gorilla. . . . Hepatitis was their number one profit-maker, and anybody that tried to come into that business, they would crush." He reasoned that it would be safer to target Hybritech's first product toward a niche market where there was less competition.[51]

Hybritech's decision to change direction was reinforced by the technical difficulties its scientists encountered in developing the hepatitis B test. Part of their problem stemmed from the fact that the Mab appeared too specific to handle the antigenic modulation the virus used as its survival mechanism. Many on the team in fact believed that the specificity of Mabs rendered them invalid for the detection of more complex organisms like viruses or bacteria. They concluded that a Mab diagnostic stood a greater chance of success if it were designed to detect simple molecules like drugs or hormones whose antigenic structures did not change.[52]

Complex regulatory hurdles further reinforced Hybritech's decision. Approval for a hepatitis test could not be obtained simply by meeting the requirements of a standard 510(k) notification to the U.S. Food and Drug Administration (FDA), because that form of notification was designed for cases where the performance of a new medical device would be judged against equivalents already on the market. A hepatitis B test necessitated the submission of a premarketing application (PMA) to the regulatory authorities, which would involve far more extensive and costly validation clinical trials and detailed documentation of the materials and procedures than was needed for 510(k).[53]

In contrast to Hybritech, Centocor decided against developing a hepatitis B test internally, and licensed instead a Mab produced by Zurawski with his colleague Jack Wand at MGH. Because this Mab had already been developed for use in an immunoassay diagnostic kit, they could—and did—pay greater attention to the ways in which Mabs worked within the kit system than did members of the Hybritech team, who became bogged down in looking at the immunochemical characteristics of the Mab itself. Aware of the complications that resulted from the antigenic modulation of the virus, Centocor's researchers painstakingly purified different hepatitis-B surface antigens from specimens collected in the Philippines, Japan, the Middle East, France, the United States, Australia, and South Africa, and soon developed a diagnostic tool that could identify the hepatitis B virus in blood. This diagnostic tool, which could be used both to prevent the transmission of the disease by blood banks and to diagnose the disease in patients, proved much more specific and effective at picking up hepatitis B than had tests using conventional antibodies. By October 1979 the Centocor team had made sufficient progress to file patent applications on the technique, the first of which was granted in June 1981.[54]

Centocor's team was also less daunted by the process of getting regulatory approval for the test than the Hybritech founders had been, because Schoemaker was already familiar with the requirements from his work at Corning. By January 1983 Centocor had gained FDA approval for its hepatitis B test, having fulfilled PMA requirements, including clinical testing of the diagnostic. This was the first Mab-based test for hepatitis approved by the regulatory authority, and it found a ready market: 600,000 tests were sold between April and December 1983.[55]

Importantly, Centocor found a way of side-stepping the diagnostic war that Hybritech had envisaged with Abbott: securing licensing agreements with companies that had well-established markets and distribution channels. One of the advantages of partnering was that it eliminated the time and expense of establishing an internal sales force and this facilitated a speedier entry into the market. Centocor deliberately set out to secure agreements with key diagnostic companies that could buy and sell the company's antibodies, either in completed test kits or for use with their own proprietary machines. Following its hepatitis-B antibody, this strategy was used for all of Centocor's diagnostic products. The arrangement helped Centocor to gain a broad market quite quickly, and to leverage its technical strength without threatening competitors. As David Holveck, who headed up Centocor's diagnostics department from 1983, put it, "Because of the marketing strategy of networking with all of the major suppliers, we insulated ourselves from competition because we were the suppliers of the reagents, and they were looking for ways of adding tests to their instrumentation." By 1983, 61 percent of Centocor's product sales were delivered by major distributors. Two years later this had increased to 74 percent.[56]

In contrast to Centocor, Hybritech's executives felt it was important to build up the company's own sales force and develop a new diagnostic platform. Their objective was to offer faster and more sensitive assays than the conventional polyclonal antibodies already on the market. Such a platform would enable the company to make its mark on the marketplace. Its platform incorporated two different Mabs to "sandwich" an antigen. The first was attached to a solid support, chosen for its power to bind to a single antigenic determinant; the second was a soluble Mab labeled with a tag, such as a radioisotope, enzyme, or fluoregenic compound, which could target different binding sites on the antigenic determinant. In August 1980, to protect its innovation, Hybritech filed an application for a patent, which was granted in 1983.[57]

Hybritech first deployed its sandwich system to develop a test for detecting allergies. Known as an IgE test, this was approved in May 1981 by the FDA, after it was shown to be equivalent to other commercially available allergy tests. This was the first Mab-based diagnostic to win FDA approval. Greene saw the approval as a major coup because it showed how small companies with few resources could compete on the stage against giants like Abbott. Importantly, Hybritech had gained the approval without a premarket application, as a result of patient negotiations with FDA regulators who were still very new to hybridoma technology. As Greene later claimed, "If Abbott had been the first one, and the FDA had come to them and said, 'We want to make this a pre-market approval,' they would have said, 'We think you're right. That's a good idea.' Right? Because all the little guys would be kept out."[58]

Hybritech went on to make several other diagnostic products using its sandwich system. In 1985 the company was given FDA authorization for its second product, a test measuring CEA antigens, which are typically found in patients with cancer of the colon, rectum, breast, or lung. The following year the FDA approved Hybritech's diagnostic to measure the PSA antigens in blood, which were considered important markers for prostrate cancer. This test, the first diagnostic for prostate cancer, became the gold standard for prostate-cancer screening. Twenty years later, however, it was shown to be a poor detector for prostrate cancer, and was criticized for encouraging unnecessary, invasive, and harmful surgeries.[59]

In addition to its cancer tests, in 1986 Hybritech gained FDA approval for its rapid home-pregnancy test. This was not the first over-the-counter pregnancy test: the first such test was approved in 1976. Nor was it the first Mab-based pregnancy test. It followed close on the heels of two other Mab-based pregnancy tests: Pregnastick, developed by Monoclonal Antibodies Inc., another Californian startup company founded in April 1979; and Clearblue, developed by Unilever, a large Dutch and British developer of consumer goods. These two tests represented a marked improvement over earlier tests—they were easier and more hygenic to use, and they were more sensitive, reducing the waiting time for results from two hours to thirty minutes. Significantly, Hybritech reduced the testing time even further, to a mere five minutes. This was achieved by the development of a new platform involving a membrane surface saturated with antibodies within an enzyme immunoassay format.[60]

Hybritech's executives claimed that their internal platforms enabled both the swift approval of their diagnostics products and differentiated Hybritech from other companies. By 1984 it had gained FDA clearance for twenty-one diagnostic products. Yet the company paid a high price for its novel platforms, both because of the costs of research and development and because of its legal battles to defend its intellectual property rights. In 1984 it became embroiled in a lawsuit against Monoclonal Antibodies Inc. for infringing on its sandwich assay patent with the creation of a pregnancy test. The case dragged on for some time. In 1985 the U.S. District Court in San Francisco declared Hybritech's sandwich assay patent invalid, sending the value of Hybritech shares tumbling on the stock market. A year later, the court judgment was overturned, but soon thereafter Hybritech mounted a costly law suit against Abbott. Overall the patent wars cost Hybritech dearly, and led to its acquisition in March 1986 by the pharmaceutical company Eli Lilly. Four years earlier, Lilly had introduced to market Humulin, the first genetically engineered drug developed by Genentech, and it was eager to capitalize on Hybritech's expertise with Mabs.[61]

In the end Hybritech developed some useful diagnostics, but failed to deliver on its long-term vision to develop therapeutics that could generate greater profits. Therapeutics demanded far greater research and development resources than Hybritech possessed, so in the end, Hybritech's executive saw the merger with Lilly as a way of delivering on this part of its vision. But the cultural clashes between the two companies, one of which started as a small, entrepreneurial venture, and the other a large hierarchical corporation, diminished the group's entrepreneurial spirit, and many of the initiatives it started stagnated and eventually ground to a halt. The dream of creating Mab therapeutics now passed on to a new company called Idec Pharmaceuticals, which was started in 1986 by Royston and Birndorf in collaboration with Ron Levy.[62]

In 1989, three years after Hybritech was acquired by Lilly, Murray, now sixty-seven and in poor health, was forced to retire and sell Sera-Lab to Porton International for £2.5 million (Figure 6.7). Porton International was a British biotechnology company set up in 1982 by Wensley Haydon-Baillie, a businessman and merchant banker, on the basis of a contract he had secured from the British government to market drugs developed at the top-secret biochemical research establishment at Porton Down in Wiltshire. While Porton Down's main objective was to create biological weapons, it had also developed antidotes and cures that Haydon-Baillie wanted to commercialize. In 1985 he received a £76 million investment from the city for the company, which had a pre-tax profit of £6.7 million and sales of £11.1 million within two years. By that time, Porton International had four hundred employees, of whom two-thirds were based in Britain and the rest mainly in the United States. The acquisition of Sera-Lab provided Porton International with an established distribution network.[63]

Although Sera-Lab was the first company to commercialize Mabs, and so left a lasting legacy, its pivotal role is often forgotten. One reason is the dominance of U.S. companies that were funded by venture capitalists and so gained greater capital and fanfare both at the time and in the

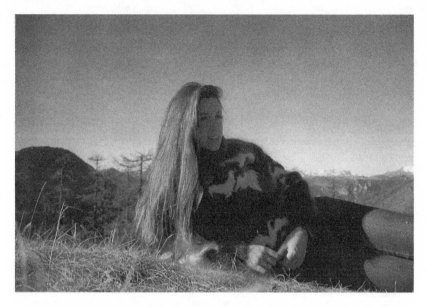

FIGURE 6.7. Jenny Murray helped direct Sera-Lab with her husband, David Murray, in the 1980s. (David Murray)

subsequent historical record. The achievements of Sera-Lab were also overshadowed by the rise of Celltech, a British biotechnology company established in November 1980 with government backing and £12 million venture capital secured from city banks. In all the British press media accounts of Celltech's establishment, no mention was made of Sera-Lab. Strikingly, when Murray approached government officials asking to get involved in the Celltech venture, they indicated that Sera-Lab would be useful only in areas where there was no patent protection. In later years Sera-Lab would be mistakenly remembered as Celltech's predecessor, and few attempts were made to uncover its true history.[64]

While Celltech's emergence initially posed a significant threat to Sera-Lab because it had the right to exploit all MRC research, the company quickly departed from a business model of supplying Mabs to researchers because that market was so small.[65] Celltech chose to concentrate instead on large-scale manufacturing of antibodies for diagnostic and therapeutic purposes. This left Sera-Lab free to continue as the leader in providing researchers with Mabs, which attracted less limelight than diagnostics or therapeutics, but were crucial in the development of such products.

In many ways, Sera-Lab was ahead of its time, although a number of companies soon followed in its footsteps. This included the British company Serotec, which was officially founded in 1982 by Ed Bernard, a former laboratory technician who started the business as an offshoot to a company he had set up to supply laboratory mice. A family-run international business, Serotec sourced and supplied its Mabs along the same lines as Sera-Lab, relying on a strong network in the academic research community. Sold to Morphosys AG for £20 million in 2006, Serotec was just another one of the many companies that emerged from advances made in the 1980s.[66]

The business of selling research Mabs would expand greatly in the early twenty-first century. Just how big the business would become can be seen by the fact that in 2012 more than three hundred companies were listed as supplying Mabs research reagents worldwide for multiple research projects in different disease areas and for a wide variety of different diagnostic formats. In 2012 the research Mab reagents market was calculated to be worth over $2 billion, with many providers having annual sales of over $100 million each year. Gone are the days when companies marketed their Mabs through catalogs and sales calls in person. Now researchers can quickly source and access the Mabs they need from the Internet. For small producers of Mabs, the rise of the Internet has afforded the possibility of direct marketing, offsetting the resource advantage that large suppliers have. But in this new marketplace, is the quality of these Mab reagents monitored enough?[67]

By the late 1980s, as Hybritech and Sera-Lab began to fade from view, Centocor went from strength to strength. Using its strategy of partnering, Centocor's team built up a profitable diagnostics line with revenues rising from $1.2 million in 1983 to $50 million in 1993. This line was highly lucrative because much of its revenue came from royalties. By the mid-1980s, Centocor was one of the very few monoclonal antibody companies making a profit.[68] It had succeeded by deliberately making its products compatible with other companies' systems, rather than by going it alone and competing with its own platform in the way that Hybritech had done.

Centocor's survival was boosted by its early success in cancer diagnostics. The company gained approval for a diagnostic test for gastrointestinal cancer in 1983, using the CA-19-9 Mab licensed from the Wistar Institute. Over the next three years it had more cancer tests authorized.

The first, CA125, licensed from the Dana-Farber Cancer Institute, was the first diagnostic available for ovarian cancer. It went on to become the standard immunoassay for monitoring ovarian cancer and evaluating a patient's response to therapy. The company also won approval for its test for breast cancer, CA15–3, which was licensed from Scripps Clinic and Research Foundation. In addition, Centocor marketed the first test for multi-drug resistance, a major problem for cancer patients.[69] All these tests are still used in clinical practice.

Centocor gained a leading role in the nascent cancer diagnostic market, securing along the way relationships with key companies in the area, including Abbott Laboratories and F. Hoffmann–La Roche. By 1990, it had captured more than a quarter of the world's market for antibody-based tests for cancer.[70] This success gave it the critical mass and support that it needed to start developing therapeutics, the goal it had envisaged from the start. As we will see, however, entering the field of therapeutics posed significant new challenges and risks, threatening the very survival of the company and the development of Mab therapeutics.

Having started with an untested technology that few in the pharmaceutical world believed had any commercial potential, Sera-Lab, Hybritech, and Centocor had shown the rewards that could be earned from developing Mab products. Other companies soon followed in their footsteps. By 1985 the FDA had approved more than seventy Mab-based diagnostic kits, accounting for sales of $30 to $50 million a year. Within four years the number of Mab diagnostic tests approved by the FDA had increased to 150. Many of these were for detecting infectious disease and monitoring cancer therapy. Others were used for determining blood concentrations of therapeutic drugs and of hormones. Nearly a third of the 150 Mabs approved were for pregnancy detection, with some enabling the diagnosis of a pregnancy as early as a week or two after conception.[71]

In the years to come, the number of Mab diagnostics reaching the market would continue to expand. By 2005, worldwide sales of Mab diagnostics were estimated to have reached $50 billion.[72] Mabs had proven themselves to be both a source of lucrative revenue as well as a means of enhancing the efficiency, accuracy, and speed of diagnostic tools. It remained to be seen, however, whether Mabs would lead to as many successful therapeutic applications.

CHAPTER SEVEN

The Challenge of Monoclonal Antibody Drugs

GIVEN THE QUICK COMMERCIALIZATION of Mab diagnostics, many assumed that Mab therapeutics would soon reach the market. These high expectations were given a boost when in June 1986 the U.S. Food and Drug Administration (FDA) approved Orthoclone (muromonab-CD3), derived from the OKT Mab series, in order to prevent kidney rejection in transplant patients. Developed by Ortho Diagnostic Systems, a subsidiary of Johnson & Johnson, Orthoclone was the first Mab approved anywhere for use as a drug in humans. Hailed as a major improvement in transplant medicine, it was approved seven years after its discovery in 1979, a shorter development time than the average of eight to ten years for most drugs. Only two other biotechnology drugs, human insulin and human growth hormone, had been approved by this time, in 1982 and 1985, respectively.[1]

With Orthoclone's approval, the future looked bright for Mab therapeutics. Yet Orthoclone was not without problems. Between 5 and 10 percent of patients on it experienced significant side effects, including fevers, thromboses, and anaphylactic shock, and these complications increased when the drug was given in multiple doses. Moreover, Orthoclone carried a risk of severe infections and cancer. Other Mab therapies tested in this period also led to complications. Part of the problem was that the antibodies were derived from mice or rats, which the human immune system treated as foreign and attacked. Such antibodies also only survived for between fifteen and thirty hours in humans, so the drugs had to be infused in high and frequent doses. Moreover, their recognition of human receptors was poor.[2]

As was the case with diagnostics, biotechnology startups led the way with Mab therapeutic development. Focusing on Centocor, the second company after Ortho Diagnostics that attempted to gain approval for a Mab therapeutic, this chapter reveals the complexities accompanying the commercialization of such drugs. Commercialization entailed far more than just a quest to understand the dynamics between Mabs and the human body and finding a Mab suitable for therapeutic use. What also mattered was the ability to negotiate both the intricacies of the stock market (to raise funds) and the regulatory hurdles (to achieve market approval).

Centocor faced much greater uncertainty in developing therapeutics than it had with diagnostics. Unlike diagnostics, therapeutics required direct absorption by humans so posed greater safety concerns. Drugs also necessitated the production of far greater quantities of Mabs than needed for diagnostics. Currently the doses of Mab drugs range from 0.5 mg to more than 5 mg/kg per treatment. This necessitates the production of between ten and hundreds of kilograms per year. Such quantities made the ten-liter fermenters used to produce Mabs for diagnostics inadequate. But scaling up fermenters to five-hundred-liter capacities posed significant challenges to manufacturing and quality control.[3]

Centocor decided it should first develop Mabs as contrast agents for diagnostic imaging procedures. While not therapies in themselves, these agents provided a way of testing the general safety of Mabs in humans and determining their therapeutic administration. The logic behind such tests was explained by the company to investors as follows: "In these tests, antibodies with radioisotopes or metals attached to them are injected into the blood stream and collected at disease sites. The location of the antibodies is then vizualised by equipment which detects the isotope or metal label. This diagnostic methodology allows a clinician to determine the extent and location of a disease area."[4]

Imaging diagnostic products were forecast by analysts to generate between five and ten times more revenue for Centocor than it had received for its blood-based diagnostics. In 1985, for example, cancer-imaging diagnostics were globally predicted to earn $200 million by 1988. Cardiac-imaging products were also projected to increase earnings from $70 million to $130 million in this time. But Centocor was not the only company deciding to enter the imaging field.[5]

The first Mabs developed by Centocor were CA-19-9 for imaging gastrointestinal cancers and CA-125 for imaging ovarian cancer. By 1983 the company had tested CA-19-9 in more than 250 suspected gastrointestinal cancer patients in the United States and Europe. The tests had shown that Mabs could detect tumors of less than one centimeter in diameter, a size not easily detected by conventional x-ray techniques. Centocor also developed a number of cardiovascular tests. The first, trade-named Myoscint, was based on a Mab licensed from Massachusetts General Hospital and was designed to locate and measure dead heart tissue caused by a heart attack. It was intended for use in tandem with conventional nuclear imaging equipment. In addition to Myoscint, Centocor worked on a test called Fibriscint to detect blood clots in patients with deep vein thrombosis (DVT) and another, called Capriscint, to detect atherosclerotic plaque, which narrows and hardens arteries and can lead to heart attacks and strokes.[6]

By 1987 Centocor had established a number of alliances with other companies, including Ortho Biotech, a subsidiary of Johnson & Johnson. The company predicted that it would have marketable imaging diagnostics within a couple of years. Progress was hampered, however, because although Mabs were good imaging agents, they did not clear from the body immediately. Thus patients had to wait for Myoscint to clear before diagnostic images could be taken and read. This prevented its use for the routine diagnosis of a heart attack in its early phase as was intended originally. It proved better for use in late presenters of suspected heart attacks, and for the detection of heart transplant rejection and myocarditis (inflammation of the heart muscle).[7]

In August 1989, Myoscint was granted European approval after trials with more than six hundred patients. It was marketed in France, Germany, Italy, Spain, and the United Kingdom. Two years later an FDA Advisory Panel recommended its approval, but a number of problems delayed final approval until January 1996. By this time other less invasive and more accurate methods had appeared. Fibriscint also proved disappointing because it would bind only to a clot with blood circulating around it, yet most patients experiencing DVT have no such circulation. In addition, Fibriscint took six hours to clear from the body, which was necessary before images could be taken. In the end, ultrasound proved less inva-sive, and provided more immediate results than Fibriscint for diagnosing DVT. As a result, Fibriscint was never commercialized.[8]

Like Centocor, many other companies struggled to market Mab im-aging diagnostics, and profits were minimal. In 1987 one financial ana-lyst predicted that Myoscint would earn $300 million annually and Fibriscint $400 million, but this was never achieved. Worldwide sales of diagnostic imaging Mab products also remained well below previous pro-jections: they were calculated to be worth just $10 million in 1998. In-come rose in the following years, but it remained negligible, totaling $15 million in 2005.[9]

While Centocor's imaging diagnostics had limited clinical and mar-keting significance, they helped develop the company's expertise in the clinical trials and manufacturing needed for drug development. Noth-ing, however, could fully prepare its executives for the risks that lay ahead: they were entering completely uncharted territory. In contrast to the na-scent industry in biotechnology therapeutics, which was then focused on genetically engineered drugs for diseases with well-established treatment protocols and markets, the therapeutic conditions that Mabs could address and the commercial sector that they could penetrate were still totally unknown.

To minimize its risk and increase its financial, scientific, and tech-nical resources as well as credibility, Centocor decided to collaborate with other companies to develop its therapeutics. By 1983 it had established partnerships with the American chemicals company FMC Corporation and the Swiss pharmaceutical company F. Hoffmann–La Roche. Cento-cor and FMC's alliance began in 1980, with FMC providing $12.4 mil-lion to the venture. Managed by a committee with a representative from both companies, the collaborators' aim was to find a way of producing Mabs from cell lines more closely resembling human antibodies, which they believed would reduce the risk of immunoreactions and enhance their therapeutic efficiency. In 1986 Centocor gained exclusive rights to the resulting technology in return for 1.35 million shares. The technol-ogy not only facilitated the production of more human antibodies than had been possible previously, but also gave Centocor a competitive edge in securing funding.[10]

Alongside its efforts to improve the safety of Mabs, Centocor began to build its own manufacturing plant for producing Mab therapeutics in Leiden, the Netherlands. Its location outside the United States was important, because until 1986 U.S. law prevented drugs made in the United States from being exported without FDA approval, even if they had European approval. Because more than 80 percent of Centocor's diagnostic products was being sold abroad, it was also a logical extension of its business to establish a plant outside of the United States. Other American-based biotechnology companies were also building manufacturing capacity abroad. By placing its plant in Leiden, Centocor hoped to get a head start in the European market, which handled over half of global healthcare sales. Leiden had a number of advantages as a location: its workforce could speak English; the Dutch government offered tax incentives to build such facilities; it was a leading center for fermentation technology, which was vital to Mab production; and it could draw on the expertise of the RIVM, a government institute based in Utrecht, in developing cell cultures for vaccine production.[11]

Scaling up Mab production for therapeutics posed several challenges. The major issue was how to mass-produce drugs at a reasonable cost. Most cell lines in the 1980s yielded only half a gram of Mabs per liter, so production was time-consuming and expensive. The ideal was to develop a hybrid cell line that could produce between five and ten grams of Mabs per liter. This demanded several steps, however, each requiring skill and patience. First was the creation of a hybrid cell, after which a clone had to be selected that secreted Mabs in high concentrations. Then a culture medium had to be developed to encourage the optimal growth of the hybridoma. Scaling up such media was not easy in terms of quality control because they contained fifty or more ingredients, and it was important to determine how many nutrients to add. Hybridomas stop secreting Mabs, for example, if given too much glucose.[12]

Just as vital to production was having a good vessel, or bioreactor, in which to grow the hybridomas. This involved complex engineering. A bioreactor needs to have the right pH balance and amount of oxygen to promote cellular growth. Its stirring mechanism also needs to have the right speed because stirring too vigorously can damage cell membranes. Given that the end product is a drug, the bioreactor must also be free from contamination. The high degree of sterility required is not easy to achieve given the many different biological ingredients it contains. In addition, many of a bioreactor's components, such as its pH probes, can be destroyed by the high temperatures required for cleaning it.[13]

Every stage of scaling up the manufacturing was a process of trial and error, requiring that Centocor not only break new ground, but also educate contractors and regulatory authorities. The whole venture was also financially draining. Any infrastructure had to be constructed and validated years before any therapeutic use was approved, and it cost money for it to function once in place. The risk was that Centocor could be burdened with expensive extra capacity should a drug not receive approval or market demand be less than anticipated. Like all startup biotechnology companies, Centocor had to tread a fine line between not having enough capacity and having too much.

Centocor's manufacturing plant in Leiden became fully operational for producing commercial quantities of therapeutic Mabs in 1988. Completing the plant had cost 20 percent more than expected. In 1989 the facility had more than two hundred staff working in three shifts. The following year Centocor expanded its production base by opening a 48,000-square-foot facility for mammalian cell culture in Saint Louis, Missouri.[14]

This expansion in manufacturing capacity was part of the firm's long-term objective to become a globally integrated pharmaceutical company. This strategy was pursued by many other biotechnology companies at the time, encouraged in part by Genentech's launch in October 1985 of Protropin, which was designed to treat growth hormone deficiency and was the first recombinant pharmaceutical product manufactured and marketed independently by a biotechnology company. To become a global integrated company, Centocor needed not only to build its own manufacturing base, but also to recruit its own sales force, because until then it had relied on other companies to market its diagnostic products.[15]

Encouraged by Wall Street advisers and board members, Centocor's executives decided to develop their therapeutics independently, financed by the high profits the company was gaining from its blood tests and the revenue collected from technology licensing and select product marketing. Centocor's total assets had increased nearly fivefold, and its sales had more than tripled between 1986 and 1988. Capital had also been raised through public stock offerings and research and development limited partnerships, a financial arrangement that allowed companies to raise funds from private investors for specific research projects off the balance sheet. In 1986 Centocor generated $91 million from research and development partnerships for the development and clinical testing of its drugs.[16]

By 1988 the firm had identified thirty new entities for drug development, including some for treating cancer. While many of its competitors were investing in the development of Mab therapeutics for cancer, Centocor's preferred lead product targeted septic shock, one of the most intractable and frequently fatal conditions in critical care. At least a third of septic-shock cases are caused by Gram-negative bacteria, which are difficult to treat with antibiotics and other drugs. Before the 1940s, Gram-negative sepsis was uncommon, but by the 1970s it had become a major problem. In 1980 it was thought to contribute between ten and fifteen cases for every thousand hospital admissions in the United States, causing mortality in 21 to 31 percent of patients overall, and 40 and 70 percent in cases complicated by organ failure. The incidence of the disease had increased with the rise in the range and administration of antimicrobial agents, and the emergence of antibiotic-resistant bacteria. Greater use of radiography and chemotherapy also appears to have increased patients' vulnerability to such sepsis.[17]

In the early 1970s William McCabe and co-workers at Boston University School of Medicine demonstrated that serum taken from patients suffering from Gram-negative sepsis contained antibodies against endotoxin (a toxin released by Gram-negative bacteria) that could help diminish the frequency of septic shock and death. Following this, in the early 1980s, Abraham Braude and Elizabeth Ziegler at the University of California, San Diego, successfully reduced the mortality of patients with Gram-negative sepsis by 37 percent using serum (labeled J5) collected from healthy male volunteers vaccinated with an inactivated strain of Gram-negative bacteria. Representing the first original line of treatment for many years, this work electrified the field. With sepsis accounting for up to $10 billion in health care expenditures annually, the market for such a treatment was predicted to exceed $300 million in 1990. Soon pharmaceutical companies and newly emerging biotechnology companies were investing millions of dollars in different serums for treating sepsis.[18]

Those in the commercial race included both Centocor and one of its competitors, Xoma, a California company founded in 1980 to exploit Mabs. Each decided to develop in-licensed Mabs. In the case of Xoma this was a murine Mab, Xomen E5, created by Lowell S. Young at the University of California, Los Angeles, who filed for a patent in April 1986. In contrast Centocor dedicated its efforts to a human Mab known as HA-1A, which was developed by the radiologist Henry Kaplan, a close friend of Braude, and Kaplan's oncologist colleague Nelson Teng, both based at Stanford University.[19]

While HA-1A (trade named Centoxin) was a promising candidate, its development posed significant challenges. Not only did the Mab necessitate extensive purification and formulation; its effects remained unknown in humans and Centocor had little expertise in therapeutic development. Even so, Centocor's executives, encouraged by Wall Street advisers and board members, decided that the company should finance Centoxin's development on its own, based on their belief that the drug could be a major breakthrough for managing sepsis and could yield sales of $400 million in the first year. They were encouraged by the fact that Amgen, a Californian biotechnology company set up in 1980 to commercialize recombinant DNA, was forging ahead on its own with what many at the time forecast would be two blockbuster drugs.[20]

Centocor's strategy was risky. Until then, most biotechnology companies that had succeeded in marketing drugs had done so by licensing their products to another company. Developing Centoxin alone required Centocor to oversee all the internal processes of development, clinical testing, and management of the regulatory reviews, as well as the recruitment and training of an internal marketing and sales force. Centocor executives estimated that to bring Centoxin to market would cost $150 million, and they launched a campaign to raise the money. Between 1986 and 1992, they secured $500 million based on Centoxin's promise and its possible superiority to Xoma's drug. This money was quickly swallowed up in clinical trials, the creation of a European and American sales force of 275 people, and the construction of its two new manufacturing plants. At the insistence of Wall Street advisers, Centocor also restructured its management team, bringing in staff from large pharmaceutical companies to help advance the company's skills in drug development and marketing. The new recruits dramatically shifted the company's culture, bringing with them new management styles, more aggressive marketing, and much higher expenditures. Centocor's research and development expenses, for example, increased by 76 percent between 1985 and 1986.[21]

In September 1988, Centocor filed a product license application for Centoxin with the FDA, the first step toward drug approval. Expectations were high. As Hubert Schoemaker and James Wavle, the company's newly appointed chief operating officer, wrote, getting Centoxin to market put Centocor at the forefront of writing "the first chapter in the story of human monoclonal antibodies, powerful new tools which will undoubtedly lead to great advances in medicine well into the next century."[22]

The drug was initially tested for its safety, pharmacokinetics, immunogenicity, and optimum dose in a pilot study involving a small sample of cancer patients who did not have Gram-negative sepsis. Soon after that, an open-label trial was launched in six American hospitals with thirty-four patients diagnosed with Gram-negative sepsis. The results were encouraging: the patients experienced no immunogenicity. The trial's results were published in January 1990, and thereafter a multicenter clinical trial, modeled on the J5 study and led by Ziegler, was initiated. Patients with sepsis or suspected Gram-negative sepsis were to be selected using strict diagnostic criteria, including a blood test, and randomly assigned either the drug or a placebo. All were to be followed after treatment for twenty-eight days or until death. Published in February 1991, the trial consisted of 543 patients, including 281 placebo recipients. Centoxin was found to reduce Gram-negative sepsis by 39 percent and the mortality of those who went into septic shock by 47 percent. Another trial, started in early 1991, demonstrated that Centoxin also helped decrease the mortality of children suffering from meningococcal septic shock (MSS), a rare but highly fatal form of meningococcal disease.[23]

The drug gained extra validation in early 1991 when the U.S. army placed an order for Centoxin, costing $2,500 a vial, for use by soldiers fighting in the first Gulf War. Following this, in March 1991, the drug received European regulatory approval for the treatment of Gram-negative sepsis and in September 1991 an FDA advisory committee recommended its approval in the United States.[24]

Based on all of these developments, expectations were running high—but it wasn't all smooth sailing. Some members of the FDA committee had expressed reservations about the validity of some of its trial results and ordered restrictive labeling for Centoxin. In late October 1991, too, a San Francisco federal court ruled that Centocor's patent for Centoxin infringed Xoma's patent for its drug E5, which Xoma was testing in partnership with the pharmaceutical company Pfizer. The decision, which came after months of bitter wrangling between the two companies, was a major blow. Patent disputes are common in the industry and can be devastating for the companies concerned. This patent dispute not only cost Centocor dearly in terms of time and finance, but also shined a spotlight on its Centoxin trial results. In late November 1991, a trial in specially bred beagles by the NIH Clinical Center's Department of Critical Care Medicine indicated that Centoxin offered no protection against sepsis and was potentially lethal. This resulted in a tempestuous meeting among the NIH, the FDA, and Centocor.[25]

The furor was heightened because medical practitioners elsewhere were expressing concerns about the drug. The most damning criticism came from Jean-Daniel Baumgartner and his colleagues in Lausanne, Switzerland, who tested HA-1A for Merieux Laboratories, which had also licensed the compound. In March 1990 Baumgartner reported that he could not reproduce the laboratory and animal results that allegedly showed Centoxin's usefulness against Gram-negative sepsis. While Centocor dismissed these findings, in July 1991 Baumgartner and his colleagues wrote a stinging attack, concluding, "Clearly, there is an urgent need for an adjunctive therapy for Gram-negative septic shock. However, it seems premature to rely entirely on a single clinical study before embarking on the large-scale use of such an expensive form of therapy, when there were possible imbalances between the study groups at entry and when the basic understanding of the specificity and the function of HA-1A is incomplete."[26]

In addition to anxieties about safety, medical practitioners also voiced concerns about the drug's high cost. Research published by Kevin Schulman in a leading American medical journal in December 1991 estimated that the average cost of Centoxin treatment for an individual patient in the United States would be $5,650. If given to all patients with sepsis it would amount to $24,100 per year of life saved. Schulman claimed that the total cost of treating septic patients would be $2.3 billion a year, of which the drug alone would account for $1.5 billion; acute hospital care would account for the rest of the costs.[27]

Schulman indicated that the cost of Centoxin would be two-thirds lower if used to treat only those diagnosed specifically with Gram-negative bacteria. No appropriate diagnostic existed, however. It could take up to two days to identify the bacteria, and sepsis can kill within a matter of hours. Clinicians working in Royal Victoria Hospital, Belfast, highlighted the problem: "In our intensive care unit Gram-negative organisms were isolated only five times in the past year (September 1990–September 1991) in a population of 500 patients, of whom 40 had severe sepsis. From the data of Ziegler et al, if only 40% of septicaemic episodes prove to be due to Gram-negative organisms, then 60% of patients with septicaemia will derive no benefit from Centoxin. For 100 patients with septicaemia this represents a wastage of £120,000 out of a total of £200,000. This wastage will continue until an accurate reliable method of identifying those patients with endotoxaemia becomes available."[28] Such concerns were not confined to Britain where the National Health Service budget constrained hospital expenditure. Duke University Hospital in North Carolina, for example, estimated that Centoxin would increase its pharmacy budget by between 10 and 40 percent. The San Francisco General Hospital, which served large numbers of nonpaying patients, also questioned whether financing Centoxin was an appropriate use of resources given its high costs and the difficulty of predicting which patients would most benefit from it.[29]

On February 20, 1992, the FDA ruled that it needed additional information about Centoxin before it could recommend approval. This shocked the financial community, and sent Centocor's shares tumbling 19 percent, representing a $675 million drop in its market value. Initially Centocor's team believed that they could resolve the problem, but three months later the FDA requested additional trials before it would consider Centoxin's approval. The day the news was announced, everything seemed to fall apart. Centocor was nicknamed "Centocorpse" by Wall Street, and shareholders saw $1.5 billion of Centocor's market capitalization disappear. Capturing the feeling, one cartoon illustrated the slope of Centocor's stock price plunging into a toilet with the title "Septic Shock." The following week, disgruntled investors filed six lawsuits against Centocor, alleging violation of federal securities laws and calling for compensation for damages.[30]

Sensitive to the calamities of one of its leading companies, the biotechnology industry suffered its own financial aftershock with the news, and many major companies lost faith in developing Mabs for therapeutic purposes. Don Drakeman, who was then chief executive officer of Medarex, a Mab-based company set up in 1987, recalled, "The Centoxin blow-up was really hard on all the antibody companies. There had been a number of prior clinical failures, and, with the high-profile Centoxin failure, Mabs became a four letter word on Wall Street. Our bankers told us to stop calling our products 'antibodies,' and just call them 'proteins.'" This disillusion was reinforced by the news that Xoma's sepsis drug had also failed to get FDA approval.[31]

The FDA's decision had not killed Centoxin, but Centocor desperately needed time and money to rescue it. To stop the company's cash burn of $50 million a quarter, many of the recently recruited pharmaceutical executives and hundreds of the sales representatives hired for Centoxin's launch were dismissed. The human cost was great. Sandra Faragalli, one of Centocor's administrators, recalled, "It was devastating to some folks. There were a number of people that were up in the higher ranks of the organization and the world just came crashing in on them. I remember . . . this gentleman literally crying, 'What am I going to say to my wife? What am I going to do? We cannot afford the home that we live in. My wife doesn't work. I have children. I have all these expenses. How are we going survive?'" Even for those who remained with the firm it was a rollercoaster year. Harlan Weisman, who headed the development of another Centocor drug, recalled, "I joined [Centocor] in January 1990 and at the time the price of the stock was just under $20. Based on the high hopes placed on Centoxin, the stock went to $50 to $55 a share by January 1991. I remember it well because it was my one-year anniversary, and I was awarded stock, which counted as income by the IRS. But when my taxes were due in 1992, the stock had fallen to $5.50 and I had to pay taxes at $55. My taxes due were higher than the value of the shares I owned. I had to borrow money from the company to pay my taxes."[32]

Unable to raise any more capital from the market, Centocor's founders began hunting for support from a suitable partner. There were other promising products in its pipeline and many leading pharmaceutical companies were keen to obtain Centoxin. In July 1992, Eli Lilly agreed to pay $100 million up front to help develop Centoxin—an unprecedented sum—in exchange for a 5 percent stake in Centocor. It also agreed to pay a further $25 million toward the development of ReoPro, a cardiovascular drug it was developing.[33]

Having rescued the company from the brink of collapse, Schoemaker resigned as chief executive officer in September 1992. Centoxin's failure to get FDA approval had taken a heavy toll on him. As his first wife, Ann McKenzie, put it, "Doing hard things like having to lay off people ripped [his] heart out." Having eroded the company's reputation with the financial market, Schoemaker recognized that it was time for Centocor to find a new face to define the company and its mission. The attitude of the investor community was summed up by one letter sent in July 1992 by one of Schoemaker's investor friends: "It is with very mixed emotions that I take up a pen to write to you now. . . . The events of the last 6 months have done irreparable damage to your own credibility with investors, who quite frankly don't believe anything you tell them any more. This is not [my] opinion, but rather a uniform consensus from numerous conversations with analysts, portfolio managers, bankers, brokers, and individual investors. Centocor desperately needs to be given a second chance by Wall Street, and this will only happen with a new hand on the helm."[34] Schoemaker was replaced by David Holveck, whom investors considered a safe pair of hands, having led the company's successful diagnostic division. Schoemaker stayed on as the company's executive chairman.

In the months that followed, Lilly and Centocor worked closely together on a new trial for Centoxin, which was launched in June 1992. Six months later, however, the trial was abandoned and European sales of Centoxin were halted because interim trial data indicated unexpectedly high mortality among patients without Gram-negative bacteria. Once again Centocor's shares fell sharply, and the disappointment was great. Long after the event Michael Melore, who headed the company's human resources, commented, "I think Centoxin does work. I read the compassionate use letters not only here but in Europe. It was unheard of: people would go into shock and then weeks later, depending on what their malady was, once again they were normal. That was unheard of. Once you got sepsis shock it was typically irreversible. There are still communities in Europe that would love to see the drug commercialised because they saw it work."[35]

Many theories were put forward for what had gone wrong with Centoxin. One explanation was that the pressure to transform Centocor into an integrated pharmaceutical company drove its executives to adopt new and more aggressive management practices that were ultimately destructive, as well as spending patterns that were unsustainable. But Kathleen Schoemaker, who was a cousin of Hubert and a member of the investment community, points out, "Nowadays a lot of CEOs have the luxury of history where they've seen what's working and what's not. . . . Centocor was one of the first big biotech companies. They were the frontiersmen in this industry. . . . At that point of time, to a lot of people it would have made sense [to build a big sales force] because when you're approved you want to get up and running. . . . Nowadays it's easy for someone to say, 'Well, that was a bad move.' But they have the luxury of hindsight."[36]

Another reason given for Centocor's failure was its fierce competition with Xoma, which had completed clinical development and submitted an application with the FDA for its Mab drug several months before Centocor. This led Centocor's executives to put undue pressure on the FDA. Michael Wall, Centocor's co-founder, explained, "When you're losing $50 million a quarter, every week [your drug is] not on the market is crucial. So you call the FDA every day."[37] The need to call the FDA was intensified by the patent lawsuit with Xoma. Centocor's executives also had no real experience of litigation and the lawsuit was totally unexpected. Xoma had the advantage of support from Pfizer, a powerful pharmaceutical company with which it was partnering to develop its septic drug. Schoemaker's initial instinct was to settle, but Wavle persuaded him to fight because a settlement could have resulted in a cross-licensing agreement between Centocor and Xoma and therefore in the loss in revenue. Their hope was to have a positive outcome like Amgen had when it was sued by Genetics Institute for a patent it held on its flagship drug, Epogen, for anemia. The dispute had started in 1988 and been a bitter and prolonged affair. Amgen had refused an out-of-court settlement because the company believed it was Epogen's rightful discoverer and saw no reason why Genetics Institute should get royalties through clever patenting. The battle ended in May 1993 with Genetics Institute having to pay Amgen $15.9 million.[38]

In retrospect, Schoemaker believed that Centocor's failure to settle with Xoma had been a major strategic error, one made worse when Centocor agreed to fight the patent litigation in California, which was Xoma's territory. Not only had Centocor lost the battle; waging it had cost the company time and money. The dispute also opened the design of the Centoxin trials and their results to public scrutiny. Significantly, the FDA received a transcript of the patent hearing, which included a submission from Pfizer outlining the errors they thought Centocor had committed. This prompted the regulators to ask tougher questions than had been asked before. One concern was the possibility that bias could have been introduced into the trial results because some of Centocor's executives had seen some unblinded interim results that had been handled by an independent committee. It was alleged that these executives, together with Centocor statisticians, had helped to change the clinical endpoints of the trial while it was still running.[39]

Centocor was further handicapped as a new company competing with a well-established pharmaceutical company, like Pfizer, that had substantially more capital and greater experience in gathering the preliminary data necessary for designing appropriate clinical trials. As a new biotechnology product, Centoxin also presented different challenges than traditional pharmaceuticals. Moreover, it was aimed at treating a poorly understood disease. Medical practitioners had little consensus about how to define sepsis and little experience with it because its incidence had risen sharply only after the 1970s. Attempts had been made in 1989 to establish a simple definition of sepsis that included the source of the infection, but clinical signs of sepsis were frequently present in patients whose blood lacked measurable levels of bacteria. Moreover, the patients presenting were often gravely ill with other diseases. That sepsis is a complex entity that affects virtually every physiological regulatory mechanism within the body further complicates its diagnosis. Managing the disease is also difficult because a large spectrum of micro-organisms (such as Gram-negative and Gram-positive bacteria and fungi) can be responsible for sepsis. This makes it difficult to diagnose the specific micro-organism prior to the administration of a drug.[40] Even so, in many ways the problems that Centocor executives faced were characteristic of the development of antibacterials in general—though at the time, Centocor had little experience with them.

The Centocor team was also entering uncharted territory in terms of trial design, which required the selection of appropriate endpoints and entry criteria, as well as the use of concomitant medications. Analysis was further complicated because the trial had multiple subpopulations, various definitions were used to determine the endpoint, and a number of approaches were used to account for patients lost to followup. In addition, too few statistical adjustments were made for the different levels of other medications, such as antibiotics, given to patients in the trial. All these factors confounded the analysis and interpretation of the results. The inadequacies exposed in the Centoxin trial design were a lesson not only for the company, but also for FDA officials who were themselves new to the manufacture, clinical testing, and regulation of Mabs. The only other Mab therapeutic, OKT3, had been approved for a much narrower and well-defined purpose. Significantly, all subsequent agents developed for sepsis failed when tested in second confirmatory trials.[41]

Probably because they had so little expertise in the therapeutics market, Centocor also made grave mistakes in pricing Centoxin. Bruce Peacock, who was Centocor's chief financing officer, recalled,

> The finance team had prepared a price for Centoxin in the U.S. reflecting the cost of the infrastructure that was needed to be put in place and utilising the E.U. price of Centoxin. We had prepared an analysis projecting worldwide sales of the drug based on this price and I said to Hubert, "Look, I am not going to be the guy to tell you what the market penetration's going to be, but even if it's as high as this, you can't make any money." Hubert said, "That can't be." We walked him through it and in classic Hubert [optimistic] fashion, he said, "All right. We'll just double the price." That was the complete pricing analysis that was done, much to the dismay of the professional marketing people. So they had this really high price, which was getting picked up in the U.S. press as a big negative coming for the U.S. hospital industry. They were saying, "How are we possibly going to pay for this?" [42]

The high price also raised FDA regulators' level of interest. As Holveck explained, "The FDA is a scientific regulatory governing body, but not without political peripheral vision. They thought it would be catastrophic to the health care system if they approved it because it would have to be on everyone's shelves and it was something like sixteen hundred dollars a bottle. We kept raising the price and that made them want to have another study before ushering it in. It put out a caution light warning that we better know damn well what we were doing."[43]

While painful, the lessons learned from the development of Centoxin helped Centocor to advance. The first application of the lessons involved its ongoing trial of Centoxin in 269 children with MSS, or meningococcal septic shock. MSS was more easily diagnosed than sepsis owing to its characteristic skin hemorrhages. Unlike adults with sepsis, children with MSS were also less likely to have underlying diseases that could confound results, and they tended to have a higher incidence of Gram-negative bacteria in their blood than adults with sepsis. All of these factors yielded a much narrower and more defined population for testing than had been the case with sepsis. In the end, however, the trial showed that while Centoxin was well tolerated, it had no significant affect on MSS.[44]

Overall Centoxin's failure marked the first of a number of commercial disappointments in the sepsis field. Significantly, the trial with MSS children indicated that the complex and multifactorial process involved in treating sepsis meant that no single treatment agent directed at only one stage of the disease would have an appreciable clinical benefit. Management of sepsis continued to be elusive into the twenty-first century.[45]

While Centocor did not win approval for Centoxin, the drug provided not only critical biological insights into sepsis as a disease, but also a stepping stone to the development of other Mab therapeutics. In December 1994, the FDA approved Centocor's cardiovascular drug abciximab (ReoPro), the second Mab drug to gain the authority's approval. ReoPro (also known as 7E3) was first developed by the cardiologist Barry Coller at the State University of New York at Stony Brook as a basic research tool for understanding the biochemistry of platelet physiology and pathology. Licensed by Centocor in 1986, much of ReoPro's early development and testing was undertaken and sponsored by Centocor, with support from Lilly from 1992.[46]

When abciximab arrived at Centocor, scientists already knew that it could help prevent blood clots, but were uncertain about how it might be deployed clinically. Centocor's team quickly set about transforming abciximab, which was rodent in origin, into a chimeric Mab, which was part mouse and part human, and therefore had less chance of causing immunoreactions.[47] The chimeric Mab was seen as potentially useful for a number of different clinical situations, including the prevention of blood clotting in people undergoing or about to suffer a heart attack. Centocor therefore decided it should be developed as a drug to prevent acute ischemic complications in patients undergoing coronary angioplasty, a common procedure to unblock coronary arteries. This would allow data on the drug's effects to be easily and thoroughly measured.[48]

Leaning on Lilly's long expertise of successful drug approvals, and learning from its mistakes with Centoxin, Centocor's investigators were determined to apply the highest possible standards to the scientific planning of ReoPro's clinical trials and for handling interim results. With the future of Centocor at stake, no chances were to be taken this time. Much to the relief of its team, results from the first trial in early 1993 indicated that ReoPro had achieved its primary endpoint. Denise McGinn, who was involved in the drug's development, recalled the moment when the initial results were analyzed:

> The data had all been entered, it had all been queried, cleaned and scrubbed. . . . The statisticians had run everything on sort of a test basis with other types of data just to make sure it would all work. The database was being held down at Duke University where the primary investigator site was. Everything was blinded which means that you didn't know which patients got the treatment and which got the placebo. We had the data, but Duke had the code, and you needed to merge the two to know the results. That's what was happening that night. . . . We all squeezed into Keaven [Anderson's] office. It was thundering and lightning outside—a huge storm. Keaven pushed the button and we all sort of stood there looking at him as he was typing. He said "Okay, I've got the primary analysis done."[49]

McGinn initially heard the wrong number and started questioning Anderson, at which point Schoemaker anxiously asked to see the bit of paper with the results. Quickly the team realized that the results were positive. The relief was enormous. As McGinn put it, "I get chills from telling this story. We had efficacy. We knew our trial had reached its primary endpoint. We had a drug that prevented heart attacks, death and recurrent angioplasty in patients who were at high risk to having these things happen. We had a drug and we knew it that night. We knew we had a company then too."[50]

The positive news, however, was only the beginning of the complex clinical development and regulatory review process, which was undergoing changes in the United States. ReoPro faced stiff scrutiny in the United States. At that time the FDA had split itself into two divisions: the biologics division, which was primarily focused on immune-response modifiers, and the traditional original drugs division. Although ReoPro was a biologic and an immune-response modifier, the FDA decided that because it was more of a cardiology drug it should go to the cardio-renal division within its traditional drugs division. The FDA cardio-renal advisory panel, however, had never previously handled or approved a biologic drug. Not wanting to repeat the same mistakes they had made with Centoxin, Centocor's executives were especially careful to maintain a collaborative relationship with the regulatory authorities and followed the FDA's advice to supply only relevant material. In the case of Centoxin, they had supplied too much paperwork, which in itself had complicated approval.[51]

Centocor submitted its application for ReoPro for review in 1993 after a team of its employees spent two and half months working seven days a week for between twelve and sixteen hours a day. ReoPro took just ten months to be approved by the European regulatory authorities and twelve months by the FDA. These approvals, which came through in December 1994, were particularly heartening given that many in the biotechnology industry had lost faith in Mab therapeutics, and few believed such a drug had merit or commercial application.[52]

ReoPro's approval marked a critical milestone for Centocor and placed Mabs firmly on the therapeutic map. It also showed that Mabs could treat acute conditions. The first therapeutic product ever to be approved simultaneously in the United States and Europe, ReoPro passed through its development phase more quickly than any other cardiovascular drug then on the market. In December 1995 its marketing potential was further boosted when clinical trials showed it to be effective in patients with unstable angina undergoing percutaneous coronary intervention; this expanded its potential market to more than a million patients. More good news followed when research in 1996 showed the drug to be cost-effective, an issue that had plagued Centoxin.[53]

By the end of 1996 Centocor was reporting that its annual sales of ReoPro were $149 million.[54] Centocor's leaders had realized their dream

of creating a marketable Mab therapeutic. The company's earlier challenges, however, are a powerful reminder that the path to the market was
neither inevitable nor straightforward for Mab drugs. They presented
major challenges both in terms of manufacturing and clinical testing
and for raising funds. For the pioneers involved in the development and
marketing of one of the first therapeutic Mabs, the journey had been
characterized by substantial risks and personal sacrifices. Not only had
they confronted major questions about the nature of disease pathology
and the appropriate therapeutic options possible with Mabs, they had
had to navigate the regulatory maze and wrestle with the volatility of the
financial market. The process had been brutal, particularly when dealing with the investors, whose fickleness had threatened the very survival
of the company.

CHAPTER EIGHT

Antibody Engineering

A RENAISSANCE FOR MAB THERAPEUTICS

AFTER THE CENTOXIN DISASTER, many in the biotechnology and pharmaceutical industry as well as the financial world viewed Mab drugs as a lost cause. This was to change in 1994 with the approval of ReoPro. Half-mouse and half-human in structure, its approval signified a major engineering revolution in Mabs since the 1980s, when various competitive and complementary engineering methods began to be developed in the academic and corporate worlds. During this era, some researchers distrusted Mabs whereas others believed that their therapeutic power and safety could be enhanced by improving their specificity and binding capabilities.

From the time of Köhler and Milstein's breakthrough, scientists had been seeking to improve the technique. Milstein captured its limitations: "All that we seem to have acquired is the potential ability to select from an animal any of the antibodies of his repertoire. It is somewhat like selecting individual dishes out of a very elaborate menu: antibodies 'à la carte'.... A gastronome worth his salt ... wants to experiment with new ingredients, new combinations. His dream is to invent new dishes and not only to taste what others are doing. I am sure our next step will be to move from the dining table, where we order and consume our antibodies 'à la carte' to the kitchen, where we will attempt to mess them up."[1]

The first Mabs were produced by fusing myeloma tumor cells taken from mice with spleen cells derived from other mice or rats previously immunized with an antigen. These Mabs were known as murine Mabs, denoting their rodent origin. While they could be made to target almost any antigen and in vast quantities, they were considered foreign by the human body. As many as half of patients treated with murine Mabs experienced immune reactions, which not only could endanger the patients, but also led to the rapid destruction and clearance of the Mab from the body before it could have its full therapeutic effect.[2]

Producing human Mabs was a major challenge. A human's immune system is intrinsically tolerant of most human antigens so will not produce many antibodies of use for therapy. Moreover, humans cannot legally be immunized and manipulated like animals and the process of immunization carries risks. One solution was to create hybridomas from antibodies isolated from the blood of individuals already exposed to particular antigens like cancer. Yet such hybridomas were unstable and stopped secreting Mabs after some time. Another approach was to fuse the Epstein-Barr virus with immortal human lymphocyte B cells taken from healthy volunteers, but this required humans to be immunized and only provided low yields of Mabs.[3]

Faced with these obstacles, scientists began wondering if genetic engineering could transform animal antibodies into human ones. One of the first people to suggest this was Milstein, who believed such a technique would free scientists from merely immortalizing naturally occurring antibodies, in the way that his and Köhler's technique did, and allow them instead to design tailor-made antibodies, including human ones. Milstein made relatively modest efforts in this area himself, but inspired others—many of them based in the Laboratory of Molecular Biology (LMB) in Cambridge, England—to take up the gauntlet.[4]

Those pursuing the task were helped by the antibody's basic uniform structure (see Figure 1.2). An antibody is a Y-shaped molecule consisting of two large, identical polypeptides, called heavy chains, and two smaller identical polypeptides, called light chains. The chains have both a variable region, located at the tip of the Y arm, which is responsible for binding different antigens, and a constant region, at the base of the Y, which is responsible for recruiting the body's other resources (including natural killer cells, macrophages, and other "effector cells") to destroy an antigen. This modular structure means that genes present on the variable region of one antibody can be cut and pasted on to the constant region of another.[5]

For those familiar with DNA recombinant technology and steeped in antibody research and immunology, shuffling genes was merely a way of mimicking the immune system's natural process, which was first described by Nobumichi Hozumi and Susumu Tonegawa at the Basel Institute of Immunology in 1976. Also known as immunoglobulins, antibodies are divided into five major classes, the main ones being IgM and IgG. Each class has a unique chemical structure and specific function. The IgM class is the first antibody produced by the immune system when it encounters a new antigen. Over time the immune system converts these into IgG antibodies. Such switching confers long-term immunity and is achieved by the rearrangement of genes between the variable and constant regions. Only three or four separate DNA segments are responsible for the vast array of antibodies that the body generates against multiple foreign invaders. Consequently, scientists could potentially combine segments of one antibody gene with the segments of another to create new antibodies.[6]

To get the ball rolling, scientists needed to find a way of engineering the appropriate rDNA for an antibody and then inserting it into a myeloma cell to facilitate transcription and translation of that gene (gene expression). The task was a major undertaking. Michael Neuberger, an immunologist and biochemist at the LMB inspired by Milstein, struggled for three years from 1980 to amalgamate the genes of the constant and variable regions. For Neuberger it was a "labor of love." He could not just pluck a standard DNA fragment from a laboratory shelf. First he needed to identify a variable region of interest, create a library of DNA fragments taken from this region, and then clone the DNA of interest. Next he had to put the DNA into a plasmid—an independent, self-replicating DNA molecule—which was inserted into a myeloma cell to express the recombinant gene and produce the antibody. Introducing DNA into myeloma cells was a challenge. Neuberger attempted various approaches, ranging from packaging the plasmid DNA into a virus, and then infecting the myeloma cell, to using different chemical treatments. He finally achieved the goal by stripping the bacterium wall that contained the plasmid and fusing the resultant "spheroplast" with a myeloma cell by using polyethylene glycol—the same strategy deployed for creating hybridomas. Introducing a plasmid containing just the DNA for the amalgamated variable and constant regions proved insufficient. Neuberger discovered he also needed to introduce DNA segments into the plasma to direct the myeloma cell to transcribe the engineered antibody gene efficiently. With little known about the DNA segments regulating antibody gene expression, this step was far from simple. Each segment had to be identified before it was inserted.[7]

Unaware of Neuberger's efforts, scientists across the Atlantic were pursuing a similar mission. They included David Baltimore, a Nobel Prize winner, and Douglas Rice, a postdoctoral fellow, both based in the Massachusetts Institute of Technology's department of biology, as well as Sherie Morrison, who was attached to Columbia University's genetics department and working with Vernon Oi, who was initially based at Stanford University, and then at Becton Dickinson Monoclonal Center in Mountain View, California. By 1984 both Neuberger and the American scientists had demonstrated the feasibility of making recombinant genes for both the light and heavy chains of an antibody and introducing them into a myeloma cell.[8]

In contrast to the painstaking and time-consuming work required to insert rDNA into a myeloma cell, the next stage proved relatively simple and quick. It involved shuffling genes from the variable to the constant regions of the antibody. This was achieved by Neuberger together with Terence Rabbitts and other colleagues at the LMB; Morrison and Oi, together with Leonard Herzenberg at Stanford University; and Gabrielle Boulianne, Marc Shulman, and Nobumichi Hozumi at Toronto University.[9] Working independently of each other, each of these academic groups took a broadly similar approach. Although they used different mammalian cell expression systems, they each linked a gene segment from a variable region of a mouse antibody to a corresponding gene segment on the constant region of a human antibody. The result, called a "chimeric antibody," possessed genes that were half-human and half-mouse, taking its name from chimera, a mythological creature made up of parts of multiple animals.[10]

In parallel with such academic endeavors, two commercial groups, the first at Genentech and the Beckman Research Institute and the second at Celltech, also developed a means of producing recombinant Mabs using bacteria expression systems. Over time these methods would bring the companies considerable revenue in royalties from the patents awarded to them. Yet the technique did not produce full and properly folded Mabs and provided a poor yield of Mabs.[11]

One advantage of the new recombinant Mabs was that their specific effector function could be selected and tailored. A Mab could thus be designed to stimulate the killing of a tumor cell by harnessing the body's natural complement system. Recombinant Mabs were also less liable to provoke immune reactions in patients. In contrast to murine antibodies, for example, chimeric antibodies were made up of only 35 percent rather than 100 percent mouse proteins. Nonetheless, such antibodies were not fully human, so scientists continued hunting for ways to make them more so.[12]

One technique that proved crucial in taking the engineering further was site-directed mutagenesis (SDM), a method first conceived of in 1971 by Clyde Hutchison III, an American biochemist and microbiologist based at the University of North Carolina at Chapel Hill and further elaborated by Herbert Scott and Hans Kössel at the University of Freiberg in 1973. The technique had been opened up for wider adoption in 1978 by Hutchinson, together with Michael Smith, a British chemist based at the University of British Columbia. SDM allowed scientists to cause a specific mutation by changing, in a very precise and specific way, part of an organism's DNA. Before SDM, the only way of achieving such a mutation was the time-consuming process of exposing organisms to radiation or chemicals and then selecting the desired mutant.[13]

Spearheading the use of SDM in antibody engineering was the LMB-based protein chemist Gregory Winter, who had learned the technique from Mark Zoller, a postdoctoral researcher in Smith's laboratory (Figure 8.1). For Winter, SDM provided an opportunity to expand the expertise he had acquired in DNA sequencing during his research to understand the pathogenic mechanism of the influenza virus. His aim was to construct a new protein by altering a gene, an idea first floated in 1978. This was a major challenge. Winter explained, "The biggest problem with building a new protein was designing it so that it would fold, and assuming it had done so and not aggregated, that it would fold in such a manner as to be functional. At a lower level was the problem of building the novel gene. At that time only small oligonucleotides were available and

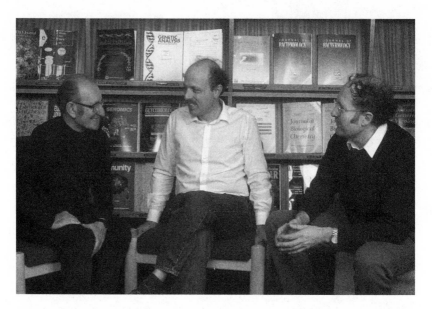

FIGURE 8.1. *Left to right:* César Milstein with Michael Neuberger and Gregory Winter. The colleagues helped reengineer Mabs to make them safer and more clinically effective. (MRC Laboratory of Molecular Biology)

they had then to be assembled into larger blocks which were then put together."[14]

Winter believed the task would be easier if he used a protein with a basic scaffold amenable to manipulation. By an ironic stroke of fate, his identification of such a protein was helped by a terrible act of violence: he was injured when an assailant smashed an iron bar over his head and twisted his arm out of its socket. After losing the use of his right arm, Winter immersed himself in learning a computer-graphics system to continue his protein chemistry research at a desk. This allowed him to investigate the 3D structure of different proteins captured with x-ray crystallography. From this, he determined that an antibody had the best scaffold. It had three loops on its heavy and light chains that could be used to hang new loops specifying new binding or catalytic activities.[15]

In 1983 Winter, encouraged by Milstein and the fact that considerable data on the DNA sequences of antibodies already existed in the public domain, began planning his experiment. Many around him were skeptical about his venture. While scientists were beginning to play around with whole variable regions of antibodies, as in the case of chimerics, few imagined that a functional antibody could be created by taking just parts of the variable region. Winter had an important advantage, however: by 1984 he was sharing an office with Neuberger, who was willing to share his newly expressed recombinant antibody genes and constructed chimeric antibodies.[16]

Winter first needed to demonstrate that the loops of one antibody's variable region could be taken off and put on to another without affecting the antibody antigen-binding function. If this worked, Winter could construct a new protein by "simply mucking around with the loops" and not worrying about the rest of the molecule. To get the ball rolling, Winter looked to create a human antibody "by stealing only the antigen-binding site (rather than the entire variable domains) from the mouse antibody." If this could be achieved, Winter would not only prove his theory, but also create a means to make rodent antibodies more humanlike. The major challenge was identifying which residues in the sequence of the mouse antibody were required for antigen binding. This task was daunting because it necessitated synthesizing DNA from the entire variable region of an antibody, and no sequence that long had been synthesized before. Winter would have to first determine the DNA sequence of the mouse antibody's variable region, then synthesize a new gene that encoded the loops from the mouse antibody and the scaffold from a human antibody. Because he did not have access to an automated DNA synthesizer, he and his technician were forced to sit for many hours at a time, turning a switch every few minutes to keep a machine running. In the end, the work took a couple of years to complete, with two people working full-time and most of Winter's laboratory resources devoted to it.[17]

By 1986 Winter and his team had demonstrated the feasibility of building a new antibody by grafting the antigen-binding loops, or complementarity-determining regions (CDRs; see Figure 1.2), from a mouse antibody into a human antibody. Their Mab was directed against a hapten, a nonprotein molecule that elicits an immune response when attached to a large carrier such as a protein. Winter's Mab had been achieved by capitalizing on Neuberger's previous development of a chimeric Mab targeting a hapten. The team filed for a patent, explaining that as the first "humanized" Mab it represented a technical breakthrough in antibody engineering. The technique, dubbed CDR grafting, reduced the mouse component of a Mab to just 5 percent.[18]

It remained to be seen, however, whether CDR grafting could be used to develop a Mab of clinical importance. Winter did not have to look far to start answering this question: just across the road, Waldmann's group was then trying to find a way to reduce the foreignness of Campath-1G, which was thought to be causing side-effects in patients. This they were doing by exploring the immunogenic effects of different therapeutic antibodies in animals and the chimerization of Campath-1G. The work was being done by the biochemist Michael Clark; Marianne Brüggemann, a geneticist and immunologist; and Mark Frewin, a technician; in collaboration with Neuberger's team. Upon learning of Winter's new humanizing approach, the team soon established a collaboration with Winter and his postdoctoral fellow Lutz Riechmann, a molecular biologist, to humanize Campath-1G. The work began in 1986 and involved first sequencing and cloning the variable region of the rat Campath-1G, then making some changes to the human antibody's basic framework in order to produce a Mab with the desired binding activity. Proceeding in painstaking steps, with each intermediate Mab being expressed and tested for activity, in 1988 the collaborators finally produced Campath-1H, the first humanized rodent antibody with therapeutic potential.[19]

When used a few months later to treat two patients with non-Hodgkin's lymphoma, Campath-1H proved a remarkably good treatment, going well beyond expectations. Within forty-three days of treatment, Campath-1H had destroyed a large part of the tumor mass in the treated patients. Just as important, it did not seem to provoke any negative immune reactions. Although the lack of immune response could have been due to the immunosuppressive nature of non-Hodgkin's lymphoma as opposed to the humanization of the Mab, the testing did demonstrate that humanization did not undermine a Mab's efficacy.[20]

Despite Campath-1H's success, researchers elsewhere initially struggled to apply CDR grafting, in part because the original scaffold of the antibody was not as static as Winter envisaged. Investigators soon discovered that inserting novel sequences of DNA within the CDR domain of an antibody could undermine the molecule's stability. One solution was developed by Cary Queen, who in 1986 helped found Protein Design Labs, a biotechnology company located in Palo Alto, California. In 1989, Queen and his colleagues reported having stabilized a Mab by restoring some of the residue sequences found outside of the CDR region. Following this breakthrough, they developed daclizumab, the first humanized Mab to win FDA approval. Designed to control the acute rejection of kidney transplants, it was marketed with the help of F. Hoffmann–La Roche. Within a short time other researchers were humanizing other potentially therapeutic Mabs, using and advancing Winter's and Queen's techniques.[21]

In 1987, Winter, not content with just humanizing rodent antibodies, launched a project to create an artificial human immune system to produce fully human antibodies. The first stage involved the generation of a large library of human antibody fragments. This was done using polymerase chain reaction (PCR), a laboratory technique first devised in 1983 that allowed for the multiple reproduction of very small samples of DNA to produce billions of copies. By 1988 Winter had adopted PCR to amplify and clone the genes of the heavy and light chain variable regions of murine antibodies, for which he filed a patent. In addition to facilitating the creation of a library of fragments, the technique eliminated the laborious and time-consuming steps involved in the sequencing and cloning of genes—steps then impeding the production of chimeric and humanized Mabs.[22]

In addition to PCR, Winter looked to phage display for his project. Originally developed to display small peptides in 1985, the technique deploys phages, viruses that infect bacteria, to connect proteins with genetic information. Upon replication, such modified viruses produce enormous, diverse libraries of proteins. Promising the rapid identification and isolation of proteins specific to any target of interest from a library of millions of different proteins bound to phages, phage display offered Winter a means to generate human antibodies. He soon discovered, however, that he had a major competitor: a large group of scientists headed by Richard Lerner and Carlos Barbas at the Scripps Research Institute, San Diego, who had been given a pre-print of Winter's work by Lutz Riechmann, who was now working at the institute. Significantly, the Scripps team had the backing of Stratagene, an American biotechnology company set up in 1984 to exploit new antibody engineering techniques.[23]

What alarmed Winter most was that the Scripps team reported that they were ready to file for a patent. Desperately needing a way to boost his resources, Winter decided to create a new company, Cambridge Antibody Technology (CAT). This he did in 1989 with the support of

Aaron Klug, then the LMB director. The company was founded not for commercial reasons, but as a means to attract financial investment in Winter's research. Joining Winter in the venture was David Chiswell, former product development and research manager at Amersham International. CAT quickly attracted investment from Peptide Technology Australia (Peptech), a biotechnology company whose founder, Gregory Grigg, had had spent time in Fred Sanger's Laboratory at the LMB. Peptech agreed to provide £750,000 in exchange for a 40 percent equity stake in CAT. Additional funds were secured through equity investments from private individuals and investment funds. Both the MRC and Winter were given a stake in the company.[24]

By 1990, Winter and his CAT colleagues had developed a platform that enabled scientists to generate enormous, diverse libraries of randomly shaped human antibodies. How the system worked was explained as follows: "A phage antibody is . . . analogous to a B lymphocyte in that it displays an antibody on its surface and carries the genes encoding that antibody. It can be selected for its ability to bind a specific antigen and subsequently amplified by reinfection of bacteria. The antibody genes can then be rescued and used to produce soluble antibody fragments or even complete antibodies."[25]

Now scientists could pour a "library" of phage antibodies through a column to which a target had been fixed that bound to specific phages. The target could be a protein expressed on a cancer cell or a molecule known to cause inflammation. Mimicking the immune system, this platform provided a means to select the most appropriate antibody fragments for a particular antigen, which could then be refined and made into a Mab. It marked a major turning point in the engineering of Mabs. Gone were the days of relying on an animal or human's natural immune system, with all their limitations. The platform provided much greater power for tailoring the specificity and affinity of the Mab and offered the possibility of building synthetic Mabs with less immunogenicity. Moreover, Mabs of interest could be generated in two weeks and the process was amenable to automation.[26]

In parallel with the development of the phage display technique, another method was emerging in Cambridge to produce human antibodies based on the research of Neuberger and Brüggemann into the regulatory mechanism underlying the generation of different antibodies.

This work involved genetically engineering a transgenic mouse to auto-matically produce human antibodies when immunized. Begun in 1986, this project was helped by Azim Surani from the Babraham Institute, Cambridge, a pioneer in animal genetic engineering. Scientists had been making transgenic mice successfully since the mid-1970s. In general terms, the technique entailed introducing foreign DNA segments into the germ line of early mouse embryos, which would then pass this recombi-nant DNA on to their offspring. The technique inactivated a mouse's own genes or introduced new genes.[27]

To start the ball rolling, the Cambridge team set about introducing gene segments from a human antibody into the DNA of early mouse em-bryos to create mice that could produce human antibodies after immu-nization. Such an idea was not new, having been floated as a possibility by Columbia University scientists in 1985. Nobody, however, had yet suc-ceeded in such an endeavor. The major challenge was that human anti-body loci are very large, containing many gene segments scattered over a few million base pairs of DNA.[28]

To make the task more manageable Neuberger and Brüggemann, with the help of Gareth Williams, set about assembling a miniature ver-sion, or minilocus, of the gene segment that codes for the heavy-chain domain from human antibodies. Making a minilocus was complex. The assembly of such genes in 1986 was much more challenging than that involved in making chimeric antibodies. As Neuberger recalls, "It meant obtaining all the various bits (multiple variable regions and joining seg-ments, synthesizing diversity segments, adding a constant region as well as what we guessed would be sufficient gene regulatory sequences) and assembling them together." The process did not require any new inven-tions, but it "was laborious and long-winded." Using existing methods for gene cloning and assembly technology, the mission took about a year to complete. The result was a hybrid mouse and human-heavy-chain minigene construct. Once made, the minilocus had to be micro-injected into mouse eggs. This was not easy because it was a large DNA molecule and needed to go down a very fine needle. To prevent the DNA from being sheared, Surani attempted various solutions, such as adding spermine to compact the DNA.[29]

The team was uncertain whether the minilocus, once inserted, could rearrange itself to generate the repertoire of different human antibody heavy chains in the mouse. Two French groups had proved in 1987 that rabbit or chicken genes for the light chain part of the antibody could assemble when injected into mice. Yet this was a far cry from what the Cambridge scientists were trying to achieve. Importantly, the minilocus for the heavy chain of an antibody was much larger, contained many more segments, and underwent more complex rearrangements than the light chain. There was no guarantee that the miniaturized version contained all the segments necessary to get successful rearrangement and expression. And moreover, once reassembled in the mouse, no one could be sure that the genes would interact with the necessary signaling components in the mouse's lymphocytes so that, following immunization with an antigen, the mouse would produce human antibodies specific to that antigen. To the team's relief, the inserted human antibody genes did indeed rearrange appropriately, enabling the expression of antibodies with human heavy chains. The group filed for a patent on the technique in 1988. Much more work was needed, however, before mice would readily produce the range of human Mabs with both heavy and light chains of human origin that would be suitable for therapeutic use.[30]

While Neuberger and Brüggemann continued developing their technique, they realized that its commercial development required far more resources than were then at their disposal. Unlike Winter, who set up his own company to advance his development of phage display Mabs, Neuberger and Brüggemann opted to provide broad nonexclusive licenses to companies prepared to take the technology further. This, they believed, would help accelerate the development of their transgenic mice and provide returns should any successful commercial products be produced. Yet few companies were prepared to invest in the technology. Even CAT, on whose scientific advisory board Neuberger served, decided not to pursue this course so as not to dilute its development of phage display. In the end only GenPharm and Cell Genesys, two Californian startups already developing their own transgenic mice, licensed the technology.[31]

By the end of 1980s it seemed that scientists would soon have transgenic mice to produce human antibodies. This was due not only to the progress in Cambridge, but also to the development of "gene-targeting technology" at the University of Utah, MIT, and Columbia University between 1988 and 1989, which allowed specific modifications to be made

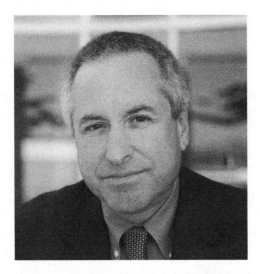

FIGURE 8.2. Nils Lonberg, n.d. (Nils Lonberg)

in the mammalian genome through the insertion of genes at precise points in an animal's DNA.[32]

Despite the optimism, certain obstacles remained. Those taking up the challenge included the team in Cambridge as well as those based at GenPharm, led by Nils Lonberg, and Cell Genesys, led by Aya Jakobovits (Figure 8.2). All three groups pursued a fairly similar strategy of creating two different strains of mice for cross-breeding. The first mouse had its genes modified to inactivate its immune system. This blocked its capacity to produce its own antibodies following immunization, and encouraged production instead by the transgenic human antibody gene. In the second mouse larger segments of the human antibody gene loci were introduced to facilitate the production of a wider range of human Mabs. Once cross-bred, transgenic mice could generate antibodies identical to human antibodies.[33]

Lonberg's experiences reveal some of the twists and turns behind the development of such transgenic mice. A chemist by training, with a Harvard University doctorate in molecular biology, Lonberg had first begun wondering about the possibilities of engineering recombinant proteins for therapeutics in 1984, when he was based at Biogen with his colleague Harry Meade. His interest was prompted by a contract that Biogen had to supply large amounts of recombinant protein. Because it was a large molecule, the protein could be expressed only through recombinant mammalian cells in roller bottles that took up an enormous amount of space. As Lonberg recalled, "Every spare closet got turned into a warm room and got filled with these roller bottles just to try to make enough protein to fulfill the company's contract." Lonberg and Meade wondered if a more efficient production system could be created by genetically engineering a cow to produce recombinant protein in its milk. Most of their Biogen colleagues, however, laughed at the proposal.[34]

In 1985 Lonberg joined the Memorial Sloan-Kettering Cancer Center, New York, as a postdoctoral scientist. Surrounded by pioneers in the generation of transgenic mice, including Elizabeth Lacy and Frank Costantini, Lonberg succeeded in genetically engineering mice to produce human proteins in their milk, which led to his being awarded the third patent ever granted for a transgenic animal. Sloan-Kettering was not only an ideal location for gaining expertise in transgenic animals; it also exposed Lonberg to Mab therapeutics. He first came into contact with them through his oncologist brother, who was also based at Sloan-Kettering. While clinically testing a mouse antibody developed by Lloyd Old and Alan Houghton for treating melanoma, his brother noted how some patients' immune responses to its mouse component were causing the rapid disappearance of the Mab in the body, thereby reducing its effectiveness. The patients with the best outcomes were those with the most delayed response to the Mab. Nils Lonberg wondered if transgenic mice could offer a way to offer this delayed response.[35]

In 1989, Nils Lonberg joined GenPharm, which provided the resources to begin developing transgenic mice to produce human Mabs. GenPharm allocated $1.3 million to the project and he secured additional NIH money. This allowed for a team of fourteen. The project involved creating two varieties of gene-modified mice. The first was to have some of its genes inactivated and the second was to have its genes modified with fully human antibody genes to facilitate production of fully IgG human antibodies. These two mice were then to be cross-bred to create a transgenic mouse with a human immune system that could generate antibodies identical to human antibodies. By late 1993, Lonberg's team had generated a mouse with a human immune system capable of producing fully human IgG antibodies with high affinities for their targets. Shortly afterward the scientists in Cambridge and at Cell Gensys reported similar success.[36]

The major advantage of transgenic mice was that scientists could now easily produce fully human Mabs with enhanced affinity for a target without spending hours humanizing or optimizing an antibody molecule. Everything could be achieved within the mouse. Following immunization, the humanized mice produced target-specific human Mabs without any subsequent manipulation. This meant that Mab therapeutics could be developed much more quickly than before.[37]

Advances in Mab engineering in the twenty years since Milstein and Köhler's invention had radically transformed the antibody molecule, helping to reduce its mouse component to almost nothing and make antibodies more compatible with the human body (see Table 8.1 and Figure 8.3). Following these developments, scientists began to investigate the possibility of using just the active portion of an antibody to create miniature Mabs. This was highly desirable because large quantities of Mabs had to be injected to achieve clinical efficacy. The high volumes needed for therapy posed significant formatting and manufacturing complications. As explained in chapter 4, Mab production required not only very large cultures of mammalian cells, but also extensive purification. All of this added to the costs of production, which raised the market price of the final therapeutics and so constrained their clinical application. If smaller fragments of antibodies could be deployed, scientists would have a means to improve production yields and the possibility of developing new and more versatile antibody formats to boost therapeutic efficacy.[38]

One of the first researchers to investigate the development of miniature antibodies was Winter, who noticed in 1989 with LMB colleagues that fragments, dubbed domain antibodies (dAbs), sometimes bound independently to antigens. These came from variable domain and heavy chains of antibodies produced from immunized animals. They hypothesized that such dAbs might have greater power to penetrate tissues. Moreover, dAbs offered the possibility of better targeting of pathogenic viruses, which remained inaccessible to full-size Mabs due to the narrow cavities on their surface antigens.[39]

The team soon discovered that dAbs could be generated without the immunization of animals. Advancing such antibodies, however, proved slow, because the single domains tended to be "sticky" and clump together.

Table 8.1

Percentage of mouse and human protein components in different forms of Mabs

FORM OF MAB	MOUSE PROTEIN	HUMAN PROTEIN
Murine	100%	0%
Chimeric	65%	35%
Humanized	5%	95%
"Fully human"	0%	100%

Source: W. R. Gombotz and S. J. Shire, "Introduction," in S. J. Shire et al., eds., *Current Trends in Monoclonal Antibody Development and Manufacturing* (New York, 2009), 3.

Furthermore, they did not always retain the affinity of their parent antibody and were not very soluble. Based on these features, dAbs seemed doomed to remain just a laboratory curiosity. In 2000, however, Winter's team finally found a way to select single-domain antibodies that did not stick together, laying the foundation for a new company, Domantis. The new antibodies offered both a more effective therapy and a means to bypass the dominant patent monopoly that by this point Genentech and other companies held on Mab engineering.[40]

While a number of different engineering methods had been developed for Mabs by the end of the twentieth century, a number of academic-based scientists remained skeptical about the advantages of one technology over another in terms of reducing immunogenicity. Clark, who had played a pivotal role in the humanization of Mabs, believed that in terms of reducing immunogenicity there was little difference among the first chimeric antibodies, humanized antibodies, or "fully human" antibodies. From his perspective the new innovations were little more than the "Emperor's new clothes." Similarly, Geoff Hale, who like Clark had helped develop the first humanized Mab for therapy, believed that the large intellectual investment in antibody engineering to eradicate the unwanted immunogenicity of Mabs had on the whole been "a distraction rather than a stimulus to progress." Neuberger, who had helped develop both chimeric antibodies and transgenic mice to produce fully human antibodies,

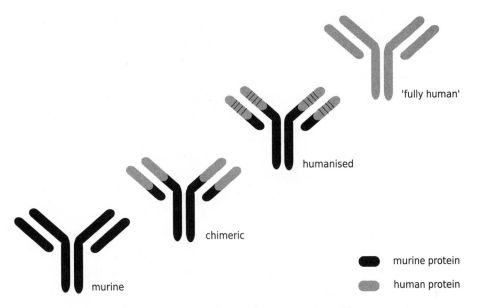

'fully human'

humanised

chimeric

murine

● murine protein

● human protein

FIGURE 8.3. Different generations of Mabs showing murine and human protein components

claims that the key reduction in immunogenicity was achieved early on with chimeric antibodies, because these replaced the constant regions of the antibody. How far the new methods—such as CDR grafting, phage antibodies, and transgenic mice, which tinkered with the variable region—further reduced the immunogenicity of Mabs is, he claims, difficult to know. The difficulty is that a properly controlled experiment to answer this question cannot be carried out.[41]

Not everyone holds such views. Lonberg, who is deeply involved in pharmaceutical development, while agreeing with Neuberger that it is difficult to perform an experiment to test how far newer techniques have reduced unwanted immunogenicity, believes that the clinical trials conducted with more recently developed CDR antibodies and with transgenic mice have shown the new techniques to have achieved significant progress in this area.[42]

One difficulty in determining how far antibody engineering has helped reduce immunogenicity is that the genes of the variable region of any therapeutic Mab, whether it be chimeric, CDR-grafted, or derived using the phage system or humanized mice, will have multiple mutations.

Consequently these genes will differ from the antibodies already existing in a nonimmunized patient and so any therapeutic Mab will be seen as slightly foreign by a patient's immune system.[43]

The debate over the relative merits of chimeric versus humanized or human antibodies is also relevant in the case of antibody fragments. While fragments permit better penetration of tissue, they can be filtered out by the kidney more easily than full-size Mabs, resulting in more rapid clearance from the body, so that they have a reduced time to work. In some circumstances, such as when they are delivering cytotoxic radioisotopes to destroy a tumor, their rapid clearance from the body can actually be advantageous. Yet in other situations it can be a disadvantage, for example when it prevents the targeted site from being sufficiently affected. Another disadvantage with fragments is that they are unable to stimulate the natural effector functions of the immune system, which sends out its own antibodies or complement in response to threats. Within the context of production, fragments can also be more likely to form undesirable clumps and be less stable.[44]

The use of the different engineering approaches has largely been driven by the accessibility to patents for each approach. In contrast to Milstein and Köhler's invention, which was never patented, the number of patents governing subsequent engineering methods is vast. Almost every particular of Mab creation and manufacture is now protected by a patent that has to be licensed if used. In 1986 it was estimated that there were only 830 patents relating to the hybridoma technology. This number grew exponentially thereafter, making the field difficult and expensive to navigate for anyone wishing to enter the space. Even for those deeply embedded in the science and the commercialization of Mabs, the abundance of patents can result in companies becoming embroiled in battles to maintain rights to their intellectual property.[45]

Some idea of the pain that patents can inflict is borne out by the example of GenPharm. In February 1994, just days before it was due to file for its initial public offering (IPO), the company was sued by its rival Cell Gensys on the grounds that it had stolen a trade secret for inactivating a mouse gene. Many within GenPharm initially did not take the legal action seriously, nor did other scientists such as Neuberger. Nonetheless, Cell Gensys was a major threat given that it had the financial backing of Japan Tobacco and had already gone public. GenPharm countered with an antitrust lawsuit and two patent lawsuits. The litigation dragged on for three long years and cost GenPharm dearly: it prevented it from going forward with its IPO, thereby crippling it financially, and it undermined efforts to find a buyer to rescue the company. GenPharm's ability to raise cash was not made any easier in the wake of the Centoxin disaster. Having raised over $75 million between 1988 and 1994, GenPharm soon found that only $15,000 remained. In order to survive, its executive was forced to get rid of all but a few of the 110 staff, as well as most of the furniture, laboratory equipment, and patents. Owing large sums of money to lawyers and banks, they thereafter turned to bartering and looking after the mouse cages of another biotechnology company in exchange for the use of a small amount of laboratory space. Eventually, in January 1997, the two companies negotiated a cross-licensing agreement. In the aftermath of the legal battle GenPharm was acquired by Medarex, an antibody company based in Annandale, New Jersey, and Cell Gensys was granted the approval for the first fully human antibody, panitumumab (Vectibix), which was produced from transgenic mice.[46]

Patents alone did not determine which new engineering methods were employed for the formulation of drugs. Also crucial was how well the Mab drugs they helped generate performed in clinical trials and navigated through the regulatory framework. Figure 8.4 highlights how quickly each method evolved from materialization of the full invention to the first marketable therapeutic. On average this process took ten to twelve years from the time when the invention first became practical. In the case of the transgenic mice the technique took much longer to mature than is suggested by the timeline. As highlighted earlier, transgenic technology was first proposed as a means to generate human antibodies as early as 1985, but it took another nine years before this was realized in practical terms and a further twelve years before a therapeutic arrived on the market. Part of this time lag is attributable to the considerable work involved in engineering the right mouse, and mouse-based experiments take time to complete. But while the transgenic technology took longer to develop than other engineering techniques, once achieved, it provided the means to produce Mab therapeutics more quickly. With murine-based Mabs, all that is needed is to immunize the transgenic animal, fuse its spleen cells with a myeloma, and then screen for the desired Mab. For this reason, transgenic mice are likely to be the preferred route for producing future Mab therapeutics.[47]

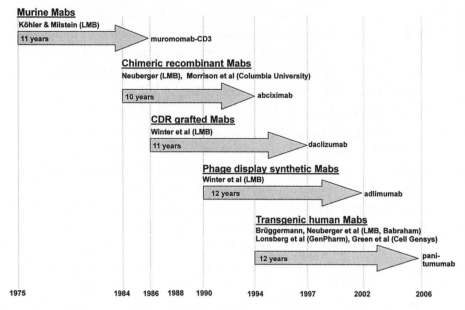

FIGURE 8.4. Timeline for Mab engineering techniques from first publication to first drug approval (Adapted from N. Lonberg, "Human Monoclonal Antibodies from Transgenic Mice," in Y. Chemojovsky and A. Nissim, eds. *Therapeutic Antibodies* [Berlin, 2008], 69–97, esp. 71, fig. 1)

Certain Mab types have dominated the therapeutic landscape. Figure 8.5 shows that the FDA initially approved only murine and chimeric Mabs, but from 1997 began also to approve humanized and human Mabs, which were first produced by CDR grafting and then by phage display and later transgenic mice. By 2009 chimeric and humanized Mabs were the predominant form of the twenty-two Mab therapeutics on the market and the twenty-eight that were then in the final stages of clinical development. Humanized and human Mab therapeutics were also the most prevalent form in phase III trials (Figure 8.6). As Figure 8.7 reveals, most of these drugs were created using murine hybridomas rather than humanized mouse hybridomas or phage display antibody libraries, although the last two methods were beginning to be used for drugs entering late-stage clinical trials. Antibody fragments were also beginning to be used in the earlier clinical development stages. Of the 450 Mabs that were in clinical development in 2009, fifty-four (12 percent) were antibody fragments.[48]

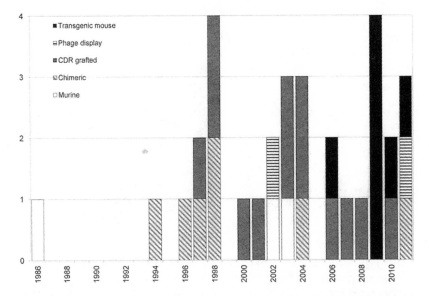

FIGURE 8.5. Number of Mab drugs approved annually by the FDA by antibody type, 1986–2011 (Adapted from N. Lonberg, "From Mouse Embryos to Antibody Therapies," paper presented to IBC, 6 Dec 2011)

Much of the rapid growth in Mabs in recent years has been in human antibodies (Figure 8.8). Transgenic mice have helped to fuel this growth. In 2010, 34 (60 percent) of the 56 transgenic-produced Mabs were generated by mice created by GenPharm and Kirin Brewery and 18 (32 percent) from the one derived from Cell Gensys.[49] Most are intended for cancer treatment. By 2011, five out of the seven approved transgenic-mice Mabs had been developed using the Lonberg and GenPharm platform.[50]

The success of human Mabs made with transgenic mice stands in contrast to those created with phage display. In 2010, fifty-six human antibodies being clinically tested originated from transgenic mice and thirty-five from phage display. Similarly, in terms of FDA approval, seven of the Mab therapeutics on the market by 2011 came from transgenic mice, while only two had been made using phage display (see Figure 8.5). The difference may be explained by the fact that many companies and academic groups are more familiar with hybridoma technology than phage display, and by CAT's restrictive licensing policy for its phage technology. Strikingly, both of the phage-display Mabs approved for the market originated from CAT, reflecting the company's dominance in this area.[51]

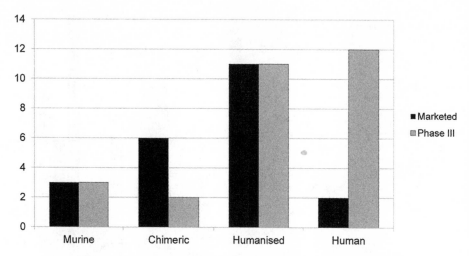

FIGURE 8.6. Number of different types of Mabs on the market or in phase III of clinical testing, 2009 (Adapted from W. R. Strohl, "Therapeutic Antibodies: Past, Present and Future," in Z. An and W. R. Strohl, eds., *Antibodies: From Bench to Clinic* [2009], 25)

What is particularly noticeable about the different antibody-engineering techniques that emerged from the 1980s is how many originated and were nurtured by LMB scientists who had been mentored by Milstein. It is also striking how active the MRC has been in guarding the intellectual property of these innovations. This stands in marked contrast to the early days when the first Mabs were deemed unworthy of patenting. The change in attitude occurred in part due to lessons the organization learned from failing to patent Köhler and Milstein's technique—a costly mistake with political fallout. It was also boosted by the Thatcher government, which encouraged the patenting of innovations arising from research funded by U.K. research bodies so as to enhance the commercial exploitation of British research and make it more competitive.[52]

In 1982, the MRC established an industrial liaison group to handle the commercial exploitation of scientific innovations. Initially, technology transfers were organized by the British Technology Group (BTG), a nonstatutory body formed in 1981 through the merger of the National Research Development Corporation and the National Enterprise Board, which had the right of first refusal to exploit research funded by research councils. In 1985, however, the British government ended the BTG's right of first refusal and gave MRC units the means to exploit their own re-

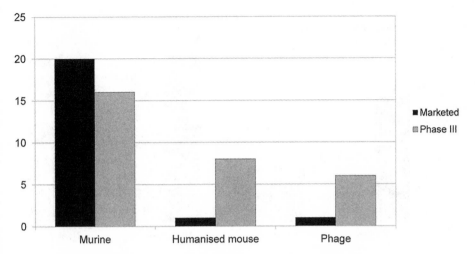

FIGURE 8.7. Number of Mabs, by source, on the market or in phase III of clinical testing, 2009 (Adapted from W. R. Strohl, "Therapeutic Antibodies: Past, Present and Future," in Z. An and W. R. Strohl, eds., *Antibodies: From Bench to Clinic* [2009])

search. This gave units like the LMB greater freedom to negotiate industrial agreements and receive greater shares in royalties. Scientists could also now expect to share in the royalties and started to found their own companies to exploit their inventions.[53]

The LMB moved quickly to patent and license out its scientists' antibody engineering techniques. First in line was the method for humanizing rodent antibodies developed by Neuberger and Rabbitts. A patent application was filed in 1984 and assigned, under an umbrella agreement, to Celltech. Second in line was the CDR grafting method developed by Winter, for which a patent application was filed in 1986. Its patent process followed a very different course because of Winter's reservations about giving away the rights to just one company. Based on the frustrations that he and other LMB colleagues had experienced with Celltech in licensing out Mabs for interferon and blood reagents, Winter opted for a nonexclusive licensing agreement. This he did with the support of the LMB and the MRC. Their model was the agreement that Stanford University had used for the Cohen-Bayer rDNA patent.[54]

The MRC established three principles for the nonexclusive license for the CDR grafting patent: first, the license should be given for the generation of a product that was to be of benefit to patients; second, no

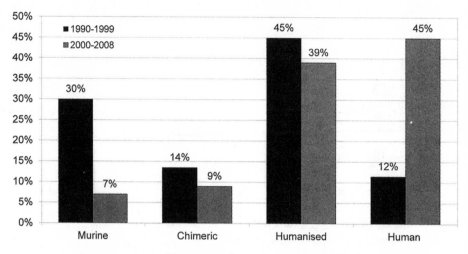

FIGURE 8.8. Percentage of four types of Mabs in clinical development, 1990–2008. Due to rounding, the total is greater than one hundred. (Adapted from figure 1, A. L. Nelson, E. Dhimolea, and J. M. Reichert, "Development Trends for Human Monoclonal Antibody Therapeutics," *Nature Reviews Drug Discovery*, 9 [Oct 2010]: 767–74)

commercial secrecy could be enforced; and third, those originally involved in the development of a method could retain the freedom to collaborate with other researchers and publish any future developments on the technology while taking care not to make needless disclosures. Overall the strategy was to license the patents nonexclusively to whomever was interested, with very little up-front payment. The rationale was that very small upfront payments would encourage cooperation. In return for licensing its patents, the MRC asked for royalties on final products. This was generally limited to 2 percent of sales. The MRC stood to benefit if the licensees achieved success.[55]

The nonexclusive licensing arrangement proved highly lucrative, signifying how widespread the LMB's antibody engineering techniques had become. Within a short time more than sixty companies worldwide had been granted nonexclusive licenses to LMB patents, and the revenue the MRC gained from these licenses more than made up for the income potentially lost from not having patented Köhler's and Milstein's techniques. Some of the greatest revenue came from the CDR grafting, but in time substantial sums also flowed from transgenic mice. In the last years of the patent for the transgenic mice, the licensing revenue exceeded £10 million per year. Much of this revenue came from sales of therapeutics based on humanized and human Mabs, which were surging. In 2006 alone, the MRC gained £127 million from the sale of human antibodies and £84 million from humanized antibodies.[56]

The income for 2006 was boosted by a £121 million deal that the MRC had made the year before with the U.S. pharmaceutical company Abbott Laboratories in lieu of royalties for Humira, the first humanized Mab to win approval. Directed toward treating arthritis, Humira was developed using the MRC's patent for phage display. Considered one of the world's largest ever intellectual property deals at the time, it marked how far the MRC had changed its patenting and licensing approach since Köhler and Milstein's first Mabs. The MRC put the money from the deal into its overall funding pot, which was then £500 million a year. By June 2012 the MRC reported that its portfolio of antibody-engineering patents had generated more than $750 million (£486 million) in royalties, which it was plowing back into medical research.[57]

The MRC has not been the only beneficiary of royalty payments; so too has the LMB. Starting in the mid-1990s, the LMB began earning just over £1 million a year in royalty income. This rose steeply in 2000, reaching approximately £6 million a year. The largest proportion of this income came from patents taken out on Winter's techniques. By 2005 the payments had reached £20 million per year, most still from Winter's patents. This exceeded the total MRC block grant to the LMB. Overall, the LMB's gross annual income was equal to that of the entire commercial income of all universities in the United Kingdom, and comparable to that of much larger U.S. academic institutions such as MIT. By 2008 the total annual royalties coming to the LMB had risen to £70 million. One indication of just how important these royalties are to the LMB is that in 2013 it was able to move into a new state-of-the-art building paid for mostly from the royalties earned from antibody-related engineering. The building was estimated to have cost over £200 million.[58]

The large royalties paid to the MRC and LMB show how far antibody engineering had transformed Mab therapeutics. With antibody engineering, scientists and clinicians now had a new form of Mab to play with. It was just the start of another part of the journey, however. Much more work lay ahead as scientists turned to the task of using Mabs to create drugs for clinical use.

CHAPTER NINE

Blockbuster Mab Drugs

THE RESHAPING OF MABS within the laboratory brought with it new hopes for the therapeutic potential of Mabs. Such optimism was boosted by the regulatory approval of the chimeric Mab called abciximab (Reo-Pro), which was used to reduce blood clots in patients who had suffered a heart attack. Granted in 1994, the approval came as a total surprise given the death knell many market analysts and others had rung for Mab therapeutics in the wake not only of the Centoxin disaster, but also of the failures between 1985 and 1993 of several murine Mabs to treat sepsis, cancer, and late-stage cardiovascular disease. Until this point, only OKT had won market approval out of a thousand candidates.

In 1995 another murine Mab reached the marketplace: edrecolomab (Panorex), which was licensed by German authorities as an adjuvant therapy—a drug given in addition to primary or main treatment—for postoperative colorectal cancer. Edrecolomab originated from the 17–1A Mab detailed in Chapter 5. First created at the Wistar Institute in the late 1970s and commercially developed by Centocor with the British pharmaceutical company Wellcome, edrecolomab was the first Mab cancer therapeutic to proceed to market. The next year, in 1996, the FDA opened the door more widely by approving four murine Mabs with radioactive tracers for use as imaging agents in humans; three murine Mabs for the treatment of cancer (small-cell lung, colorectal, and prostate); and one murine Mab to help alleviate myocardial infarction. The overall track record for murine Mab therapeutics, however, was poor, and their clinical development decreased significantly by the mid-1990s, so that by 2003 no therapeutics were in the patent-application pipeline.[1]

Murine antibodies soon faded into the background with the emergence of new engineered Mabs. Following abciximab's approval, in 1997 another chimeric drug, rituximab (Rituxan), was authorized by the FDA to treat B-cell NHL. A year later, the FDA licensed three more Mab therapeutics, one a humanized Mab and two chimeric ones. Thereafter, the FDA authorized between one and four new Mabs each year between 1997 and 2011 and European regulatory authorities between one and six Mabs a year.[2] Table 9.1 lists the first drug approvals by FDA and European authorities between 1986 and 2014. It shows that from the late 1990s the bulk of Mabs approved were chimeric, humanized, or human. Many were licensed for autoimmune disorders, a striking development given the early investment directed toward cancer therapeutics (see Chapter 5 and Figure 9.1). Significant numbers were also approved for multiple indications (Table 9.2), because Mabs had helped to reveal that these diseases shared a common pathway: the immune system.[3]

This chapter explores the development of rituximab and infliximab, two of the best-selling Mab therapeutics today. The evolution of these drugs not only illustrates how a single Mab therapeutic came to be used for multiple indications, but also shows the significant role that Mabs have played in fostering new understandings of the causes of cancer and autoimmune disorders, thereby opening avenues to more effective care. Their stories also show how the development of Mab drugs shifted from prioritizing rare diseases to treating more lucrative common illnesses. Although each drug took a different path to the clinic, they encountered similar hurdles along the way. These included not only the challenge of scaling up production for newly engineered antibodies, and getting Mabs through clinical trials and regulatory approval, but also securing enough funding. All of this required a complex alliance among academic researchers, industry leaders, and financiers as well as the consent of patients.

Rituximab's foundation was laid by the work of the oncologist Lee Nadler at the Dana-Farber Cancer Institute of the Harvard Medical School in Boston. In 1977 Nadler began looking for ways to create a Mab to treat non-Hodgkin's lymphoma (NHL), a subset of blood cancers that begin

Table 9.1

Monoclonal antibody drugs with their first approval dates from the FDA and European regulatory authorities, 1986–2014

COMPANY	TRADE NAME (GENERIC)	ANTIBODY TYPE	FIRST INDICATION (EXPANDED INDICATIONS)	DATE OF FIRST APPROVAL BY FDA (EUROPEAN)
Ortho Biotec	Orthoclone OKT3 (muromonab)[a]	murine	organ transplant	1986 (NA)
Centocor	Centoxin (Nebacumab)[a]	humanized	septic shock	NA (1991)
Centocor/Eli Lilly	ReoPro (abciximab)	chimeric	prevent blood clots in angioplasty	1994 (1995)
Centocor/GSK	Panorex (edrecolomab)[a]	murine	CRC	NA (1995)
Idec/Genentech	Rituxan (rituximab)	chimeric	NHL (RA, DLBC, NHL)	1997 (1998)
Roche	Zenapax (Daclizumab)	humanized	organ transplantOR[g]	1997 (1999)
Novartis	Simulect (basiliximab)	chimeric	organ transplant	1998 (1998)
MedImmune	Synagis (palivizumab)	humanized	RSV	1998 (1999)
Centocor	Remicade (infliximab)	chimeric	CD (RA, AS, PA, UC, PP)	1998 (1999)
Genentech	Herceptin (trastuzumab)	humanized	BC[f]	1998 (2000)
Immunex/Wyeth-Ayerst	Enbrel (etanercept)	chimeric	RA	1998 (NA)
Wyeth-Ayerst/Pfizer	Mylotarg (gemtuzumab ozogamicin)[a]	humanized	AML	2000 (NA)
Genzyme/Ilex Oncology	Campath/Lemtrada (alemtuzumab)	humanized	B-CLL (B-CLL[d], MS)	2001 (2001)

Idec	Zevalin (ibritumomab tiuxetan)	murine	NHL	2002 (2004)
CAT/Abbott	Humira (adalimumab)	human	RA (JIA, PA, AS, CD, PP)	2002 (2003)
Biogen Idec	Amevive (alefacept) [a]	chimeric	P	2003 (NA)
Corixa	Bexxar (tostiumomab)	murine	NHL (NHL[c])	2003 (NA)
Tanox/Genentech	Xolair (omalizumab)	humanized	AA	2003 (2005)
Genentech	Raptiva (efalizumab)[a]	humanized	PS	2003 (2004)
BMS/Imclone	Erbitux (cetuximab)[e]	chimeric	CRC[f] (SSCHN, CRC[f])	2004 (2004)
Genentech	Avastin (bevacizumab)	humanized	CRC[f] (NSCLC, HER2-BC)	2004 (2005)
Elan/Biogen Idec	Tsabri (natalizumab)	humanized	MS, CD	2004 (2006)
Genentech	Lucentis (ranbizumab)	humanized	AMD	2006 (NA)
Amgen	Vectribix (panitumab)	human	CRC[f]	2006 (2007)
Alexion	Soliris (eculizumab)	humanized	PNH	2007 (2007)
UCB	Cimzia (certolizumab pegol)	humanized	CD (RA)	2008 (2009)
Centocor/Schering Plough	Simponi (golimumab)	human	RA, PA, AS	2009 (2009)
Novartis	Ilaris (canakinumab)	human	FCAS and MW	2009 (2009)
Centocor/Ortho Biotec	Stelara (sutekinumab)	human	PP	2009 (2009)
Genmab/ GSK	Arzerra (ofatumumab)	human	CLL	2009 (2010)
Roche	Actemra (tocilizumab)	humanized	RA	2010 (2009)
Amgen	Prolia, Xgeva (denosumab)	human	OE	2010 (2010)

(continued)

Table 9.1 (continued)

Monoclonal antibody drugs with their first approval dates from the FDA and European regulatory authorities, 1986–2014

COMPANY	TRADE NAME (GENERIC)	ANTIBODY TYPE	FIRST INDICATION (EXPANDED INDICATIONS)	DATE OF FIRST APPROVAL BY FDA (EUROPEAN)
HGS/GSK	Benlysta (belimumab)	human	SLE	2011 (2011)
BMS	Yervoy (ipilimumab)	human	M[f]	2011 (NA)
Seattle Genetics	Adcetris (brentuximab vedotin)	chimeric	HL	2011 (NA)
Roche/ ImmunoGen	T-DM1 (trastuzumab emtansine)	humanized[b]	HER2-BC	2012 (NA)
HGS	Abthrax (raxibacumab)	human	anthrax	2012 (NA)
Genentech	Perjeta (pertuzumab)	humanized	HER2-BC	2012 (NA)
Roche	Kadcyla (trastuzumab emtansine)	humanized	HER2-BC	2013 (2013)
Millennium Pharmaceuticals	Entyvio (vedolizumab)	humanized	UC, CD	2014 (2014)
Eli Lilly	Cyramza (ramucirumab)	human	gastric cancer	2014 (in review)

Glycart Biotechnology AG/Biogen Idec/Chugai Pharmaceutical/ Roche	Gazyva (obinutuzumab)	humanized	CLL	2014 (in review)
Janssen Biotech	Sylvant (siltuximab)	chimeric	Castleman disease	2014 (2014)

Source: K. Stein, "FDA-Approved Monoclonal Antibody Products," unpublished paper, 2010; A. Scolnik, "mAbs: A Business Perspective," *mAbs* 1, no. 2 (Mar./Apr. 2009): 179–84, 180–81; J. M. Reichert, "Marketed Therapeutic Antibodies Compendium," *mAbs* 4, no. 3 (May/June 2012): 414, table 1; J. M. Reichert, "Therapeutic Monoclonal Antibodies Approved or in Review in the European Union or United States," available online at http://www.antibodysociety.org/news/approved_mabs.php (accessed 3 Oct. 2014).

Note: AA—allergic asthma; AMD—age-related macular degeneration; AML—acute myeloid leukemia; AS—ankylosing spondylitis; BC—breast cancer; B-CLL—B-cell chronic lymphocytic leukemia; BMS—Bristol-Myers Squibb; CD—Crohn's disease; CLL—chronic lymphocytic leukemia; CRC—colorectal cancer; DLBC—diffuse large B-cell lymphoma; FCAS—familial cold autoinflammatory syndrome; GSK—Glaxo-Smith Kline; HGS—Human Genome Sciences; HL—Hodgkin's lymphoma; JIA—juvenile idiopathic arthritis; M—melanoma; MS—multiple sclerosis; MW—Muckle-Wells syndrome; NA—no approval; NHL—non-Hodgkin's lymphoma; NSCLC—non-small-cell lung carcinoma; OE—osteoporosis; OR—organ transplant; PS—psoriasis; PA—psoriatic arthritis; PNH—paroxysmal nocturnal hemoglobinuria; PP—plaque psoriasis; RA—rheumatoid arthritis; RSV- respiratory syncytial virus; SLE—systemic lupus erythematosus; SSCHN—squamous cell carcinoma of head and neck; UC—ulcerative colitis; UCB—

[a] drug later withdrawn or discontinued
[b] antibody conjugate
[c] refractory to chemotherapy
[d] single agent
[e] combination therapy
[f] metastatic
[g] prophylaxis
[h] first-line therapy

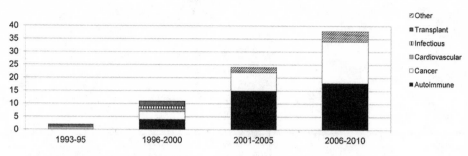

FIGURE 9.1. Number of Mab drugs approved by FDA by different categories, 1993–2010 (includes first and supplementary approvals) (Adapted from K. Stein, "FDA-Approved Monoclonal Antibody Products," unpub. paper, 2010)

in the lymph system. Many around him, including his mentor, Stuart Schlossman, were skeptical that he would succeed. In 1979, however, he formed a collaboration with his former classmate Phil Stashenko, a dentist and immunologist who had learned how to produce Mabs in Milstein's laboratory and had attempted to produce them against strep mutants (tooth bacteria) for use in mouthwash. By 1980, the two scientists, funded by NIH grants, had generated some murine Mabs specific to human B lymphocytes. One of these, B1, reacted strongly to a subset of B-cell NHL when tested on tumor cells obtained from nineteen patients with acute and chronic leukemias and twelve patients with NHL. The Mab bound to an antigen, later labeled CD20, that is only present on the surface of all benign or malignant B cells and not mature plasma cells or very early B cells formed in the bone marrow. This opened up a new avenue for treating lymphoma. A Mab that targeted only the CD20 antigen gave clinicians the tool they needed to target B-cell lymphoma while leaving untouched the very early B cells forming in the bone marrow, thereby allowing the regeneration of healthy B cells. Moreover, B1 was found to harness the immune system by binding to human complement, which could destroy lymphoid B cells.[4]

After their discovery, Nadler treated a fifty-four-year-old lymphoma patient unresponsive to standard or experimental chemotherapy with a customized Mab (Ab 89) directed against the CD20 antigen on the patient's tumor cells. While Ab 89 failed to improve the patient's condition, it temporarily decreased his tumor cells without causing toxicity. It was also encouraging that no antigens shed into the patient's plasma to block the Mab, which was targeting the lymphoma cells.[5]

Table 9.2

Percentage of Mab drugs approved for first and additional indications by the FDA, 1996–2010

	AUTOIMMUNE DISORDERS			CANCER		
	TOTAL	FIRST APPROVAL	ADDITIONAL APPROVALS	TOTAL	FIRST APPROVAL	ADDITIONAL APPROVALS
1996–2000	4	2 (50%)	2 (50%)	3	3 (100%)	—
2001–2005	15	5 (33%)	10 (67%)	7	5 (71%)	2 (29%)
2006–2010	18	5 (27%)	13 (72%)	16	2 (12%)	14 (87%)

Source: K. Stein, "FDA-Approved Monoclonal Antibody Products," unpublished paper, 2010.

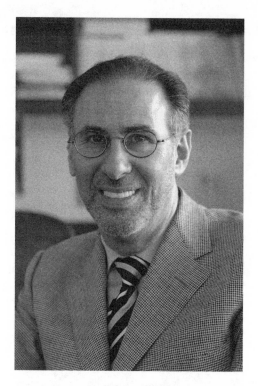

FIGURE 9.2. Lee Nadler's delivery of the first Mab to a patient with B-cell lymphoma laid the foundation for the development of rituximab. (Dana-Farber Cancer Institute)

Excited by his findings, Nadler began hunting for pharmaceutical support (Figure 9.2). Most company executives he approached, however, believed the market was too limited, since only thirty thousand to forty thousand new cases of B-cell lymphoma were being diagnosed each year. Assuming that they could charge only a few thousand dollars for each dose of a Mab therapeutic, they could not see how such a drug could achieve the $300 million revenue generally expected from a pharmaceutical product.[6]

This negative attitude was not unusual. Ron Levy, the second oncologist whose work helped lay the foundations for rituximab, experienced similar difficulties obtaining backing for his patient-specific idiotype Mabs, which he was creating at Stanford University to treat B-cell lymphoma patients (see Chapter 5). Out of frustration, Levy and his colleague decided to found a biotechnology company, Biotherapy Systems, in Mountain View, California, in 1985. A year later they merged it with Idec Pharmaceuticals, a company established along similar lines in San Diego in 1984 by Ivor Royston, Levy's former Stanford colleague.[7]

In contrast to pharmaceutical executives, the biotechnology entrepreneurs believed a lymphoma drug had the potential to be commercially viable. The disease was incurable and its patient base was rapidly expanding. The age-adjusted incidence of NHL in the United States, for example, was increasing by 3 to 4 percent annually, resulting in a near doubling of the rate. Similar rises were happening globally. In part, this increase was attributable to diagnostic improvements and the growth of lymphomas related to acquired immunodeficiency syndrome (AIDS). For the most part, however, the rise remained unexplained.[8]

Lymphoma has three grades: low, intermediate, and high. These relate to how fast the lymphoma develops. The most common form of NHL is diffuse large B-cell lymphoma (DLBCL) and the second most common is low-grade follicular lymphoma (FL). Idec aimed to target FL because its progress is slower, providing a window of opportunity for making a customized anti-idiotype antibody. By the late 1980s, Idec had developed with Levy some customized anti-idiotype antibodies, and over half of those patients treated went into remission. Thereafter, a selection of antibodies made for individual patients were screened against a panel of idiotypes compiled from other newly diagnosed patients to find one that targeted an idiotype shared by patients. This yielded seventeen anti-idiotype Mabs, but these proved disappointing when tested on new cases, so the company continued with its customized approach.[9]

Based on the promise of its customized anti-idiotype Mabs, Idec was valued at just over $50 million in its initial public offering in 1991. Just two years later, however, Idec's executives decided to abandon developing customized antibodies, despite promising results from late-stage clinical trials. Their rationale was that a patient-specific therapy had no commercial future. Much of the company's strategy to date had been driven by a belief that patients with lymphomas expressed the same or identical idiotypes. Yet idiotypes were found to overlap less frequently than anticipated. Any product developed, therefore, would treat only a small fraction of patients.[10]

Those championing Idec's change in strategy were the company's chief executive officer, William Rastetter, a former MIT academic and

Genentech employee, and its head of research, Nabil Hanna, a former NCI researcher and employee of the pharmaceutical company Smith-Kline & French Laboratories. Instead of producing customized Mabs, they advocated creating a standardized drug for use by many patients, which they believed would be more cost-effective and could be achieved by generating a Mab specific to B cells. To this end, in August 1990 two of the company's scientists, Darrell Anderson and Alice Cox, began immunizing mice with a human B-cell line. One of the Mabs they produced turned out to be an IgG antibody that by chance recognized the CD20 antigen. This was highly fortuitous. Not only had Nadler demonstrated the clinical utility of an anti-CD20 Mab against lymphoma, so too had clinicians at the University of Washington and Fred Hutchinson Cancer Research Center in Seattle, who had treated four patients with B-cell lymphomas using a high-dose murine Mab.[11]

The creation of the Mab was the first step in a long process. First it needed to be transformed from a murine antibody into a chimeric one so as to reduce its immunogenicity and increase its circulating half-life. This would facilitate the repeated administration of the Mab and in lower doses. A chimeric Mab, because it contained human-constant regions, was also more likely to activate the patient's immune system to produce complement to destroy cancer cells. The work was headed by Mitchell Reff, who joined Idec in 1990 after working at Smith Kline & French Laboratories.[12]

In addition to chimerization, efforts were poured into developing a mammalian cell expression system for large-scale production. This was important because until now production had been geared toward murine rather than chimeric Mabs. To get the ball rolling, a tool known as an expression vector was developed to insert a specific gene into a target living cell in order to facilitate building a recombinant antibody. This was done by adapting expression vectors that Reff and colleagues had developed at Smith Kline & French. It was a painstaking task that involved nineteen additional cloning steps. The aim was to develop a versatile expression platform for producing any reengineered antibody that Idec wanted to develop, whether it be chimeric, humanized, or human.[13]

In addition to generating an expression vector, a suitable mammalian cell had to be found. Two mammalian cells were currently deployed for expressing Mabs. The first, frequently used by academic laboratories, was a mouse myeloma cell line derived from a tumor of a mouse B cell (Sp2/o). The second was a Chinese hamster ovary (CHO) cell line which, while used for the large-scale production of many other recombinant protein drugs, only expressed small quantities of antibodies. Eventually the CHO cell line was settled on, in part because genetic engineering of the cell line had helped to increase the quantities of antibodies produced. Work soon began on adapting a mutant CHO cell line originally developed in 1986 by Larry Chasin at Columbia University and modified by a technique devised at Smith Kline. This was led by Andrew Grant, a process science engineer. The task was difficult because he and his team had no prior experience of working with the CHO cell line for large-scale mammalian cell culture—and cells frequently change the properties of their secreted proteins when scaled up from a research laboratory to large-scale manufacturing.[14]

Alongside efforts to boost production, clinical development began, directed by Antonio Grillo-López, a hematologist-oncologist and former employee of DuPont Merck Pharmaceutical Company and Warner Lambert's Parke Davis. Early in vitro studies indicated that rituximab killed B cells associated with NHL by inducing one or more of three immune responses: complement-dependent cytotoxicity, antibody-dependent cell-mediated cytotoxicity, and/or apoptosis. The pharmacokinetics, safety, immunogenicity and B-cell depleting potency of rituximab was also tested in four cynomolgus monkeys. These monkeys showed no adverse reactions to the drug.[15]

In December 1992, Idec submitted an investigational new drug application to the FDA to launch human trials with rituximab. Several uncertainties underlay its testing. Among the questions being asked was whether rituximab's depletion of both malignant and benign B cells could lead to infections or even additional tumors in patients. Of particular concern was the fact that the depletion of normal, helper T-cells was known to promote AIDS.[16]

The first trial, conducted by Levy with Idec, consisted of four doses of 375 mg/m^2 of rituximab, given intravenously to outpatients. The dose was determined by the fact that it was the maximum amount Idec could then manufacture. Much to the team's surprise, including Levy, the trial revealed that normal B cells could be attacked and depleted without prompting immune deficiency or infections. While patients experienced mild fevers, chills, respiratory symptoms, and occasionally hypotension upon first receiving the drug, they did not experience an increase in IgG antibodies or infection beyond what was expected. The trial also indicated that rituximab spared B cells in the bone marrow and that patients naturally replenished their supply of B cells within six months of completing treatment.[17]

Despite these promising results, Idec lacked the resources to launch further trials. The venture needed far more than the $10 million that Idec had raised in 1994 from selling its shares. The additional funds would be hard to generate given the general unpopularity of Mab therapeutics and limited size of the lymphoma market. In addition, the company was rapidly burning through its funds. By 1994, Idec had less than six months of cash reserves and its stock was trading around two dollars a share, representing just 14.2 percent of its IPO value three years earlier.[18]

Nearing bankruptcy, Idec's fortunes changed in March 1995 when Genentech reversed its earlier decision not to enter an alliance with Idec. This came about from a chance encounter between Levy and David Ebersman, Genentech's business development officer, at a conference set up by Stanford University to connect academic scientists with industry. The partnership with Genentech provided Idec with not only the financial resources for extending clinical trials, but also the expertise necessary for obtaining regulatory approval and marketing. Genentech was already involved in the development of other Mab therapeutics, having launched clinical trials for Herceptin to treat breast cancer in 1992. The alliance was timely for Genentech, as well: it gave it the means to fend off a buyout by the Swiss-based company F. Hoffmann–La Roche, which had acquired a 60 percent stake in Genentech in 1990 with an option to buy further stakes in 1995. Genentech agreed to give Idec $14.1 million upfront to finance rituximab's development in return for co-marketing rights in the United States. Idec was to receive a share of sale profits, and Roche received the rights to conduct further development and commercialization of the drug outside the United States (with the exception of Japan, where these rights were assigned to Zenyaku Kogyo Company).[19]

Once the Genentech deal was signed, further clinical testing ensued. This included a multicenter phase II trial undertaken with thirty-seven patients suffering from low-grade or follicular NHL. All the patients had relapsed after chemotherapy, and 54 percent of them had failed to benefit from aggressive therapy. Encouragingly, 46 percent of the patients experienced a clinical remission of their disease during the trial. Three separate phase II trials conducted with rituximab in combination with CHOP (cyclophosphamide, doxorubicin, vincristine, and prednisone) chemotherapy, interferon alfa-2a, and IDEC-Y2B8 also suggested that the drug was effective.[20]

In late 1995 Idec, in consultation with the FDA, convened a conference with a panel of three lymphoma experts in order to produce a consensus statement defining the response criteria for lower-grade FL. The statement established guidelines for evaluating rituximab that were endorsed by the FDA and European NHL experts. The protocol was important for forthcoming phase III trials because no standard criteria existed for evaluating the clinical response of drugs in NHL patients.[21]

In April 1995, Idec launched a phase III trial involving thirty-one different American and Canadian medical centers. The first results, reported in December 1996, showed that 48 percent of the patients had responded to the treatment, which was comparable to results with single-agent cytotoxic chemotherapy. Encouragingly, only one patient had developed an immune response, and all infections suffered by patients were modest. The drug had proven effective when given at both the $375mg/m^2$ dose and much lower. Based on these findings, Idec submitted an application to the FDA in February 1997 for the drug to be approved for market at $375mg/m^2$. The drug was formally approved as Rituxan in November 1997. Six months later, in June 1998, it was approved as Mabthera in Europe.[22]

Rituximab's approval was seen as a major achievement in America because it was the first Mab to receive FDA authorization as a cancer treatment. Capturing some of the sentiment, one commentator wrote, "We are no longer firing blanks, we finally have a magic bullet!"[23] Critically, rituximab demonstrated that in some circumstances a Mab that targeted an antigen present on both tumor and normal cells did not cause havoc in the rest of the body. Going forward, researchers would no longer need to search for pure tumor-specific targets when developing Mabs for cancer therapeutics.[24]

While at times the prospects for a Mab therapeutic against cancer had seemed an unobtainable goal, the actual development of rituximab was remarkably fast, taking just seven years from discovery to approval.

This was helped by the strict criteria established at the start of the pivotal phase III trial for evaluating clinical responses to the drug. Equally important was the fact that the drug was directed toward a rare medical condition, or what was known as an "orphan" disease, which lowered the threshold for the number of patients expected to complete clinical trials for gaining regulatory approval. Idec obtained regulatory approval with a trial consisting of just 166 subjects, thus reducing both the time and costs of the clinical trial process. The orphan status of the drug also offered Idec tax benefits and market exclusivity for some years following approval.[25]

Although rituximab was originally targeted to a small market niche, it was soon generating sales beyond the expectations of Idec's executives (Figure 9.3). Much of its success was due to its status as the first new single agent for the treatment of NHL in a decade. The positive safety profile and efficacy of the drug in NHL patients also encouraged its expansion into other forms of cancer. Idec and Genentech rapidly began testing rituximab in patients with immediate and high-grade NHL, chronic lymphocytic leukemia (CLL), and multiple myeloma. In addition, they studied how rituximab fared in patients newly diagnosed with lymphoma as opposed to those who had not responded to chemotherapy. This opened up scope for the drug to be a first-line treatment and thus administered to more patients. CLL, for example, is the most common form of leukemia in adults in Western countries, accounting for approximately 30 percent of all leukemias in the United States.[26]

Rituximab was also tested in combination with other drugs. Multiple chemotherapy drugs, rather than single agents, had been used for the treatment of lymphomas since the 1960s. In 2006, the FDA approved rituximab as a firstline treatment in combination with CHOP or other anthracylcine-based chemotherapy regimens in patients with diffuse large B-cell, CD20 positive NHL. This approval was granted on the basis of data collected from three multicenter studies involving the use of rituximab in combination with other treatments in 1,854 previously untreated patients with the condition.[27] In 2010, the drug was further approved for use in combination with fludarabine and cyclophosphamide for previously treated and untreated patients with CD20-positive CLL.

Today, rituximab is the best-selling biologic drug in oncology. In part, this achievement reflects the degree to which it has improved cancer care.

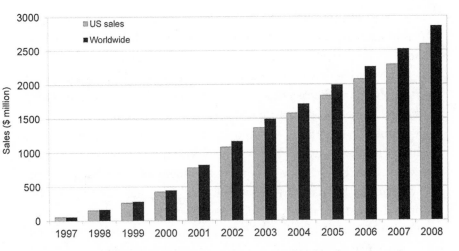

FIGURE 9.3. Sales of rituximab in the United States and worldwide, 1997–2008 (Genentech, Rituxan Historical sales)

Its greatest success has been in NHL patients. In 2007, for example, data from large randomized clinical trials indicated that the addition of rituximab to standard chemotherapy regimens helped improve both response rates and survival outcomes in patients with FL and DLBCL. Data from a U.S. Surveillance, Epidemiology and End Results program also showed that while the incidence of NHL had continued to rise following the drug's introduction in 1997, mortality from NHL declined 2.8 percent each year to 2003.[28]

Soon after rituximab began making its mark in cancer, it was found to be beneficial for rheumatoid arthritis (RA). One of the first indications that rituximab could be useful for such a disease came from the case of a British man treated for NHL lymphoma, first reported by a team based at University College London (UCL) Centre for Rheumatology. This patient had first developed lymphoma symptoms in 1989 at the age of fifty-four and had received a combination of different chemotherapies over the years. In 1993 he began experiencing musculoskeletal symptoms associated with RA, which gradually worsened, spreading from shoulder pain to swelling and pain in his elbows, knees, wrists, and ankles. By July 1998 his condition had become so debilitating that he required a wheelchair. To the man's surprise and that of his clinicians, his condition significantly improved following rituximab treatment for his lymphoma. Within weeks he noticed some improvement in his joint pains and stiffness and after three months he was virtually symptom-free and could walk up to five miles a day. He remained symptom-free from RA for another four months. By contrast, CT scans showed no change in his lymphoma.[29]

The finding that a drug intended for cancer could help a patient with an autoimmune disease like RA was not unusual. As early as 1956, for example, methotrexate, a drug first used to treat childhood leukemia, had been noted to have positive effects in patients with RA and psoriasis, a chronic immune-mediated disease that affects the skin. By the mid-1980s methotrexate had become a common treatment for RA. That a Mab directed toward B cells could help with RA was nonetheless intriguing, because during the late 1990s most assumed the condition was not an antibody-mediated disorder and was predominately a T-cell mediated disease in which B cells played no role. Following the lymphoma case, UCL researchers, led by the rheumatologist Jonathan Edwards, began investigating the effects of rituximab in other RA patients. This provided an opportunity to test their newly formulated hypothesis that a specific subset of auto-reactive B lymphocyte cells capable of self-perpetuation was essential to the persistence of RA. They were hoping to establish whether RA was the manifestation of B cells producing antibodies that stuck to normal joints, thereby encouraging an attack by a patient's T cells.[30]

By 2002, the UCL team had administered rituximab, both alone and in combination with other drugs, to twenty-three patients, the majority of whom experienced a marked clinical improvement, many for as long as thirty-three months. To confirm these observations, they launched a randomized control phase II trial with twenty-six rheumatology centers in eleven countries (Australia, Canada, Israel, and eight European countries). In the trial 161 patients who had active RA despite treatment with methotrexate were randomly assigned to one of four treatments. The symptoms of patients treated with rituximab, given either alone or in combination with cyclophosphamide or methotrexate, improved significantly more than those of the control group given only methotrexate. This result not only confirmed that rituximab was an effective treatment for RA, but also reinforced the hypothesis that B cells helped promote the disease.[31]

In February 2006, the FDA approved rituximab for use in combination with methotrexate in patients with moderate to severe RA. This approval was granted on the basis of positive data from three randomized, double-blinded, placebo-controlled studies of patients with active RA. What proved pivotal was a study of 499 patients whose RA had failed to respond adequately to other disease-modifying anti-rheumatic drugs. In this study 51 percent of those who were given methotrexate with rituximab achieved a 20 percent improvement in their condition, as opposed to 18 percent of those who took methotrexate with a placebo.[32]

The FDA's decision opened up another commercial avenue for rituximab and marked how far it had come from its first days as a drug perceived as unworthy of investment because it was intended for only a small subset of cancer patients. Now the Mab was targeting a chronic condition affecting approximately 1 percent of the world's population.[33] In 2008 the worldwide pharmaceutical market for arthritis was estimated to generate the vast sum of $15.9 billion in revenue. That year the revenue from rituximab totaled $5.53 billion, of which $746 million came from RA sales.[34]

RA was just the first of many autoimmune diseases investigated with rituximab. Early research, for example, also suggested that it could help treat idiopathic thrombocytopenia purpura, a platelet disorder. Similarly, open-label retrospective studies indicated its effectiveness in treating lupus, although its use for this disease was not pursued due to poor results in two randomized trials. More success was achieved in the case of Wegener's granulomatosis and microscopic polyangiitis, two rare conditions that cause inflammation in blood vessels. In April 2011, the FDA approved rituximab in combination with a steroid to treat both diseases. The approval was granted on the basis of a single control trial with 197 patients. It represented the first FDA-approved therapy for the two orphan diseases.[35]

Rituximab's approval for different autoimmune disorders was eased by a path already well trodden by infliximab, the first Mab ever approved for treatment of an autoimmune condition. Infliximab initially gained FDA endorsement in 1998 for Crohn's disease, a rare but chronic condition that involves severe inflammation of the bowel. At the time of approval just over 800,000 patients were thought to be Crohn's sufferers worldwide. Crohn's can strike at any age, but mostly commonly occurs in fifteen- to twenty-five-year-olds. It can cause a variety of symptoms, including abdominal pain, diarrhea, vomiting, weight loss, and serious intestinal complications such as bowel obstruction, bowel perforation, fistulae, intestinal hemorrhage, and cancer of the bowel and small and large intestines. Skin rashes, arthritis, inflammation of the eye, tiredness, and lack of concentration are also common.[36] In November 1999, the FDA approved infliximab for RA, and thereafter for other forms of inflammatory arthritis, ankylosing spondylitis (2004), and psoriatic arthritis (2005). U.S. approval was also granted in 2005 for treatment of the inflammatory bowel disease known as ulcerative colitis, and a year later for plaque psoriasis.

Infliximab originated from the laboratory of Ján Vilček, a virologist who migrated from communist Czechoslovakia to New York University (NYU) School of Medicine in 1964 (Figure 9.4). Interested in soluble mediators that regulate the immune system, Vilček had been investigating the workings of cytokines, hormone-like proteins produced by the body to control infection and tumors. In 1982 he was joined by Junming Le, a postdoctoral scientist who had picked up some training in producing Mabs at the Memorial Sloan Kettering Institute. Together, Vilček and Le set out to develop Mabs as a tool to differentiate different proteins. While making one against the cytokine interferon, they noticed that cells taken from human white blood cells, when manipulated and put into culture, could under certain conditions produce not only interferon, specifically gamma interferon, but also tumor necrosis factor alpha (TNFα). This was another cytokine understood to turn tumors black and destroy them. It had been first identified in 1975 by the immunologist Lloyd Old together with Elizabeth Carswell at the Memorial Sloan Kettering Cancer Center in New York. By the early 1980s some researchers had begun to connect TNFα with both cancer and some autoimmune diseases, but its investigation remained limited, with only about twenty-five people working on the cytokine worldwide in 1984.[37]

In 1983 Michael Wall, co-founder of Centocor, invited Vilček to collaborate with the then fledgling company to develop the Mab that he and Le had produced against gamma interferon as a diagnostic reagent—as well as Mabs against TNFα and lymphotoxin, another cytokine. In return for financing Vilček's research, including Le's salary, Centocor would be entitled to license any Mab products made in Vilček's laboratory and NYU would receive royalties from any products sold.[38]

Initially, Vilček and Le struggled to produce Mabs against TNFα, because they lacked access to TNFα in its pure form.[39] In late 1988, how-

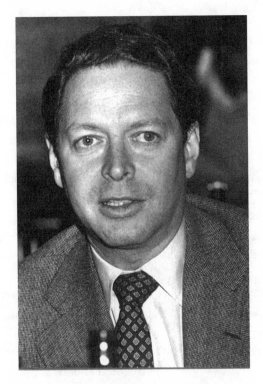

FIGURE 9.4. Ján Vilček, ca. 1980. Vilček and Junming Le created the first Mab against tumor necrosis factor alpha (TNFα) approved for the treatment of autoimmune diseases and inflammatory disorders. (Ján Vilček)

ever, they finally achieved their objective, helped by the cloning of TNFα genes and the making of recombinant TNFα by Genentech in 1985, which Vilček received because he was currently collaborating with Genentech. One of the Mabs they generated, called "A2," proved to be capable not only of binding to TNFα with a high affinity and selectivity, but also of neutralizing it.[40]

With TNFα implicated in the pathogenesis of sepsis in 1985, A2 stirred immediate interest from Centocor, which was then, as Chapter 7 has highlighted, looking to develop a drug against sepsis. Given A2's therapeutic promise, Centocor was quick to transform the murine antibody into a chimeric one, labeled "cA2." Following evaluation in cell cultures and animal models, the Mab was then tested in patients with septicemia in a phase

I–II trial in 1991. While well tolerated in patients, the drug, however, proved unsuitable for use against sepsis, and was cast aside as a result.[41]

The situation was to change as a result of a request to use cA2 to treat RA patients. Marc Feldmann, a Polish-born Australian immunologist at the Kennedy Institute for Rheumatology in London, made the request through Jim Woody, his former doctoral student who had become a scientific director at Centocor. Together with Ravinder Maini, an Indian-born rheumatologist, Feldmann had been investigating the cause of autoimmune diseases since 1984, and by 1990 had determined that several cytokines triggered inflammatory reactions associated with RA (Figure 9.5). This was based on investigations of tissue taken from the joints of RA patients using immunohistochemical staining with Mabs and complementary and RNA probes. Subsequently undertaking tests on mice in 1991, it was demonstrated that blocking just one cytokine, TNFα, could halt the inflammation provoked by other various cytokines. Feldmann and Maini believed that cA2 provided a tool for determining whether the same was true in humans.[42]

The proposal to use cA2 to treat RA patients contradicted the scientific consensus that a single molecule would not be able to neutralize the complicated process of inflammation. It also challenged the prevalent view that therapeutic antibodies were unsuitable to treat chronic diseases. This was because repeated administration of Mabs increased the likelihood of immunogenic reactions. Many also feared that disruption of the cytokine system could exacerbate inflammation. The use of a Mab to treat RA, however, was not new. Since 1989 a number of murine and chimeric Mabs directed against specific subsets of T cells had been tried in patients with the disease.[43]

The first trial with cA2 was conducted in 1992 with twenty severely incapacitated RA patients who had been unresponsive to other therapies. Fearing that cA2 could trigger harmful side effects in already very ill patients, the investigators were greatly relieved to witness dramatic improvements following the drug's administration. Thomas Schaible, then director of Clinical Immunology Research at Centocor, recalled a video of one young woman barely able to walk down stairs before treatment and then able to do so between two and four weeks after receiving her first two infusions of cA2. He recalled, "It was remarkable . . . you could hardly

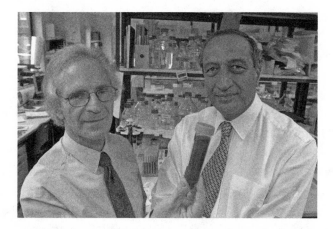

FIGURE 9.5. Marc Feldmann (*left*) and Ravinder Maini helped pioneer the development of Mab therapeutics for treating rheumatoid arthritis. (Imperial College London)

believe it was the same woman. She actually pranced down those steps." Corresponding data confirmed vast improvement in her joints.[44]

The small-scale trial indicated that blocking TNFα did not cure the disease, with a number of patients experiencing a recurrence of their symptoms after finishing treatment, but cA2 appeared safe and well tolerated. Various physiological tests also confirmed that it caused a retreat of the disease. Based on this, Centocor funded a phase II study of cA2 with three arms of treatment. Two groups of patients were to receive the drug in different doses, and one group, which was to act as the control, was to receive a placebo. Overall seventy-three patients were enrolled from four different European centers. Results from the study, published in 1994, indicated cA2 to be an effective and safe short-term treatment for RA.[45]

News that cA2 could be an effective treatment for RA was particularly welcome for Centocor's executives, who were still reeling from the pain of having cut the company's workforce after the Centoxin disaster. With an estimated six million patients undergoing treatment for RA in the United States and Western Europe, a third of whom would be candidates for treatment, the drug's potential market was vast. The key question for Centocor's management was how to take the drug forward. Having faced near-bankruptcy by attempting to develop Centoxin—which had also been considered a potential blockbuster—alone, the board of directors was unlikely to agree to internal development of cA2. Even staff within Centocor were dubious about cA2's potential. In the end, Centocor opted for internal development for the U.S. market and partnering for markets elsewhere.[46]

Just as Centocor's executives were pondering how to take cA2 forward for the treatment of RA, they received news of its benefits for Crohn's disease. This was reported by Sander van Deventer, a gastroenterologist at the Academic Medical Center in Amsterdam, who had participated in Centoxin's sepsis trials. He had first requested access to cA2 in 1993 to treat a fourteen-year-old girl with very severe Crohn's disease whose life was in jeopardy and who had failed to respond to all other treatments. His idea of using cA2 was based on his observation that tissue samples taken from the gastrointestinal tract of other Crohn's disease patients showed an elevated level of TNFα. Given to van Deventer to administer on compassionate grounds, the drug brought about rapid clinical improvement in the young girl which lasted for three months before her symptoms recurred. Soon after this, ten other patients with Crohn's disease were treated in Amsterdam with cA2, again with positive results.[47]

By 1996 cA2, by now called CenTNF, had been found to be beneficial for both RA and Crohn's disease in phase II trials. This posed an agonizing dilemma for Centocor's executives. The key question was which disease to devote resources to, so as to gain regulatory approval. Their decision was not easy because both diseases were profoundly debilitating and no effective treatment existed for either. Finally, they opted for Crohn's, motivated by the fact that it was a rare disease so would need fewer patients in a phase III trial and thus be less expensive to develop. Positioning CenTNF as an orphan disease treatment also offered tax benefits and increased its prospects for fast-track regulatory review. Furthermore, no competing therapeutics existed for the disease.[48]

Crohn's also permitted the drug's testing to be directed toward a much narrower and more defined endpoint. This was important, because Centoxin's failure to win regulatory approval had been attributed to the primary endpoints of its clinical trials being too broad and ill-defined for its efficacy to be assessed. The aim now was to target a specific subset of patients among the five hundred thousand U.S. patients suffering Crohn's: two hundred patients with moderate-to-severe Crohn's disease for whom conventional therapy was known to have failed. This small population reinforced the drug's orphan status for FDA review.[49]

Centocor established two phase III studies. The first involved 108 patients with moderate-to-severe, treatment-resistant Crohn's disease randomly assigned to four different courses of treatment. The purpose was to compare the effects of three different doses of the drug, now known as infliximab, with a placebo, and this first trial showed both that infliximab offered significantly stronger clinical improvement than a placebo and that the best results were achieved with five milligrams of the drug. The second study, designed to compare infliximab with a placebo, enrolled ninety-four patients with Crohn's disease who had enterocutaneous fistulae, a complication affecting between 40 and 60 percent of Crohn's sufferers. Such a condition is highly painful, caused by deep openings from the bowel wall through to the skin surface that lead to drainage of mucous and/or fecal matter. Results from the second trial were similarly positive: 62 percent of those taking infliximab experienced a closure of at least 50 percent of their open fistulae for at least a month, compared with 26 percent of those taking a placebo, and total closure occurred in 46 percent of those given the Mab compared with just 13 percent of those receiving the placebo.[50]

In December 1997, Centocor filed an orphan application for the drug on the basis of an unmet medical need. Granted an expedited review, an FDA Gastrointestinal Advisory Committee discussed the drug in an open public meeting in May 1998. Those present included Centocor representatives, FDA officials, industrial and academic specialists, Wall Street analysts, and patients. The event was nerve-wracking for Centocor's research team and executives. Schaible, who presented the data for the company, recounted, "Going into [the meeting], we understood that getting a recommendation was not going to be a slam dunk. It wasn't our data that would hurt us. We knew that [infliximab] worked effectively, if not profoundly, in these patients. Our concern was that the committee would not think we had enough clinical trial experience." A nonrecommendation could delay the drug's approval by many months, and would cost the company approximately $10 million per month. This would be a major setback given that Centocor was still wrestling to survive financially.[51]

In the end, the meeting voted unanimously for the FDA to approve infliximab (marketed as Remicade) for two narrow indications: as a single-dose therapy for the treatment of patients with moderate to severe inflammatory disease resistant to conventional therapy; and as a three-dose infusion regimen for patients with actively draining external fistulae. According to Schaible, what helped swing the decision was a handful of Crohn's patients attending the hearing. Grabbing the floor from the start, they detailed the complex and debilitating effects of the disease on their quality of life. This put into perspective everything that would follow. As Schaible put it, these patients' "stories put a face on the disease. . . . They were not statistical data—they were real people with faces." Crucially, "they were saying, 'This is a terrible disease, and now we have a drug that can really make a difference. Please don't take it away from us. It works and we desperately need it.'" Their plea resonated strongly given that no new treatment had been approved for Crohn's disease in three decades. Asher Kornbluth, a gastroenterologist attending the day-long hearing, summed up the scene, "At least one Wall Street analyst was seen engrossed in a financial analysis titled 'The Crohn's Population and Market Penetration,' as a 23-year-old woman described her experience with her penetrating fistulizing disease."[52]

Those attending the meeting reviewed the safety issues extensively. These included side effects reported among patients tested with both Crohn's disease and other indications, including RA. Overall, data from 453 patients were surveyed. Disconcertingly patients who received infliximab had experienced a higher incidence of infection (mostly minor), infusion reactions, and malignancy than those who received a placebo. A spirited debate also ensued over whether the short-term improvements witnessed with infliximab could be sustained and whether it should be used solely as a bridge to a longer-acting agent. This was difficult to answer given the newness of the drug. What reassured the committee was Centocor's promise to conduct postmarketing surveillance of patients who received the drug.[53]

In August 1998, the FDA gave the go-ahead for marketing infliximab for treating Crohn's disease. This marked a major milestone. It signified that a Mab drug was of benefit to patients with a chronic illness and could be used repeatedly over time. According to David Holveck, Centocor's chief executive officer at the time of the approval, the FDA's decision had been helped by the careful attention paid to finding the appropriate dose and intervals for giving the drug in trials. These steps helped the drug to maintain its efficacy over time and prevented patients from developing negative immune responses to the Mab. It also reduced infusion reactions and hypersensitivity.[54]

Having strategically positioned infliximab's development for an orphan disease for which the market was limited, Centocor would soon achieve its goal of tapping into the much wider and lucrative RA market. In November 1999, the FDA approved infliximab for RA and the following year the European regulatory authorities followed suit. Permission was granted for the drug to be used in combination with methotrexate for the treatment of patients who had an inadequate response to methotrexate alone. The decision was based on results from a multicenter, multinational phase III trial involving 428 patients. In this randomized control trial, 52 percent of the subjects who received infliximab and methotrexate experienced a reduction in their signs and symptoms compared to 17 percent of those given methotrexate alone.[55]

Infliximab was not the first Mab to receive approval for treating RA. In November 1998, Centocor had been beaten by Immune, a biotechnology company based in Seattle, in partnership with Wyeth-Ayeth Pharmaceuticals, which gained FDA approval for etanercept (Enbrel). Like infliximab, etanercept was designed to treat RA by blocking the action of TNFα. Infliximab soon had other competitors. One of its strongest rivals was adalimumab (Humira). Approved by the FDA in 2002, adalimumab was the third TNFα inhibitor and the first fully human Mab to win regulatory approval. Developed as part of a collaboration between Cambridge Antibody Technology (CAT) and BASF Bioresearch Corporation, the Mab had been created using phage display technology. In contrast to infliximab, which is administered intravenously, etanercept and adalimumab are administered with a subcutaneous injection.

Despite this competition, infliximab soon captured a large proportion of the market. In 1998, the year the FDA licensed the drug for Crohn's disease, its U.S. sales were $27.5 million. Sales increased following the drug's authorization for RA and other indications (Table 9.3 and Figure 9.6). By November 2007 the drug had been approved in eighty-eight countries for fifteen inflammatory disease indications and was being used to treat more than one million patients worldwide. In 2008, infliximab

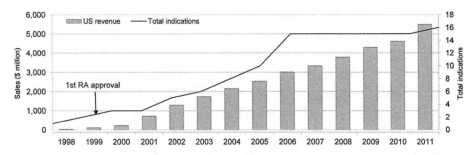

FIGURE 9.6. Annual U.S. sales of infliximab with number of approved indications (clinical uses). Note the first approval of infliximab for rheumatoid arthritis (RA) in 1999. (From Centocor, *Annual Report* [1998]; *New Jersey Citizen Action and United Senior Action of Indiana v. Johnson & Johnson and Centocor*, 11 Apr. 2002; Johnson & Johnson, *Annual Reports* [2002–11])

commanded 23 percent of the arthritis drug market, putting it in second place after adalimumab, which had a share of 28 percent. That year infliximab generated $5.9 billion in revenue worldwide. It would generate $8 billion in 2010, making it the third medicine ever to top $8 billion in annual sales, and the best-selling biological medicine in the world for that year.[56]

By 2008 Mab drugs were dominating the market for arthritis therapies, in part because they worked so much better than the competition. Prior to their emergence, the mainstay of therapy had been non-steroidal anti-inflammatory drugs designed to ameliorate the symptoms rather than address their cause. Aimed at controlling pain and inflammation, such treatments did little to alter the structural progression of the disease and the long-term disability that accompanied it. Therapies were also deployed to slow the disease process, but mostly only after there was radiographic evidence of joint damage. Such drugs often produced only a slow response and had a high level of toxicity. By contrast, Mab-based drugs offered a more rational approach based on understanding and modifying the underlying mechanism triggering the disease. As can be seen in the case of infliximab, Mabs played a pivotal role both as a laboratory tool for investigating the pathogenesis of the disease and as a device to treat the disease. In this context Mabs helped raise the bar in the quest to achieve disease remission and joint and bone healing in RA. Most encouraging was the speed with which Mabs acted and that the

Table 9.3

FDA-approved blockbuster Mabs by indication, path to market and sales, 2007

TRADE NAME (GENERIC)	INDICATIONS		REGULATORY PATH TO APPROVAL	YEARS TO APPROVAL	U.S. SALES, IN BILLIONS	% OF TOP 20 BIOTECH DRUG SALES
	FIRST	LATER				
Remicade (infliximab)	CD	RA, AS, PA, UC, PP	O, A, P, F	4.6	$5	9.84
Rituxan/Mabthera (rituximab)	NHL	RA, DLBC, NHL[c]	O, P	5.1	$4.9	9.62
Herceptin (trastuzumab)	BC[b]	BC	F, P	7.5	$4.3	8.45
Avastin (bevacizumab)	CRC[b]	CRC[b], NSCLC, HER2-BC[a]	F, P	7.1	$3.6	7.15
Humira (adalimumab)	RA	RA, JIA, PA, AS, CD, PP	O	3.7	$3.1	6.04
Erbitux (cetuximab)	CRC[b]	SCCHN	A, P	9.7	$1.4	2.73
Lucentis (ranbizumab)	AMD		P	6.8	$1.2	2.39
Synagis (palivizumab)	RSV		P	3.6	$1.1	2.25

Source: P. A. Scolnik, "mAbs: A Business Perspective," *mAbs* 1, no. 2 (Mar./Apr. 2009): 179–84, table 1.

Note: A—accelerated approval; AMD—age-related macular degeneration; AS—ankylosing spondylitis; BC—breast cancer; CD—Crohn's disease; CRC—colorectal cancer; DLBC—diffuse large B-cell lymphoma; F—fast-track; JIA—juvenile idiopathic arthritis; NHL—non-Hodgkin's lymphoma; NSCLC—non-small-cell lung carcinoma; O—orphan indication; P—priority review; PA—psoriatic arthritis; PP—plaque psoriasis; RA—rheumatoid arthritis; RSV—respiratory syncytial virus; SSCHN—squamous cell carcinoma of the head and neck; UC—ulcerative colitis.

[a] conditional

[b] metastatic

[c] first line therapy

clinical improvements were sustained. The availability of infliximab and other similar drugs not only helped to reduce symptoms and structural damage, but also improved physical function.[57]

Yet Mab therapy was not a total panacea. Patients could develop negative immunogenic responses to such drugs; the very mechanism of action that made the TNFα-blocking agent so effective increased the risk of infection. In the case of infliximab, tuberculosis and other opportunistic infections, as well as sepsis, were observed early on in patients given the therapy. Similarly malignancies, including lymphoma, appeared among those taking the drug. The question was whether these complications were a direct consequence of the therapy, or merely the manifestation of a latent disease. To address the issue, Centocor established a postmarketing mechanism to survey all patients prescribed the drug. Done with the aid of patient registries set up in partnership with academics to collect data, Centocor's surveillance strategy was ahead of its time. Only later would the FDA and European Medicines Agency (EMEA) oblige companies to implement postmarketing surveillance as part of the approval process for drugs.[58]

Over a decade has now passed since rituximab and infliximab were first licensed. Since then, many more Mab drugs have entered the clinical trial phase. Based on calculations for two-year running averages, the number of Mab drugs entering clinical study per year fluctuated from twelve to fourteen between the late 1980s and 1996 and rose to thirty-four candidates in the years from 1997 to 2006.[59] Not all of these drugs succeeded, but as Table 9.1 shows, many have made their way to market for a variety of conditions since the late 1990s. Just how far Mab drugs had come by the 1990s can be seen from the subsequent fate of Centocor, which in 1999 Johnson & Johnson bought for $5.2 billion, one of the largest biotechnology deals at the time, as a means to strengthen its pipeline of new drugs. Much of Centocor's attraction was its Mab technology, expertise, and growth potential. In 1998 alone, Centocor generated $192 million in profits on sales of $317 million. This represented a profit margin of around 60 percent—which was particularly striking given that just four years earlier the company had been on the verge of collapse.[60]

More than thirty Mab drugs have been marketed since 1986 and hundreds more are in clinical study. Since the advent of infliximab and rituximab, the number of therapeutic Mabs has grown exponentially. Between

January 2000 and June 2005, more than 130 therapeutic Mabs entered clinical study, with at least thirty of them in phase II or phase III trials in 2010.[61] One of the reasons for Mabs' success is that they have proven highly versatile. This versatility was greatly helped by the improvements made to the technology through the genetic and biological engineering techniques outlined in Chapter 8, which provided a large variety of full-size Mabs and alternative antibody formats. By 2007 Mab therapeutics had an estimated annual growth rate of more than 35 percent, outstripping both the growth and profitability of small molecule drugs, which were estimated to have a growth rate of less than 8 percent. That year eight of the Mab therapeutics on the market accounted for nearly $25 billion in sales, and almost half of the top twenty biotech treatments on the market that year. Three of these drugs were for cancer, two were for autoimmune disorders, one was for both oncology and autoimmune indications, and the remaining two for age-related macular degeneration and the prophylaxis of respiratory syncytial virus (RSV) infections in children.

Table 9.3 shows the lucrative sales of the eight blockbuster Mabs approved by the FDA on the market in 2007, the short time they took to win approval, and their rapid label expansion. Palivizumab achieved the fastest time to market, taking just 3.6 years from an application for approval to the final go-ahead. As with other biotechnology drugs, inventors of Mab therapeutics first secured approval to test and market the drug for treatment of an orphan disease and thereafter sought supplementary approvals to expand the market.[62]

Many of the approved Mabs have used FDA programs that were created in 1992 to streamline the process of drug approval. The FDA has a number of schemes in place. These include priority review, granted where a drug offers the possibility of a major advance in treatment or provides treatment where there is no adequate therapy. Another is accelerated review, which is given where a surrogate endpoint or clinical endpoint is used other than survival or irreversible morbidity. (An endpoint is a laboratory measurement or physical sign that represents a clinical meaningful outcome, such as survival or symptom improvement.) Postmarketing trials are mandatory in the case of accelerated review to verify anticipated clinical benefits. Yet another path, fast-track, is used for drugs addressing serious or life-threatening diseases or conditions with an unmet medical need. In 2008, one or more of these regulatory mechanisms had been

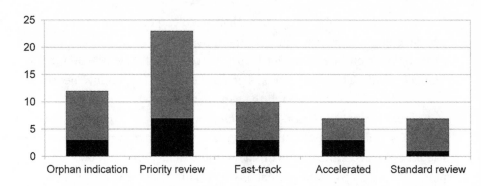

FIGURE 9.7. Number of FDA-approved Mab drugs from 1986 to 2012 according to their regulatory path. The Orphan Drug Act of 1983 offered tax incentives for medicines designed to address rare diseases, and so offered a pathway for approval for some Mab therapeutics. (FDA approvals)

used during the development of the majority (67 percent) of FDA-approved Mab therapeutics.[63] Figure 9.7 highlights the high number of Mab drugs expedited to market on the basis of FDA priority review between 1986 and 2012. Each was considered a major advance in treatment or was aimed at conditions for which there was an unmet medical need.

The large proportion of Mab therapeutics expedited for FDA approval is not a case of drugs being rushed to market. In 2008 the average clinical phase for all twenty-one U.S.-approved Mab drugs on the market was 80.8 months, with a range of 37.3 to 140.3 months. Mab drugs targeting cancer took somewhat longer in the clinic, 90.8 months. Those for autoimmune conditions took slightly less time—76.2 months. In fact, drug candidates that utilized at least one FDA mechanism for quicker approval took significantly longer on average in clinical trials than did their non-designated counterparts.[64]

While Mab therapeutics take time to develop clinically, their success rate is noticeably higher than other new chemical entities. Chimeric and humanized Mabs have been especially successful in this respect. By 2005, 21 percent of chimeric Mabs and 24 percent of humanized Mabs had made it to market (Table 9.4). This compares with the 11 percent of all therapeutic compounds that made it to market in 2004. The success rate was higher for cardiovascular drugs, 20 percent, than for therapeutics for on-

Table 9.4

Approval success rates for Mab drugs, up to 2005

MAB TYPE AND AREA OF APPLICATION	TOTAL NUMBER OF MABS	NUMBER DISCONTINUED	NUMBER FDA APPROVED	COMPLETION[a] (%)	APPROVAL SUCCESS[b] (%)
Chimeric Mabs, all products	39	19	5	62	21
Oncological chimeric Mabs	21	9	2	52	18
Immunological chimeric Mabs	9	7	2	100	22
Chimeric Mabs, 1987–97	20	12	5	85	29
Humanized Mabs, all products	102	41	9	49	24
Oncological humanized Mabs	46	13	4	37	24
Immunological humanized Mabs	34	17	4	62	19
Humanized Mabs, 1988–97	46	24	9	72	27

Source: J. M. Reichert, et al. "Monoclonal Antibody Successes in the Clinic," *Nature Biotechnology* 23, no. 4 (Sept. 2005): 1073–78, esp. 1077, table 2.

Note: Based on dataset compiled by Tufts Center for the Study of Drug Development. This dataset contains 355 therapeutic products in clinical study sponsored by more than one hundred commercial companies.

[a] Percentage of products with a known fate in a given cohort.

[b] Based on phase I to U.S. FDA approval.

cology and central nervous system disorders (5 and 8 percent, respectively). In the case of oncology products, both chimeric and humanized Mabs had higher approval rates than those for new chemical entities in 2004 (18, 24, and 5 percent, respectively). Overall, Mabs directed toward hematological malignancies have been more successful than those directed toward solid tumors.[65]

So far, slightly fewer chimeric and humanized Mabs have been approved than other biologically based therapies. Recombinant protein therapeutics that entered clinical study during the 1980s had a 26 percent U.S. approval rate. This trend, however, is being overturned. By 2007 the investment in Mab therapeutics had turned into what one observer called a "Gold Rush." That year alone two hundred biotechnology companies were developing Mab drugs for clinical use and there were more Mabs at each stage of the process—from research and development, to preclinical and phase I–III trials, and on to application for approval as a new drug—than for all other biologics combined. Mabs were the dominant type of protein therapeutic in clinical study, with about 50 percent of these devoted to cancer, 25 percent to immune-inflammatory diseases, and 10 percent to infectious diseases.[66]

The surge in interest in Mab therapeutics in recent years can be partly attributed to how much such drugs have helped to transform the management of disease, notably cancer and autoimmune disorders. Yet this is not the whole story. Many companies have embraced Mabs as a means to boost their dwindling portfolio of profitable drugs in the face of the imminent expiration of key patents and the rise of generic medicines. Unlike patents on many other drugs, including other biological therapies, which will soon expire, Mab patents still have a long time to run. Furthermore, generic Mabs are still in their infancy. Just how significant Mabs have become can be seen from the $46.8 billion paid in 2009 by Roche, a leading pharmaceutical company, for Genentech, a biotechnology giant with one of the strongest and most lucrative portfolios of Mab drugs. The previous year Genentech had received approximately $13.4 billion from its Mab cancer drugs.[67]

Given that initially many pharmaceutical companies had turned down Mabs as unprofitable, clearly few imagined the billions of dollars that Mabs would generate. But while such drugs have helped improve the care for many diseases previously considered untreatable, their arrival has radically increased the price tag for treatments for these same life-threatening and seriously debilitating diseases. This surge in cost has prompted fierce debates about who should be given access to such drugs and who should pay for them.

CHAPTER TEN

A Quiet Revolution

THE LEGACY OF MONOCLONAL ANTIBODIES

SIX OF THE TEN BEST-SELLING DRUGS in the world today are Mab therapeutics. One of these, adalimumab (Humira), a treatment for rheumatoid arthritis and other autoimmune conditions, was listed as the top-selling drug across the globe in 2012, with an annual revenue of $9.3 billion. Adalimumab's sales are predicted to surpass the peak sales of Lipitor, a cholesterol-lowering drug that has been the biggest selling drug historically.[1]

By 2012 there were more than thirty Mab drugs on the world market. Of these, ten had achieved blockbuster status, generating profits of more than $1 billion. These included three marketed for cancer by the Roche Group: bevacizumab (Avastin), rituximab (Rituxan), and trastuzumab (Herceptin), which collectively raised $17 billion in annual revenue in 2009. In 2012 antibody therapies generated $55 billion globally. Mab drugs currently make up a third of all new medicines introduced worldwide, and attract strong interest by investors. Companies with Mab platforms, for example, significantly outperformed the NASDAQ Biotechnology Index between 2008 and 2010. Even during the financial downturn after 2008, many Mab developers raised substantial capital from the stock market. In 2009, for example, Seattle Genetics, a biotechnology company developing Mab therapeutics for cancer, raised $136 million, and in 2010, ImmunoGen, also a developer of anticancer Mab drugs, raised

$77.6 million.[2] The lucrative Mab therapeutic market today contrasts powerfully with the early entrepreneurs' struggle to obtain investment in the 1980s, and serves as a reminder of how far Mabs have changed the healthcare landscape.

Some of the benefits of Mab drugs for patients are illustrated by the experiences of "Marianne," who at age sixteen developed ulcerative colitis, an autoimmune disorder similar to Crohn's disease that causes inflammation of the large intestine and can cause colon cancer. Marianne's symptoms included bloody diarrhea and terrible stomach cramps five or six times a day, and sometimes even more frequently. She recalled, "I had to run to the bathroom frequently. I didn't want to socialize. I couldn't be far from the bathroom at any time. I always worried about where the bathrooms were. I had to have my driving route mapped out so I knew where all the bathrooms were on the way . . . [so I could] pull over easily." Her condition did not improve with steroids or other medications, though they led to substantial weight gain. She became so irritable and depressed that she needed antidepressants. Her desperation reached a tipping point when she attended a debutante ball at the age of eighteen. She recalled, "That night I just had enough. I was [in the bathroom] the entire evening. It was supposed to be a fun time—you dance with your dad, you have fun [with] friends—and I was absolutely miserable the whole time. I couldn't enjoy myself." Having spent two years on medication, Marianne decided then and there to have her colon removed surgically. As she put it, "I knew it was the only option, since there was no cure. If you remove a diseased colon, you no longer have the disease . . . I wanted to have the surgery so that I didn't have to deal with the side effects of all the medications any more."[3]

Instead of surgery, Marianne's consultant suggested that she participate in a clinical trial for infliximab (Remicade) that had just been launched. To Marianne's great surprise the drug was immediately effective. She recalled, "After the first infusion, I believe the next day, I went out and got some pizza. I wanted pizza so bad. I was tired of restricting my diet. I wanted to just see what would happen—probably not the smartest thing. I was able to eat it, which I couldn't do for years without having horrible stomach ache and diarrhoea. I was able to eat whatever I wanted without any symptoms, which was great." By the time Marianne turned nineteen she had completed her infliximab treatment and her disease had gone into remission. For her, the drug had been a lifesaver. As she remembered, "After taking Remicade I didn't have to worry about running to the bathroom in the middle of a college lecture and having all these people turn around and stare at me because I got up three times. I didn't have to worry about playing lacrosse at other colleges, and running off the field in the middle of the game to use the bathroom. Remicade gave me more freedom in what I could do, and what I could eat. I could be up late studying and order Chinese take-out like everybody else." With infliximab, Marianne gained much more energy and no longer needed to take steroids. As she said, with infliximab "essentially my life was back to normal."[4]

Infliximab, however, did not provide a total cure. Marianne was still on medications that lowered her resistance to colds and infections. Five years after receiving infliximab, her symptoms of ulcerative colitis also resurfaced. This time infliximab gave her little relief and had neurological side effects. Another Mab drug also proved futile. While Marianne was eventually forced to have her colon removed surgically, she still believes that infliximab transformed her life. If she had not taken the drug when she did, she asserts, "I'd still be where I was or worse. I wouldn't have seen that life can be good. I would have given up hope and just resigned myself to taking medications that may or may not have worked forever, and just kept dealing with the symptoms. Remicade showed me that there's light at the end of the tunnel."[5]

In the early 1990s when Marianne first took infliximab, Mab drugs were still experimental. Since then they have become more established. Yet starting in the early 1990s when Centoxin was developed for septic shock, their high price has triggered much discussion about their cost-effectiveness and benefits.

Take a more recent controversy around trastuzumab (Herceptin), a humanized Mab commercialized by Genentech for treating metastatic breast cancer. Approved for the market in the United States in 1998 and in Europe in 2000, trastuzumab is intended for patients who test positive for human epidermal growth factor receptor 2 (HER2/neu), a protein found on the surface of tumor cells. Approximately 15 to 20 percent of women with metastatic breast cancer are likely to test positive for HER2. Those with the marker have half the survival time of other metastatic breast cancer patients, whose survival is usually between eighteen and twenty-four months after diagnosis. Designed to target and inhibit HER2, trastuzumab significantly improves the chances of women with HER2-positive metastatic cancer. Nonetheless, it is not a cure and many patients suffer a return of their cancer after initially responding well to treatment. The drug can also cause side effects, the most serious being life-threatening heart problems. In addition, the drug is very expensive. In 2005 trastuzumab was estimated to cost £30,000 per patient per year in Britain.[6]

Initially, trastuzumab was licensed to treat advanced breast cancer. In May 2005, however, data collected from four large multi-center randomized clinical trials with more than thirteen thousand cancer patients indicated that trastuzumab halved the chances of recurrence in those women with early breast cancer who have a high risk of rapid relapse, and significantly increased their chances of survival. The results electrified medical oncologists. One *New England Journal of Medicine* editorial claimed they were so "revolutionary" they would "completely alter our approach to the treatment of breast cancer." Data from two additional trials reported in December 2005 backed these earlier findings.[7]

News of trastuzumab's effectiveness in early breast cancer spread quickly as newspapers and other media trumpeted tales about the "wonder drug." Following this, a string of stories were published in Britain about patients fighting for access to the drug, although it had not yet been approved by regulatory authorities for use in early breast cancer. By presenting the personal and traumatic experiences of young women with children, the media caught public attention—and increased sales of the drug. Such coverage also helped spur several campaigns in 2005 by British women calling for it to be made available to all who needed it. Provision was patchy, though, because local health authorities had no obligation to fund the drug before it had been officially licensed for early breast cancer.[8]

As patients' demands for trastuzumab began to mount, healthcare providers faced an increasing ethical dilemma over resource allocation. In Britain the total annual bill for providing trastuzumab to all the five thousand women diagnosed each year with early stage breast cancer would have been an estimated £109 million. This amount was substantially higher than the £17 million allocated in 2002 to treat 1,950 patients with late-stage metastatic cancer.

Central to the debate was how much would have to be spent to save a life. One oncologist, Karol Sikora, summed up the challenge in 2006:

"The data suggest that you have to give [trastuzumab] to eighteen women to get one life saved. So the cost is over £400,000 for that one life. If you're the woman whose life is being saved then, of course, it's a wonder drug for you. The other seventeen don't know whether it's going to be or not, but obviously with the drug there they want the best possible treatment. That's the conundrum, you have to give it to a lot of people to get the 6% benefit overall."[9]

Extending trastuzumab's use to early breast cancer was not only controversial in Europe. In New Zealand, where the government's health authority had funded its use for advanced breast cancer from 2002, major concerns began to be voiced from 2006 about extending access to early breast cancer sufferers. Andy Simpson, chairman of the New Zealand Association of Cancer Specialists, for example, estimated that providing trastuzumab treatment for every one patient would delay chemotherapy for another three cancer patients. This reflected the additional costs of staff time in pathology testing, cardiac monitoring, pharmacy preparation, and infusion. Trastuzumab required between seventeen and eighteen intravenous infusions a year. Overall, Simpson believed that extending trastuzumab to early cancer patients would compromise the life-saving treatment of a thousand other patients.[10]

Initially, New Zealand's health authority refused to fund trastuzumab for early stage breast cancer. Mirroring what happened in Britain, this decision prompted a major campaign by women, who began filing lawsuits and petitioning parliament. It included a publicity stunt called "Bikers for Boots" involving pink-clad motorbike riders circling the North Island. The media was also filled with stories about women mortgaging their homes and using their retirement savings to pay for treatment. Funding was finally permitted in 2007, but was limited to three treatments or nine weeks of treatment instead of the recommended twelve-month period. This was partly dictated by the fact that a year's funding would cost NZ$20–25 million per year, which seemed exorbitant given that the country's entire cancer budget was NZ$35–45 million. Funding for a year's course of treatment was finally agreed to in December 2008, following a heated election campaign to ensure this funding and a change of government.[11]

The New Zealand government's reluctance to fund a full year of treatment in part reflected the complete lack of evidence for what the optimal duration and dose of trastuzumab was for treating early breast cancer. The gap in information was meaningful not just for patients, but also for the public coffers. British health economists, for example, calculated in 2006 that trastuzumab's cost could be reduced from £20,000 to £2,000 if given at a fifth of the standard dose and for just nine weeks. The optimal duration and dose of trastuzumab to be given continued to be debated for some time. Two closely watched clinical trials were launched to investigate the issue. The first, conducted by the French National Cancer Institute, explored whether half a year of treatment would be as good as one year, and the second, sponsored by Roche, the drug's manufacturer, tested whether two years of treatment would be better than one. The studies had major financial implications. One analyst claimed that sales of trastuzumab would decrease by $2.6 billion if given for six months, but increase by $5 billion if given for two years. In the end, the research, published in 2012, indicated that neither a shorter nor longer duration of the drug was better at preventing a recurrence of cancer than the standard one year.[12]

As one of a myriad of highly priced new designer drugs that have come to market, trastuzumab highlights some of the questions raised about the cost-effectiveness of such therapeutics. At issue is not only the drug's actual cost. While Mab therapeutics tend to be milder and have fewer toxic side effects than other chemotherapy drugs, they have to be infused into patients, which can create complications. Any complication increases the nursing time required and the time that patients may have to take off from work.[13]

Even where the health benefits of Mab therapeutics are proven, controversies will continue about their economic viability because of their expensive price. High prices, however, are generally associated with early innovative treatments, and Mabs are not the only drugs to have staggering prices. The cost of cancer treatments, for example, has more than doubled in the past two decades, leading to an outcry by many European and American cancer specialists. Another reason that the Mab drugs are so expensive is that many are still protected by patents. A drug's patent life is twenty years from the date of filing, in order to help developers recoup some of the research and development costs involved in getting to a drug to market. Some of the patent life is in fact reduced because some of that time, on average eight years, is taken up by clinical trials and regulatory approval.[14]

The total amount that companies spend on drug development has been fiercely contested. Figures for the years 1997 to 2011 show that twelve leading pharmaceutical companies spent on average $802 billion to gain approval for just 139 drugs ($5.8 billion per drug). One major expenditure in drug development is clinical trials, which as a result of increasingly labyrinthine regulations have needed to be larger and more complex in recent years. Between 1999 and 2005, the average length of a clinical trial increased by 70 percent, the average number of routine procedures rose by 65 percent, and the average clinical trial staff work burden surged by 65 percent. Enrollment criteria and trial protocols have also become more stringent. This has meant that 21 percent fewer volunteers have been admitted into trials and 30 percent have dropped out before completion of the tests. The most costly clinical trials are those undertaken at the phase III stage, which is used to confirm a drug's effectiveness and monitor its mid- to long-term side effects in large groups of patients. These trials represent about 40 percent of a drug's research and development costs.[15]

More traditional small-molecule drugs often become cheaper once they are off patent and can be produced as generic medicines. Whether this will happen in a similar way for Mab therapeutics is uncertain. One of the obstacles is the complexity of Mab drugs, which makes them difficult to replicate perfectly—and any inadvertent chemical modifications can affect their performance and safety. As a result, regulatory authorities require clinical trials for biosimilar Mabs to demonstrate their equivalence for efficacy. (This is not the case with small molecule generics.) In order to be sure that the biosimilar version is close enough to the original drug to provide a safe, effective treatment, these clinical trials need to be very large. For example, the biosimilar Mab infliximab, approved in Korea in 2012 and in Europe in 2013, underwent clinical testing in 874 patients in twenty countries across 115 sites. In addition to the costs of clinical testing, producing biosimilar Mabs requires state-of-the-art manufacturing technology, which is both expensive and cumbersome. Overall, analysts expect that the complexities involved in manufacturing and testing biosimilar Mabs will keep costs high and that their price will only be between 20 and 30 percent less than their patented counterparts. This is much less savings than for small molecule drugs, which cost between 80 and 90 percent less once off patent.[16]

Another contributing factor to the high cost of Mab therapeutics is their low potency. Unlike most other drugs, including other biologicals, which are mostly given in milligram quantities, Mab drugs generally need to be administered in grams. Large volumes of Mabs—ranging from tens to hundreds of kilograms per year—are therefore needed to meet market demand. Manufacturing such quantities has been a major challenge until very recently. Unlike traditional small molecule drugs, which can be mass-produced through chemical synthesis for less than a dollar per gram, or simpler biological drugs (such as genetically engineered human insulin) that can be made efficiently and cheaply in bacterial hosts like *E. coli,* Mabs are large, complex, multi-component proteins that can only be produced in mammalian cells. Mammalian cells have certain limitations: they grow slowly and have very low expression yields. When Mab therapeutics were initially developed in the 1980s, the expression levels were generally 100 to 500 milligrams per liter, and these yields continued to be low for some time. Antibody titers in excess of one gram per liter were rare in 2002, with many drugs being launched using production cell lines and manufacturing processes that yielded only approximately 0.5 to 1 gram per liter of Mab. The low yield made Mab production expensive. At the time when the first Mab therapeutic was licensed in 1986, one gram of Mab cost between $2,000 and $5,000. During the late 1990s, manufacturing constituted about 20 to 25 percent of the sale price.[17]

By the end of the twentieth century, large-scale manufacturing had become a particularly urgent matter, and it reached a crisis in 2000, when the demand for etanercept (Enbrel), an antibody fusion protein approved for treating rheumatoid arthritis, exceeded production capacity. The shortage in capacity, as well as a need to reduce costs, triggered major efforts to improve the efficiency of manufacturing. Many of these efforts centered on selecting and genetically modifying mammalian cells to facilitate their maximum growth and productivity and to improve the conditions in bioreactors by optimizing the culture media and introducing advanced ways of refreshing those media in order to feed the cells as efficiently as possible. Multiple bioreactors were also installed to increase output. Currently multiproduct facilities can span up to 500,000 square feet with total bioreactor capacities of up to 200,000 liters, usually achieved with more than one 25,000-liter bioreactor. Some idea of the numbers and capacity of bioreactors now in operation can be seen in Table 10.1. Improvements

Table 10.1

Capital investment costs for Mab facilities using mammalian cells

MANUFACTURING FACILITY	DATE FACILITY COMPLETED	CAPITAL INVESTMENT (MILLIONS)	AREA (SQ. FEET)	PRODUCTION BIOREACTOR CAPACITY		
				NUMBER	SIZE (LITERS)	TOTAL (LITERS)
Genentech—Vacaville, CA	2000	250	310,000	8	12,000	96,000
Imclone BB36, Branchburg, NJ	2001	53	80,000	3	10,000	30,000
Biogen LSM, Research Triangle Park, NC	2001	175	245,000	6	15,000	90,000
Boehringer Ingelheim, Biberach, Germany	2003	215	—	6	15,000	90,000
Lonza biologics expansion, Portsmouth, NH	2004	207	270,000	3	20,000	60,000
Amgen BioNext, West Greenwich, RI	2005	500	500,000	9	20,000	180,000
Genentech NIMO,** Oceanside, CA	2005	380	470,000	6	15,000	90,000
Imclone BB50, Branchburg, NJ	2005	260	250,000	9	11,000	99,000
Biogen Idec, Hillerød, Denmark	2007*	350	366,000	6	15,000	90,000
Lonza biologics, Tuas, Singapore	2007*	250	—	4	20,000	80,000
Genentech expansion, Vacaville, CA	2009*	600	380,000	8	25,000	200,000

Source: S. S. Farid, "Process Economics of Industrial Monoclonal Antibody Manufacture," *Journal of Chromatography,* vol. 848 (2007): 8–18, table 1.

* Expected completion date.

** Originally built by Biogen Idec and sold to Genentech in 2005.

were also made in the purification process so as to increase the yield of the end product. Purification in itself requires a number of steps, including chromatography and filtration. Over the last twenty years, advances in these separation media have improved the productivity and efficiency of downstream processing, ensuring the removal of possible contaminants such as viruses.[18]

Between 1994 and 2009 the total global cell-culture capacity increased more than a hundredfold and production began to outstrip market demand. Nonetheless, while productivity has continued to improve, building a mammalian cell-culture facility remains costly and time-consuming. Such a facility takes five years on average to build, and costs several hundred million dollars, an outlay that is made well in advance of clinical trials or the receipt of drug approval. Other costs include the royalties that companies have to pay for intellectual property rights in Mab production and in the technology for humanization of the Mabs, as well as the raw materials needed for Mab production. Protein A affinity resin, for example, which is used in the purification process, cost $17,000 a liter in 2009. Production also remains time-consuming, with each batch of Mab therapeutics taking between eight and ten weeks to produce. The lengthy manufacturing process of Mabs and its associated costs have prompted scientists to explore other means of production, including plants and transgenic dairy animals. Progress in this area, however, has so far been limited.[19]

More promising are recent developments to enhance the potency and efficacy of Mabs, so as to make it possible to prescribe lower doses and potentially reduce costs. A number of approaches have been adopted to augment the efficacy of Mabs. One of the most encouraging is the use of genetic engineering to remove glycosylation sites from the variable domain of the antibody. This enhances the effector function of Mabs, such as antibody dependent cell-mediated cytotoxicity (ADCC), which activates the patient's innate immune cells to kill a target cell like cancer. Glyco-engineering also produces Mabs that are both less likely to provoke an unwanted immune response than Mabs created by protein engineering and more chemically homogeneous, which makes them are easier to develop (and replicate) as drugs.[20]

By 2012 fifteen glyco-engineered Mabs had entered late-stage clinical trials and one, mogamulizumab, had been approved for the Japanese market for relapsed or refractory adult T-cell leukemia/lymphoma, and was being investigated for treating asthma. The compound was created by Kyowa Hakko Kirin, a Japanese company using a platform that it had developed as a result of finding, serendipitously, that a Mab it had produced with reduced fucose in its sugar chains exhibited much higher ADCC. This discovery led the company to seek to genetically modify a Chinese hamster ovary cell (CHO) line to produce antibodies with no fucose content. After many years of painstaking work, this goal was finally achieved by knocking out the FUT8 gene in the CHO cell line. The advantage of glyco-engineered antibodies is that they are not rejected by the human body because it naturally produces fucose-free antibodies.[21]

When Kyowa Hakko Kirin started on its venture, many in the pharmaceutical industry doubted whether the project would result in antibodies with clinical efficacy. Indeed, there was much debate about the importance of ADCC to the clinical efficacy of therapeutic antibodies. Attitudes changed as a result of research on the genetic polymorphism of cancer patients, which demonstrated a strong correlation between ADCC response and long-term survival rates in patients with metastatic cancers who took rituximab and trastuzumab. Today a number of companies are investing in ADCC-enhancing technology as a way of hopefully optimizing and maximizing the clinical efficacy of therapeutic antibodies at reduced doses and cost. Where ADCC is generating some of the greatest excitement is in the field of cancer and autoimmune disorders.[22]

While the new generation of Mabs may greatly enhance the treatment of cancer and autoimmune disorders, which are well-established disease targets for Mab therapeutics, it remains to be seen whether Mab therapeutics will be effective in other areas. Nowhere is this question more urgent than in the case of infectious diseases. To date, only two anti-infective Mab drugs have been licensed: the first, palivizumab, was approved in 1998 for the prevention of respiratory syncytial virus (RSV) in high-risk premature babies and the second, raxibacumab, was approved in 2012 for the treatment of inhalation anthrax, a rare and lethal disease that is potentially spread by biological weapons.

The slow progress of Mab therapeutics for infectious diseases can in part be attributed to the large arsenal of other anti-infective drugs such as vaccines and antibiotics. Because they are specific to a single pathogen, Mab drugs are also commercially less attractive than traditional drugs because they cover a narrower spectrum of patients. In addition, Mabs need to be administered by intravenous or subcutaneous injection, unlike other anti-infectives, which can be taken orally, so they are unsuitable for patients in developing countries who have limited access to healthcare. Mabs are also more effective at preventing infection rather than treating established ones, and unlike vaccines provide only short-term prophylaxis. And finally, the high development and manufacturing costs associated with Mabs, and their poor record in winning approval for treating infectious diseases, lessen their commercial appeal.[23]

According to the immunologist Arturo Casadevall, the adoption of Mabs for infectious diseases requires a paradigm shift back to earlier forms of treatment before the arrival of sulphonamides in 1935. Most antimicrobial drugs before 1935 were pathogen-specific, that is, they were used to treat only one or two kinds of infections after a microbial diagnosis. Sulphonamides and subsequent antibiotics, by contrast, worked against a broad spectrum of pathogens and could be used for the immediate treatment of bacterial infections without the need to identify pathogens beforehand. While highly effective, these drugs disturb the host's microbial flora and encourage drug resistance. Casadevall thus advocates a return to administering pathogen-specific drugs after microbiological diagnosis and to using therapies to enhance a patient's own immunity. He points out that Mabs offer an effective way of generating pathogen-specific drugs and therapeutics for boosting the immune system.[24]

Caution is needed going forward, however, because the success of Mabs will greatly depend on access to appropriate diagnostics. Remember the case of Centoxin described in Chapter 7: its downfall was linked in part to the inability of clinicians to identify Gram-negative bacteria before its administration. This failure not only hindered the selection of an appropriate patient cohort to demonstrate the drug's efficacy against sepsis, but also meant that many more patients received the drug than was necessary, thereby raising its cost to the point where healthcare providers were unable to cover it. Clearly any future development of Mab therapeutics for infectious diseases will require major advances in diagnostic microbiology in order to avoid this same outcome. These will not be easily achieved, but diagnostics are already improving rapidly, helped by recent technological advances with PCR, DNA typing, antigen detection, and nucleic acid hybridization.[25]

That a Mab therapeutic is pathogen-specific could hinder its use for treating mixed infections. One solution might lie in the use of a cocktail of Mabs to target the diverse range of antigens that viruses carry. Such a strategy would effectively mimic the natural immune response: once infected, the body tends to develop several antibodies in response to the antigens presented by a virus, each of which attaches to one of the different antigens. It is this diversity of antibodies that helps the immune system fight the invader. The use of a cocktail of Mabs is already being investigated for the treatment for rabies. The disease has been handled hitherto by giving infected patients a combination of a rabies vaccine with rabies immune globulin (RIG), which is derived from sera pooled from either human donors or horses vaccinated against rabies. RIG is derived from sera containing different antibodies and has been proven effective. Nonetheless, it is very expensive and in short supply, particularly in the developing world where the vast majority of rabies fatalities take place—55,000 to 70,000 deaths a year. A cocktail of Mabs could be an alternative way to deliver these various antibodies to patients all at once.[26]

In many ways, the Mabs cocktail is an extension of serum therapy, which employed blood serum taken from immunized animals and was commonly used to treat infectious diseases until the late 1940s. While serum therapy largely fell out of favor with the rise of antibiotics, it did not disappear completely. Several antibody (immunoglobulin G) preparations, for example, were licensed in the 1980s to prevent and treat viral diseases, including measles, rubella, hepatitis (A, B, and C), cytomeglovirus, respiratory syncytial virus, rabies, vaccinia, varicella-zoster virus, and West Nile, Ebola, and corona viruses. Because they are derived from pooled sera taken from survivors of various viral epidemics, however, such products contain a vast number of antibodies, many of which are incapable of neutralizing a viral infection but instead can trigger the release of other, unrelated antibodies and so impede treatment. They also carry the risk of pathogen transmission and are difficult to standardize.[27]

Recent advances in Mab engineering have opened up new opportunities for serum therapy. Importantly, Mabs offer the means to prepare standardized agents that when combined in a cocktail can yield a product that is more precise and more potent than traditional serum therapy.[28] In addition, a cocktail of Mabs provides a means to augment the host's recovery system without directly killing a microbe. This minimizes the chance that the pathogens will rapidly mount their resistance.

To date the development of anti-infective Mab products has attracted little commercial investment. In part this is because infectious diseases are short-lived and therefore have a limited market. This is in contrast to chronic conditions like cancer and autoimmune diseases, which require regular treatment and therefore have greater profit potential. Nonetheless, the pharmaceutical climate is changing, fueled by concern over the rise in new pathogens (such as West Nile and corona viruses), the reemergence of old pathogens (like tuberculosis), increasing antibiotic resistance among micro-organisms and the rise of superbugs like MRSA, as well as the growing epidemic of patients who are immuno-compromised as a result of HIV infection, organ transplantation, chronic degenerative diseases, and improvements in cancer care. Fears about bioterrorism are also a factor.

These heightened concerns are leading both the public and private sectors to reexamine in a more positive light the development of Mabs for infectious diseases. This trend may be boosted by the availability of public funding from the U.S. government, which in 2004 passed the Project Bioshield Act, which allocated $5.6 billion to encourage companies to develop innovative therapeutics to counter diseases spread by biological weapons. The National Institutes of Health also offers grants to support the production, preclinical studies, and early clinical studies of innovative products against infectious diseases.[29]

Although the development of Mab therapeutics for infectious diseases poses many challenges, the rewards are potentially high. For example, worldwide sales of palivizumab (the anti-infective Mab directed at preventing serious lower-respiratory-tract disease in high-risk premature babies exposed to outbreaks of RSV in the winter months) exceeded $900 million in 2012. The drug took eight years of intensive work to develop, and is very expensive to administer, but it has helped to reduce the number of infants needing hospitalization and the cost of their care.[30]

While the future is uncertain for employing Mab therapeutics for infectious diseases, Mabs have already transformed the diagnostic landscape for such diseases. As Chapter 3 outlined, Mabs have been used in a variety of diagnostic formats since the 1970s, including immunohistochemistry on tissue samples, enzyme-linked or fluorescence-based immunoassays of tissue extracts or bodily fluids, and a range of other simple tests, such as particle agglutination. In such tests, the Mabs act as probes either to detect antigens characteristic of particular infectious agents, or to determine whether a patient has had an immune response to an infection. Identifying whether a patient has made antibodies against an infection is particularly valuable in the case of viral infections, where antigen detection can be difficult. In this situation, tests are carried out to see whether a patient has IgM antibodies, which are characteristic of an early infection, or IgG antibodies, which develop at a later stage.[31]

Overall, Mabs laid the foundation for the development of simple, cheap, fast, and accurate diagnostics that were easily adapted for mass screening and automation. As Chapter 6 highlighted, these tests were quickly commercialized by entrepreneurs who seized upon Mabs as a means of competing against already well-established diagnostic companies and as a stepping stone to the development of Mab therapeutics. By the mid-1980s numerous Mab kits were being marketed for the diagnosis of infectious diseases including herpes, chickenpox, hepatitis B, rabies, and legionellosis.[32]

Traditionally, diagnosis of an infection required the identification of the organism either directly from infected material, or more commonly, from a culture made with the infected material. One of the advantages of Mab-based immunoassay tests is that they permit the determination of disease directly from clinical samples, bypassing the need for laborious and time-consuming culturing of a causative microbial agent. For example, prior to the arrival of Mabs, diagnosis of human sexually transmitted diseases required an initial culturing of the causative bacteria, which took between two and six days, followed by confirmatory testing. By contrast, a Mab test can be performed on a clinical sample and completed within minutes. By 1991, the Mab diagnostics market was generating approximately $1.9 billion, of which $55 million was spent on nonsexually transmitted diseases and $245 million on sexually transmitted diseases.[33]

Mab tests have proven useful not only in the diagnosis of viruses and bacteria, but also in the detection of other types of parasites that are difficult to grow in culture, such as unicellular and multicellular organisms, fungi, mycoplasma, and chlamydia. Used in tandem with microscopy and flow cytometry, Mabs have also offered far more refined differential diagnoses, providing for the more certain identification of an infectious agent. Such tests can be particularly beneficial in the case of immunocompromised patients, such as those with AIDS, who suffer from a disproportionately higher instance of fungal infections.[34]

Mabs have played a particularly important role in preventing the transmission of infectious diseases through blood transfusions. The Mab diagnostic for hepatitis B, as Chapter 6 showed, was one of the earliest developed for this purpose, gaining approval in 1983. By the late 1980s, a Mab test had also been developed for the detection of HIV. This test was later superseded by a test using recombinant HIV proteins produced from bacterial sources. Mabs, however, continued to be important in the management of AIDS; they are deployed for the quantitative measurement of CD4 cells in blood, the primary criterion for the diagnosis of AIDS.[35]

In addition to helping diagnose sexually transmitted diseases, Mabs are critical to the public health surveillance of influenza. While most influenza outbreaks are self-limited, the disease is highly contagious and annually kills between 500,000 to one million people worldwide. Over the past twenty years influenza-associated deaths, 90 percent of which occur in the elderly, have increased substantially. One challenge with the disease is that its clinical presentation is similar to other respiratory illnesses. Furthermore, different viruses cause influenza. Laboratory diagnosis of influenza commonly involves first culturing the virus, which can take between two and fourteen days, followed by a quick test known as the hemagglutination test (a serological method based on an observation made by George Hirst in 1942 that serum containing flu antibodies inhibits the clumping together of blood cells that normally occurs in the presence of the influenza virus). Mabs began to be incorporated into hemagglutination tests in the early 1980s. While such diagnostics are not sufficiently quick enough to help with the management of individual patients, they are crucial for confirming the arrival of influenza in the community, thereby helping to control the spread of infection. They are also pivotal for the identification and control of novel highly pathogenic influenza strains. It was used, for example, in the detection of the human H5N1 influenza virus in Hong Kong in 1997. In addition, they are instrumental to vaccine development for forthcoming influenza seasons.[36]

The use of Mabs for the routine testing of common conditions like influenza highlights how revolutionary Mabs have been since their development in 1975 as a laboratory tool to understand the diversity of antibodies. Little could the two Cambridge University scientists, Milstein and Köhler, have foreseen how much their innovation would spread. Today Mabs are no longer merely tools deployed at the laboratory bench, but also critical components in tests used across many areas of healthcare, including blood typing for transfusions, tissue typing for transplantations, early diagnosis of myocardial infarction, determination of blood T-cell levels in HIV-infected patients, analysis of tissue biopsies for cancer and other disorders, tests that patients can purchase over the counter for self-diagnosis of ovulation and pregnancy, as well as tests to detect drug abuse in sports or at work. Performed originally with polyclonal antisera drawn from immunized animals, Mabs have permitted a much higher degree of standardization and accuracy in these tests, and have allowed them to be carried out on a scale that was unthinkable just a few decades ago.

Mabs have also opened up new frontiers in our understanding of the pathways of disease. As Chapter 3 points out, Mabs quickly proved to be highly versatile probes for learning about the functions of the brain and the central nervous system—and the discoveries made possible by these Mabs in turn paved the way for new understandings of what causes neurological disease and for possible neuropharmacological interventions. Likewise, Mabs have been used to investigate and treat cancer, providing powerful tools for identifying and targeting different antigens on tumors. Although these applications did not quickly translate into successful Mab therapeutics for cancer, in more recent years Mab therapeutics have offered alternatives to drugs with a broad spectrum and high toxicity. This has transformed the care of cancer patients, who no longer face the prospect of losing hair and the other serious side effects associated with other cytotoxic drugs. The advantage of Mabs is that they can be given as maintenance therapies. This is reshaping our perceptions of some cancers from what was once seen as inevitably fatal to a chronic condition. Mabs have also enabled the prescription of specific therapeutics for particular tumor antigens in individual patients. This allows a greater degree of personalization in the management of cancer than was possible in the past. Indeed, Mab therapeutics are expected to be an increasingly important component in personalized cancer therapies. This trend has been helped by the rise in molecular diagnostics since the late 1990s, which made it possible to measure the levels of proteins, genes, or specific mutations in tumors into clinically relevant subtypes and thus better predict a patient's response to a particular drug. One example of this partnership is the Mab trastuzumab, which is marketed with a diagnostic test for Her2/neu. The diagnostic test has proven important in establishing both the efficacy of the drug as well as its cost-effectiveness for a specific patient. Another Mab therapeutic used in the personalized treatment of cancer is rituximab, which targets patients with CD20-positive B-cell non-Hodgkin's lymphoma.[37]

As we have learned, Mabs have not only helped advance cancer research and treatment, but also transformed the management of autoimmune disorders. Mabs have provided a major tool for understanding the onset and progression of autoimmune diseases and revealed new therapeutic possibilities. Importantly, they facilitated a paradigm shift in the treatment of autoimmune diseases away from just treating symptoms to targeting and preventing their cause.

Another area where Mabs have had a major impact has been in the development of stem cells. Stem cells are unspecialized cells found in all multicellular organisms that under the right conditions can self-replicate and give rise to the mature, functional cells that make up the different organs of the body, such as the heart, skin, muscle, and liver. Part of the attraction of stem cells is that they provide a powerful tool for understanding the signals and mechanisms of cell differentiation and offer a means to replace cells and heal damaged tissues in the body—an approach referred to as regenerative medicine. More than a thousand clinical studies are now under way to investigate how stem cells could be used to treat diseases like Parkinson's, heart disease, and diabetes. In addition, cancer stem cells are being used to screen potential anti-tumor drugs and develop new approaches for treating cancer. The ability to generate large numbers of specialized cells from stem cells has also prompted their use for testing the safety of new medicines in the hope that they can reduce the need for animal testing experiments by the pharmaceutical industry.

Mabs were instrumental historically in the identification and utilization of hematopoietic stem cells (HSCs), immature cells found in bone marrow, to improve the treatment of leukemia. One of the key figures in this research was Curt Civin, a pediatric oncologist who, together with colleagues at Johns Hopkins University, began developing Mabs in the early 1980s as a tool to isolate HSCs from the millions of cells found in the bone marrow. By 1984 the team had discovered an antigen, initially called My-10 and later CD34, which enabled the isolation and extraction of HSCs from the bone marrow cells. This allowed for the transplant of thousands of purified stem cells, thereby paving the way to safer cancer therapy since before this innovation, transplanted bone marrow contained cancerous cells. The Mabs developed by Civin and his team also provided a means of isolating the rarer and more informative stem cells while weeding out the more numerous, but less useful, mature cells. This method provided a means to produce stem cells on a large scale.[38]

In addition to Mabs' legacy for health, the early promise and success of Mabs generated great wealth for individual venture capitalists and facilitated investment in other newly emerging technology platforms. Medical research has benefited as well from the millions of dollars gained from royalties on Mab patents, which have been paid to universities and nonprofit organizations. In 2005, for example, Ján Vilček pledged $105 million of his royalty earnings from infliximab to New York University School of Medicine to further basic science. In the same year, the U.S. pharmaceutical company Abbott Laboratories paid the British Medical Research Council over $100 million in lieu of future licensing royalties for adalimumab, which had been approved for market in the United States in 2002 for the treatment of RA.[39]

Mabs have gone only some way to fulfilling Paul Ehrlich's late nineteenth-century dream that antibodies could provide a "magic bullet" for treating disease. And they have generally received less public fanfare than other forms of biotechnology such as genetic engineering and stem cells. But Mabs have nonetheless quietly helped unlock our power to understand and diagnose disease—and to bring relief to millions of sufferers around the world. In a world of antibiotic-resistant "superbugs" and an aging population grappling with autoimmune disorders and cancer, Mabs offer the potential for new, targeted treatments and drugs that can offer personalized care—and a window into the complex, overlapping conditions that underlie human disease.

NOTES

Details regarding all interviews, archived personal papers, and email correspondence are provided in the Bibliography. In addition, materials frequently cited have been identified by the following abbreviations:

ANN REV IMMUNOL	*Annual Review of Immunology*
ARTHRITIS RHEUM	*Arthritis & Rheumatology*
BMJ	*British Medical Journal*
CLIN CHEM	*Clinical Chemistry*
CLIN INFECT DIS	*Clinical Infectious Diseases*
EJI	*European Journal of Immunology*
EMBO J	*The EMBO Journal*
FASEB J	*Federation of American Societies for Experimental Biology Journal*
HS-PP	Hubert Schoemaker Papers
J BIOL CHEM	*Journal of Biological Chemistry*
J HIST BIOL	*Journal of the History of Biology*
J IMMUNOL METHODS	*Journal of Immunological Methods*
J INFECT DIS	*Journal of Infectious Diseases*
JEM	*Journal of Experimental Medicine*
JI	*Journal of Immunology*
MSTN	Milstein Papers, Churchill College Archive Centre, Cambridge, Eng.
NAT BIOTECHNOL	*Nature Biotechnology*
NAT IMMUNOL	*Nature Immunology*

NAT REV DRUG DISCOV   *Nature Reviews: Drug Discovery*
NEJM   *New England Journal of Medicine*
NEW SCI   *New Scientist*
PHIL TRANS R SOC LOND B *Philosophical Transactions of the Royal Society B:*
                        Biological Sciences
PNAS   *Proceedings of the National Academy of Sciences*
SCI AM   *Scientific American*

PREFACE

The following works are cited in the Preface: D. Margulies, "Monoclonal Antibodies: Producing Magic Bullets by Somatic Hybridization," *Journal of Immunology* 174, no. 5 (2005): 2451–52; Transparency Market Research, "Monoclonal Antibodies Market—Global Industry Size, Share, Trends, Analysis and Forecast, 2012–2018," available at http://www.transparencymarketresearch.com/mono clonal-antibodies.html; RnRMarket Research, and "Monoclonal Antibody Industry 2013 Global and China Market Analysis" (Feb. 2013), available at http://www .rnrmarketresearch.com (both accessed 17 Sept. 2014); E. Buxbaum, *Fundamentals of Protein Structure and Function* (New York, 2007), 137–51; J. L. Marx, "Monoclonal Antibodies and Their Applications," in J. L. Marx, *A Revolution in Biotechnology* (Cambridge, Eng., 1989), 145–59; S. O'Brien and T. Jones, "Humanization of Monoclonal Antibodies by CDR Grafting," in M. Welschof and J. Kraus, eds., *Methods in Molecular Biology*, vol. 27: *Recombinant Antibodies for Cancer Therapy: Methods and Protocols* (Totowa, N.J., 2003), 81; T. G. Berman, "Today's Biotech Breakthroughs Are Saving the Lives of Patients," letter to the editor, *Financial Times* (18 Nov. 2004); C. Arnst and A. Weintraub, "Biotech, Finally," *Business Week* (13 June 2005); S. Smith Hughes, *Genentech: The Beginnings of Biotech* (Chicago, 2011); M. A. Firer and G. Gellerman, "Targeted Drug Delivery for Cancer Therapy: The Other Side of Antibodies," *Journal of Hematology and Oncology* 5, no. 70 (2012); J. M. Reichert and E. Dhimolea, "Foundation Review: The Future of Antibodies as Cancer Drugs," *Drug Discovery Today* 17, nos. 17–18 (2012), 954–63; A. Scott, J. D. Wolchok, and L. J. Old, "Antibody Therapy of Cancer," *Nature Reviews: Cancer* 12 (2012), 278–87.

CHAPTER 1. HUNTING FOR THE ELUSIVE "MAGIC BULLET"

1. A. Silverstein, *A History of Immunology* (San Diego, 1989), ch. 1.
2. C. P. Gross and K. A. Sepkowitz, "The Myth of the Medical Breakthrough: Smallpox, Vaccination, and Jenner Reconsidered," *International Journal of Infectious Diseases* 3, no. 1 (1998): 54–60; S. Riedel, "Edward Jenner and the History of Smallpox and Vaccination," *Baylor University Medical Center Proceedings* 18, no. 1 (2005), 21–25; P. Debré, *Louis Pasteur* (Baltimore, 2000), chs. 14–15.
3. Silverstein, *History*, 18, 29, and ch. 2; L. Chernyak and A. I. Tauber, "The Idea of Immunity: Metchnikoff's Metaphysics and Science," *J Hist Biol* 23, no. 2 (1990): 187–249; L. Chernyak and A. I. Tauber, "History of Immunology:

The Birth of Immunology; Metchnikoff, the Embryologist," *Cellular Immunology* 117 (1988): 218–33.

4. Silverstein, *History*, 30–32; A. Silverstein, "Cellular versus Humoral Immunology: A Century-Long Dispute," *Nat Immunol* 4–5 (2003): 425–28; A. C. Hüntelmann, "Two Cultures of Regulation? The Production and State Control of Diphtheria Serum at the End of the Nineteenth Century in France and Germany," *Hygiea Internationalis* 6, no. 2 (2007): 99–120; U. Klöppel, "Enacting Cultural Boundaries in French and German Diphtheria Serum Research," *Science in Context* 21, no. 2 (2008): 161–80.

5. J. E. Alouf, "A 116-year Story of Bacterial Protein Toxins (1888–2004): From 'Diphtheric Poison' to Molecular Toxicology," in J. E. Alouf and M. R. Popff, eds., *The Comprehensive Source Book of Bacterial Protein Toxins* (Waltham, Mass., 2006): 3–4; U. Lagerkvist, *Pioneers of Microbiology and the Nobel Prize* (London, 2003), 91.

6. F. Winau and R. Winau, "Emil von Behring and Serum Therapy," *Microbes and Infection* 4 (2002): 185–88; D. S. Linton, *Emil von Behring: Infectious Disease, Immunology, Serum Therapy* (Philadelphia, 2005), 28–37, 58–63; J. Simon, "Emil Behring's Medical Culture: From Disinfection to Serotherapy," *Medical History* 51 (2007): 201–18.

7. Kitsato and Behring did not use the term antitoxin. Behring viewed the agent as a form of disinfectant. See J. Lindenmann, "Origin of the Terms 'Antibody' and 'Antigen'," *Scandinavian Journal of Immunology* 19, no. 4 (1984): 281–85; A. Cambrosio, D. Jacobi, and P. Keating, "Ehrlich's "Beautiful Pictures" and the Controversial Beginnings of Immunological Imagery," *Isis* 84, no. 4 (Dec. 1993): 662–99, esp. 666–67; Simon, "Emil"; Linton, *Behring*, 108–109.

8. P. Gronski, F. R. Seiler, and H. G. Schwick, "Discovery of Antitoxins and the Development of Antibody Preparations for Clinical Uses from 1890–1990," *Molecular Immunology* 28, no. 12 (1991): 1321–32; A. Mendelsohn, "Cultures of Bacteriology: Formation and Transformation of a Science in France and Germany, 1870–1914," Ph.D. diss., Princeton University, 1996, 299–309; Winau and Winau, "Behring"; J. Simon, "Emil Behring's Medical Culture"; Lagerkvist, *Pioneers*, 93–95.

9. The word "antibody" took time to be established. See Lindenmann, "Origin."

10. A. M. Silverstein, "Paul Ehrlich's Passion: The Origins of His Receptor Immunology," *Cellular Immunology* 194 (1999): 213–21; Linton, *Behring*, 105–106.

11. The term "antigen," a label used to denote a foreign invader, originated from research into antagonist products of bacteria in France from 1893. See Lindenmann, "Origin."

12. Ehrlich's immunity theory drew on his earlier discovery that dyes have side chains relating to their coloring properties and that each side chain had specific functions and affinity. See Silverstein, "Paul"; S. H. E. Kaufmann, "Elie

Metchnikoff's and Paul Ehrlich's Impact on Infection Biology," *Microbes and Infection* 10, nos. 14–15 (2008): 1417–19; C. R. Prüll, "Part of a Scientific Master Plan? Paul Ehrlich and the Origins of His Receptor Concept," *Medical History* 47 (2003): 332–56. Prüll argues that Ehrlich took time to develop his side-chain theory because as a Jew he could not obtain secure employment. See also T. Travis, "Emil Fischer and the Key to Specificity," *Chemistry and Industry* (18 Apr. 1994).

13. Silverstein, *History*, chs. 4–7, p. 14; A. M. Moulin, *Le dernier langage de la médicine: Histoire de l'immunologie de Pasteur au SIDA* (Paris, 1991), 67–97; Cambrosio, Jacobi, and Keating, "Ehrlich's 'Beautiful Pictures'"; E. Crist and A. I. Tauber, "Debating Humoral Immunity and Epistemology: The Rivalry of the Immunochemists Jules Bordet and Paul Ehrlich," *J Hist Biol* 30 (1997): 321–56.

14. A. Petterson, ceremony speech, Nobel Prize in Physiology or Medicine 1919, available at http://nobelprize.org/nobel_prizes/medicine/laureates/1919/press.html (accessed 17 Sept. 2014); A. B. Laurell, "Jules Bordet—A Giant in Immunology," *Scandinavian Journal of Immunology* 32, no. 5 (1990): 429–32; Crist and Tauber, "Debating"; C. Schmalstieg and A. S. Goldman, "Jules Bordet (1870–1961): A Bridge between Early and Modern Immunology," *Journal of Medical Biography* 17, no. 4 (2009): 217–24.

15. J. Drews, "Paul Ehrlich: Magister Mundi," *Nat Rev Drug Discov* 3 (2004): 1–5; H. P. Vollmers and S. Brändlein, "The 'Early Birds': Natural IgM Antibodies and Immune Surveillance," *Histology Histopathology* 20 (2005): 927–37; J. Drews et al., "Drug Discovery: A Historical Perspective," *Science* 287 (2000): 1960–64; D. D. Boyden, *An Introduction to Music* (London, 1959), 339.

16. U. Lagerkvist, *Pioneers of Microbiology and the Nobel Prize* (London, 2003).

17. N. Jerne, "Waiting for the End," *Cold Spring Harbor Symposium on Quantitative Biology*, 32 (1967): 591–603; Silverstein, *History*, 60–61; I. Löwy, "The Epistemology of the Science of an Epistemologist of the Sciences: Ludwik Fleck's Professional Outlook and Its Relationships to His Philosophical Works," in R. S. Cohen and T. Schnelle, eds., *Cognition and Fact: Materials on Ludwik Fleck* (Dordrecht, 1986), 421–24.

18. Silverstein, *History*, 65–67; L. E. Kay, "Molecular Biology and Pauling's Immunochemistry: A Neglected Dimension," *History and Philosophy of the Life Sciences* 11 (1989): 211–19, esp. 216; D. R. Forsdyle, "The Origins of the Clonal Selection Theory of Immunity," *FASEB J* 9 (1995): 164–66; P. D. Hodgkin, W. R. Heath, and A. G. Baxter, "The Clonal Selection Theory: 50 Years since the Revolution," *Nat Immunol* 8, no. 10 (2007): 1019–23, esp. 1019.

19. Löwy, "Epistemology," 433–44; I. Löwy, "Immunology in the Clinics: Reductionism, Holism, or Both?" in K. Kroker, P. Mazumdar, and J. Keelan, eds., *Crafting Immunity: Working Histories of Clinical Immunology* (Aldershot, 2008), 165–77.

20. L. Van Epps, "Michael Heidelberger and the Demystification of Antibodies," *JEM* 203, no. 1 (2006): 5; J. Carneiro, "Towards a Comprehensive View of the

Immune System," Ph.D. diss., Unité d'Immunobiologie Institut Pasteur, 1996, 11; M. Heidelberg, "A 'Pure' Organic Chemist's Downward Path: Chapter 2—The years at P. and S," *Annual Review of Biochemistry* 48 (1979): 1–21; H. L. Van Epps, "How Heidelberger and Avery Sweetened Immunology," *JEM* 202, no. 10 (2005): 1306; J. Cruse, "A Centenary Tribute: Michael Heidelberger and the Metamorphosis of Immunologic Science," *JI* 140 (1988): 2861–63.

21. Kay, "Molecular Biology and Pauling's Immunochemistry," 216; L. E. Kay, *The Molecular Vision of Life* (Oxford, Eng., 1993), 174–85; D. M. Knowles, *Neoplastic Hematopathology* (Philadelphia, 2001), 44; A. Cambrosio, D. Jacobi, and P. Keating, "Arguing with Images: Pauling's Theory of Antibody Formation," *Representations* 89 (2005): 94–130; T. Söderqvist, *Science as Autobiography: The Troubled Life of Niels Jerne* (London, 2003), 176; Silverstein, *History,* 72–76.

22. M. Cohn, "Reflections on the Clonal-Selection Theory," *Nature Reviews: Immunology* 7 (2007): a23–a30; Söderqvist, *Science,* 167–85; A. M. Silverstein, "Splitting the Difference: The Germline–Somatic Mutation Debate on Generating Antibody Diversity," *Nat Immunol* 4, no. 9 (2003): 829–33; D. R. Forsdyke, "The Origins of the Clonal Selection Theory of Immunity," *FASEB J* 9 (1995): 164–66; J. M. Cruse and R. E. Lewis, "David W. Talmage and the Advent of the Cell Selection Theory of Antibody Synthesis," *JI* 153 (1994): 919–24.

23. Silverstein, *History,* 75–76, 79–80.

24. C. Viret and W. Gurr, "The Origin of the 'One Cell-One Antibody' Rule," *JI* 182 (2009): 1229–30.

25. Silverstein, *History,* 80–88; Silverstein, "Splitting."

26. Silverstein, *History,* 75–76.

27. C. A. Janeway, "The Discovery of T Cell Help for B Cell Antibody Formation: A Perspective from the Thirtieth Anniversary of This Discovery," *Immunology and Cell Biology* 77 (1999), 177–79.

28. A. Silverstein, "The Clonal Selection Theory: What It Really Is and Why Modern Challenges Are Misplaced," *Nat Imunol* 3 (2002): 793–96.

29. A. C. Hüntelmann, "Diphtheria Serum and Serotherapy: Development, Production and Regulation in Fin-de-Siècle Germany," *Dynamis* 27 (2007): 107–31; Linton, *Behring,* ch. 4.

30. Z. An, ed., *Therapeutic Monoclonal Antibodies* (Hoboken, N.J., 2009), 21; Linton, *Behring,* 121–47; A. Glatman-Freedman and A. Casadevall, "Serum Therapy for Tuberculosis Revisited: Reappraisal of the Role of Antibody-Mediated Immunity against Mycobacterium Tuberculosis," *Clinical Microbiology Review* 11, no. 3 (1998): 514–32.

31. Rockefeller University, "The First Effective Therapy for Meningococcal Meningitis," n.d.; Semp Inc., "Texas Cerebrospinal Meningitis Epidemic of 1911–12: Saving Lives with New York City Horse Immune Serum"; Anon., "The Specific Antibodies of Anti-Pneumococcal Sera," *American Journal of Public*

Health 14, no. 9 (1924): 767–68; Anon., "Medicine: Pneumonia Cure?," *Time* (May 19, 1924); H. F. Dowling, "The Rise and Fall of Pneumonia-Control Programs," *J Infect Dis* 127, no. 2 (1973): 201–206; S. H. Podolsky, *Pneumonia before Antibiotics: Therapeutic Evolution and Evaluation in Twentieth-Century America* (Baltimore, 2006), ch. 1; H. Marks, *The Progress of Experiment: Science and Therapeutic Reform in the United States* (Cambridge, Eng., 2000), 62–67.

32. A. Cassadevall and M. D. Scharff, "Return to the Past: The Case for Antibody-Based Therapies in Infectious Diseases," *Clin Infect Dis* 21 (1995): 150–61, table 1; Cruse, "Centenary Tribute to Michael Heidelberger"; Gronski, Seiler, and Schwick, "Discovery;" Linton, *Behring,* 328–40, 423–24; An, *Therapeutic,* 21; M. B. Llewelyn, R. E. Hawkins, and S. J. Russell, "Discovery of Antibodies," *BMJ* 305 (1992): 1269–72.

33. Gronski, Seiler, and Schwick, "Discovery of Antitoxins"; L. Harris, "Public Health Administration: Progress in the Treatment of Pneumonia," *American Journal of Public Health* (1924): 620; Anon., "Medicine: Pneumonia Cure?"; Carneiro, *Towards,* 11.

34. C. Nicolle, "Investigations on Typhus: Nobel Lecture," 1928; C. F. McKhann and F. T. Chu, "Antibodies in Placental Extracts," *J Infect Dis* 52, no. 2 (1933): 268–77; C. F. McKhann and F. T. Chu, "Use of Placental Extract in Prevention and Modification of Measles," *American Journal of Diseases of Children* 45 (1933): 475–79; E. J. Cohn et al., "The Characterization of the Protein Fractions of Human Plasma," *Journal of Clinical Investigation* 23, no. 4 (1944): 417–432; C. W. Ordman, C. G. Jennings, and C. A. Janeway, "The Use of Concentrated Normal Human Serum Gamma Globulin (Human Immune Serum Globulin) in the Prevention and Attenuation of Measles," *Journal of Clinical Investigation* 23, no. 4 (1944): 541–49; J. Stokes, E. P. Maris, and S. S. Gellis, "The Use of Concentrated Normal Human Serum Gamma Globulin (Human Immune Serum Globulin) in the Prophylaxis and Treatment of Measles," *Journal of Clinical Investigation* 23, no. 4 (1944): 531–40; H. Ganguli and S. N. Mukherjee, "Placental Globulin in the Prevention of Measles," *BMJ* (11 Dec. 1954): 1395–97; A. N. H. Creager, "Producing Molecular Therapeutics from Human Blood: Edwin Cohn's Wartime Enterprise," in S. de Chadarevian and H. Kamminga, eds., *Molecularizing Biology and Medicine: New Practices and Alliances, 1910s–1970s* (Amsterdam, 1998), 107–139.

35. W. H. Manwaring, "Biochemical Relativity," *Science* 72, no. 1854 (1930): 23–27; W. H. Manwaring, "Renaissance of Pre-Ehrlich Immunology," *JI* 19, no. 2 (1930): 155–63; Gronski, Seiler, and Schwick, "Discovery," 1329; Silverstein, *History,* 67–68, 84.

36. Kay, "Molecular Biology," 216; Kay, *Molecular Vision,* 174–75; D. M. Knowles, *Neoplastic Hematopathology* (Philadelphia, 2001), 44, 176.

37. Cassadevall and Scharff, "Return," 151; A. Cassadevall, D. L. Goldman, and M. Feldmesser, "Antibody-Based Therapies for Infectious Diseases: Renaissance for an Abandoned Arsenal," *Bulletin de l'Institut Pasteur* 95 (1997): 247–57.

38. S. Deshpande, *Enzyme Immunoassays: From Concept to Product Development* (1996), 8–9.

39. Löwy, "Epistemology," 424–25; H. G. Kunkel, R. J. Slater, and R. A. Good, "Relation between Certain Myeloma Proteins and Normal Gamma Globulin," *Proceedings of the Society for Experimental Biology and Medicine* 76 (1951): 190–193; R. J. Slater, S. M. Ward, and H. G. Kunkel, "Immunological Relationships among the Myeloma Proteins," *JEM* 101 (1955): 85–108; J. B. Natvig and J. D. Capra, "Henry J. Kunkel," available online at the National Academies Press website, http://www.nap.edu/openbook.php?record_id=12042&page =224 (accessed 17 Sept. 2014); Rockefeller University, "Henry G. Kunkel (1916–1983), 1975 Albert Lasker Basic Medical Research Award, available online at http://www.rockefeller.edu/about/awards/lasker/hkunkel (accessed 17 Sept. 2014); Rockefeller University, "The Discovery of the Classes and Structures of Immunoglobulin Molecules," available online at http://centennial.rucares.org/index.php?page=Immunoglobulin (accessed 17 Sept. 2014); K. Eichmann, *Köhler's Invention* (Basel, 2005), 39–40.

40. R. G. Lynch, "Plasmacytomas and Basic Immunology," in R. Lynch, ed., *Milestones in Investigative Pathology* (Bethesda, Md., 2009), 17–18. This work was an extension of work that Potter had begun in 1956. See Albert Lasker Basic Medical Research Award to Köhler, Milstein, and Potter, 1984, available online at http://www.laskerfoundation.org/awards/1984_b_description .htm (accessed 17 Sept. 2014); K. Horibata and A. W. Harris, "Mouse Myelomas and Lymphomas in Culture," *Experimental Cell Research* 60, no. 1 (Apr. 1970): 61–77; Eichmann, *Köhler's*, 26, 42; A. Cambrosio and P. Keating, *Exquisite Specificity: The Monoclonal Antibody Revolution* (Oxford, Eng., 1995), 26–27, A. Cambrosio and P. Keating, "Monoclonal Antibodies: From Local to Extended Networks," in A. Thackray, *Private Science: Biotechnology and the Rise of the Molecular Sciences* (Philadelphia, 1998), 165–81, 175; A. Cambrosio and P. Keating, "Between Fact and Technique: The Beginnings of Hybridoma Technology," *J Hist Biol* 25, no. 2 (1982): 175–230, 208–12.

41. N. K. Jerne and A. A. Nordin, "Plaque-Formation in Agar by Single Antibody Producing Cells," *Science* 140, no. 3565 (26 Apr. 1963): 405.

42. T. Staehelin, "Pittsburgh 1962, no. 63 Revisited: Too Many Antibodies, Too Few Ribosomes?" *Scandinavian Journal of Immunology* 62, supp. 1 (2005): 23–26.

43. Interviews with Ivan Lefkovits. Other plaque tests were successfully developed soon after the one devised by Jerne and Nordin. See Söderqvist, *Science*, 236–37; Eichmann, *Köhler's*, 21.

44. G. Chedd, "Nobel Prizes for Antibody Structure," *New Sci* (19 Oct. 1972): 142–43; L. A. Steiner, "Rodney Robert Porter (1917–1985)," *Nature* 317, no. 6036 (1985): 383; G. M. Edelman, "The Evolution of Somatic Selection: The Antibody Tale" (Dec. 1994), in J. F. Crow, ed., *Perspectives on Genetics: Anecdotal, Historical, and Critical Commentaries* (Madison, Wis., 2000), 426–32.

45. Chedd, "Nobel"; Edelman, "Evolution"; Steiner, "Porter"; Eichmann, *Köhler's*, 6–8, 40–41.

46. BII, *Annual Report* (1972), introduction by N. K. Jerne, reprinted in I. Lefkovits, ed., *A Portrait of the Immune System: Scientific Publications of NK Jerne* (London, 1996), 745–52.

47. Interviews with Lefkovits; Söderqvist, *Science*, 258–60, 268.

48. N. K. Jerne, "The Immune System," *Sci Am* (July 1973): 52–60; N. K. Jerne, "Towards a Network Theory of the Immune System," *Annales d'Immunologie* 125C (1974): 373–89; K. Eichmann, *The Network Collective: Rise and Fall of a Scientific Paradigm* (Basel, 2008), ch. 9; Söderqvist, *Science*, 269–73.

49. Söderqvist, *Science*, 274; Moulin, *Dernier*, 12; Eichmann, *Network*, 87–88; Eichmann, *Köhler's*, 23–24.

50. M. Cohn, "Natural History of the Myeloma," *Cold Spring Harbor Symposium on Quantitative Biology* 32 (1967): 211–12; W. Gerhard, T. J. Braciale, and N. R. Klinman, "The Analysis of the Monoclonal Immune Response to Influenza Virus. I. Production of Monoclonal Anti-Viral Antibodies in Vitro," *EJI* 5 (1975): 720–25; G. Köhler and C. Milstein, "Continuous Cultures of Fused Cells Secreting Antibody of Predefined Specificity," *Nature* 256, no. 5517 (1975): 495–97; C. Milstein, "Monoclonal Antibodies," *Sci Am* 243 (1980), 66–75; Eichmann, *Köhler's*, 8–9, 40; Cambrosio and Keating, *Exquisite*, 28.

51. G. Barski, S. Sorieul, and F. Cornefert, "Production of Cells of a "Hybrid" Nature in Cultures in Vitro of Two Cellular Strains in Combination," *Comptes rendus hebdomadaires des seances de l'Academie des sciences* 251 (1960): 1825–27; Eichmann, *Köhler's*, 49–53; R. Cotton, "The Road to Monoclonal Antibodies," unpublished paper in Milstein's papers, MSTN, file D112, Churchill College Archives Centre, Cambridge, Eng.

52. A hapten is partial antigen that can act with a previously existing antibody, but it cannot stimulate more antibody production unless combined with other molecules.

53. J. G. Sinkovics et al., "A System of Tissue Cultures for the Study of a Mouse Leukemia Virus," *J Infect Dis* 119 (1969): 19–38; J. G. Sinkovics, "Early History of Specific Antibody-Producing Lymphocyte Hybridomas," *Cancer Research* 41 (1981): 1246–47; J. G. Sinkovics, "An Interesting Observation Concerning Specific Antibody-Producing Hybridomas," *J Infect Dis* 145 (1982): 135; A. R. Williamson and B. E. G. Wright, "Selection of a Single Antibody-Forming Cell Clone and Its Propagation in Syngeneic Mice," *PNAS* 67 (1970): 1398; A. R. Williamson and B. A. Askonas, "Senescence of an Antibody-Forming Cell Clone," *Nature* 238 (11 Aug. 1972): 337–39; B. A. Askonas and A. R. Williamson, "Factors Affecting the Propagation of a B Cell Clone Forming Antibody to the 2,4-Dinitrophenyl Group," *EJI* 9 (1972): 487; B. A. Askonas, "From Protein Synthesis to Antibody Formation and Cellular Immunity," *Ann Rev Immunol* 8 (1990): 1–21; Interview with Andrew McMichael; Askonas evidence in T. Tansey and P. Caterall, "Technology Transfer in Britain: The Case of Monoclonal Antibodies," in T. Tansey et al., eds., *History of Twentieth Century Medicine Witness Seminars, 1993–1997*, vol. 1 (London, 1997), 1–31, 6–17.

54. R. Klinman, "Antibody with Homogeneous Antigen Binding Produced by Splenic Foci in Organ Culture," *Immunochemistry* 6, no. 5 (1969): 757–59.

55. Interview with Walter Gerhard.

56. W. Gerhard, "The Analysis of the Monoclonal Immune Response to Influenza Virus, II: The Antigenicity of the Viral Hemagglutinin," *JEM* 144 (1976): 985–95; Gerhard, Braciale, and Klinman, "Analysis of the Monoclonal Immune Response"; T. J. Braciale, W. Gerhard, and N. R. Klinman, "Analysis of the Humoral Immune Response to Influenza Virus in Vitro," *JI* 116 (1976): 827–34; H. Koprowski, W. Gerhard, and C. M. Croce, "Production of Antibodies against Influenza Virus by Somatic Cell Hybrids between Mouse Myeloma and Primed Spleen Cells," *PNAS* 74, no. 7 (1977): 2985–88; P. C. Doherty, "Challenged by Complexity: My Twentieth Century in Immunology," *Ann Rev Immunol* 25 (2007): 1–19; Cambrosio and Keating, *Exquisite*, 15–16; R. Vaughan, *Listen to the Music: The Life of Hilary Koprowski* (New York, 2000), 172–73.

57. R. Levy and J. Dilley, "The In Vitro Antibody Response to Cell Surface Antigens, I: The Xenogeneic Response to Human Leukemia Cells," *JI* 119, no. 2 (1977): 387–93; R. Levy and J. Dilley, "The In Vitro Antibody Response to Cell Surface Antigens, II: Monoclonal Antibodies to Human Leukemia Cells," *JI* 119, no. 2 (1977): 394–400; R. Levy, R. Wartnke, R. Dorfman, and J. Haimovich, "The Monoclonality of Human B-Cell Lymphomas," *JEM* 145 (1977): 1014–28; B. Azar, "Profile of Ronald Levy," *PNAS* 107, no. 29 (2010): 12745–46; interviews with Ron Levy and Zenon Stepleswki.

58. Milstein, "Monoclonal."

59. Milstein and his team learned tissue culturing from Abraham Karpas, who was then based in a laboratory next to Milstein at the LMB. Milstein and Cotton had become involved in the fusion of cells primarily to study the activation or expression of antibody genes. By fusing two cells it was hoped that they could find out what controlled the expression of genes in antibodies. By creating a hybrid cell from two different parental antibody cells, Milstein and Cotton wanted to know if the fused antibody would express the two sets of genes from the parental cells, or if only one set of genes would be expressed from the parental cell. The fused antibody was found to express both sets of genes. See A. Karpas, "César Milstein (1927–2002): A Somewhat Personal Reflection," *Trends in Immunology* 23 (2002): 321–22; R. G. H. Cotton and C. Milstein, "Fusion of Two Immunoglobulin-Producing Myeloma Cells," *Nature* 244 (1973): 42–43; Cotton, "Road"; C. Milstein, "Inspiration from Diversity in the Immune System," *New Sci* (21 May 1987): 54–58; Interview with David Secher; J. Schwaber and E. P. Cohen, "Human X Mouse Somatic Cell Hybrid Clone Secreting Immunoglobulins of Both Parental Types," *Nature* 244, no. 5416 (1973): 444–47; J. Schwaber and E. Cohen, "Pattern of Immunoglobulin Synthesis and Assembly in a Human-Mouse Somatic Cell Hybrid Clone," *PNAS* 71, no. 6 (1974): 2203–207; Cambrosio and Keating, "Between."

60. Milstein, "Monoclonal."

61. Waldmann learned the plaque test from Lefkovits. See interview with Herman Waldmann; H. Waldmann, H. Pope, and I. Lefkovits, "Limiting Dilution Analysis of Helper T-Cell Function," *Immunology* 31 (1976): 343–52. Secher made the X63 cell line as part of his and Milstein's investigation of the somatic mutation in B cells thought to determine the specificity of antibodies. Interview with Secher; Cambrosio and Keating, "Between," 209, 211, 214; Eichmann, *Köhler's*, 52–53.

62. M. Goldberg, *Cell Wars: The Immune System's Newest Weapons against Cancer* (New York, 1989), 15.

63. N. Wade, "Hybridomas: The Making of a Revolution," *Science* 215 (1982): 1073–75, 1074; Eichmann, *Köhler's*, 67.

64. Köhler and Milstein, "Continuous"; Milstein, "Monoclonal"; Eichmann, *Köhler's*, 55–70.

CHAPTER 2. A HESITANT START

1. A. Cambrosio and P. Keating, *Exquisite Specificity: The Monoclonal Antibody Revolution* (Oxford, Eng., 1995), 15.

2. Milstein to Vickers, 10 July 1975, MSTN, file C324.

3. J. Newell, "Living Factories—New Drugs from Hybrid Cells," unpublished paper, BBC External Services, 12 Aug. 1975, MSTN, file A/2/A.7; G. P. Winter and K. James, "Antibody Engineering," *Proceedings of the Royal Society B, Biological Sciences* 324, no. 1224 (1989): 537–47.

4. Roche had helped found and sponsor the BII. Interviews with Ivan Lefkovits and Theo Staehelin.

5. Interview with César Milstein; J. Finch, *A Nobel Fellow on Every Floor: A History of the Medical Research Council Laboratory of Molecular Biology* (Cambridge, Eng., 2009), 238; E. M. Tansey and P. Caterall, "Technology Transfer in Britain: The Case of Monoclonal Antibodies," in E. M. Tansey et al., eds., *History of Twentieth Century Medicine Witness Seminars, 1993–1997*, vol. 1 (Apr. 1997): 1–34, 25.

6. Trigwell to Hamlyn, 7 Oct. 1976; Hamlyn to Milstein, 28 Oct. 1976; Milstein to Trigwell, 21 Mar. 1979. All in MSTN, file C324.

7. J. Gowans in Tansey and Caterall, "Technology," 16.

8. Ibid., 8–9, 25–29; S. de Chadarevian, *Designs for Life: Molecular Biology after World War II* (Cambridge, Eng., 2002), 356–57; R. Bud, "From Applied Microbiology to Biotechnology: Science, Medicine and Industrial Renewal," *Notes and Records of the Royal Society* 64 (2010): S17–S29; R. Bud, "Penicillin and the New Elizabethans," *British Journal for the History of Science* 31, no. 3 (1998): 305–33; K. Eichmann, *Köhler's Invention* (Basel, 2005), 91–93; D. Dickson, "California Set to Cash in on British Discovery," *Nature* 279 (1979) 663–64.

9. Anon., "Patent Failure Doomed the NRDC," *New Sci* (1988): 31; T. A. Springer, "César Milstein, the Father of Modern Immunology," *Nat Immunol* 3, no. 6 (2002): 501–503; Interview with John Ashworth; de Chaderevian, *Designs*,

354–55; Bud, "From Applied Microbiology"; M. Sharp et al., "The Management and Coordination of Biotechnology in the U.K., 1980–88," *Proceedings of the Royal Society B, Biological Sciences* 324, no. 1224 (1989): 509–23; ACARD/Advisory Board of Royal Council/Royal Society, *Biotechnology, Report of the Joint Working Party* (London, 1980), 28, MSTN, file C324; Milstein to Thatcher, 17 Apr. 1989, MSTN, file C337; Interview with Milstein; L. Marks, "The Story of César Milstein and Mabs," 2013, available online at http://www.whatisbiotech nology.org/exhibitions/milstein/patents (accessed 18 Sept. 2014).

10. Milstein recorded sending a sample of the cell line X63.Ag8 to Koprowski on 7 Sept. 1976, based on a request the month before; MSTN, file C282, MSTN, file C285. See also H. Koprowski, W. Gerhard, and C. Croce, "Process for Providing Viral Antibodies by Fusing and Viral Antibody Producing Cell and a Myeloma Cell to Provide a Fused Cell Hybrid Culture and Collecting Viral Antibodies" (filed 15 June 1977, issued 1 Apr. 1980), U.S. Patent 4,196,265; H. Koprowski and C. Croce, "Method of Producing Tumor Antibodies" (filed 28 Apr. 1978, issued 23 Oct. 1979), U.S. Patent 4,172,124.

11. N. Wade, "Hybridomas: A Potent New Biotechnology," *Science* 208, no. 4445 (1980): 692–93; G. Fjermedal, *Magic Bullets* (New York, 1984), 185–88; R. Vaughan, *Listen to the Music: The Life of Hilary Koprowski* (New York, 2000), 178; Fjermedal, *Magic*, 180–84.

12. H. Koprowski and C. Croce, "Hybridomas Revisited," *Science* 210, no. 4467 (1980): 248; Vaughan, *Listen*, 177; Koprowski to Milstein, 22 Apr. 1977, MSTN, file C285; Milstein to Koprowski, 4 May 1977, with penciled note, MSTN, file C324; Pressman to Koprowski, 28 Feb. 1978, MSTN, file C283, folder 2; U.S. Patents 4,172,124 and 4,196,265.

13. Interview with Walter Gerhard; Koprowski to Milstein, 19 Nov. 1976; Koprowski to Milstein, 6 July 1978; Milstein to Koprowski, 17 July 1978; Koprowski to Milstein, 1 Aug. 1978, all in MSTN, file C324.

14. Milstein's penciled note on Tridgell to Milstein, 16 Mar. 1979; Milstein to Tridgell, 21 Mar. 1979, both in MSTN, file C324.

15. Vaughan, *Listen*, 178. Koprowski had form as a risk-taker. In 1986 controversy arose over some field trials that he had conducted with a recombinant-based rabies vaccine in cattle without the Argentinian government's approval and without informing farm workers of the vaccine's potential risks. Koprowski argued that the vaccine was safe and saw the fuss as disproportionate and tied up with Argentinian politics. Vaughan, *Listen*, 198–200. See also D. Finley, *Mad Dogs: The New Rabies Plague* (College Station, Tex., 1998), 43–45.

16. Interview with Michael Clark; Kemp to Milstein, 11 Jan. 1979, MSTN, file C281; Scharff to Milstein, 17 Oct. 1977, MSTN, file C284; Anon. to Milstein, 15 Apr. 1982, MSTN, file 306, folder 2.

17. Milstein to Farnborough, 30 May 1977, MSTN, file C285; Anon. to Milstein, 15 Apr. 1982, MSTN, file 306, folder 2; Kemp to Milstein, 11 Jan. 1979, MSTN, file C281.

18. Interview with Hilary Koprowski; Koprowski and Croce, "Hybridomas." The Wistar team's mindset is discussed in detail in A. Cambrosio and P. Keating, "Between Fact and Technique: The Beginnings of Hybridoma Technology," *J Hist Biol* 25, no. 2 (1992): 175–230; Cambrosio and Keating, *Exquisite*, 14; Vaughan, *Listen*, 174–75; Eichmann, *Köhler's Invention*, 51–52.

19. Trucco to Milstein, 24 Feb 1982, MSTN, file H135; Reiter to Milstein, 25 May 1978, MSTN, file C283, folder 2; Reinisch to Milstein, 16 May 1980, MSTN, file C324.

20. The ability to patent research conducted in institutions funded by the U.S. government was formalized in December 1980 with the Bayh-Dole Act. Vaughan, *Listen*, 146.

21. Tansey and Caterall, "Technology," 9; Interview with Milstein; S. Smith Hughes, "Making Dollars Out of DNA: The First Major Patent in Biotechnology and the Commercialization of Molecular Biology, 1974–1980," *Isis* 92 (2001): 541–75; D. J. Kevles, "Diamond v. Chakrabarty and Beyond: The Political Economy of Patenting Life," in A. Thackray, ed., *Private Science: Biotechnology and the Rise of the Molecular Sciences* (Philadelphia, 1988), 66–79.

22. D. Dickson, "Wistar Denied Monoclonal Antibody Patent in U.K.," *Science* 222, no. 23 (1983): 1309; Editorial, "Spin-off from Cell Fusion," *Lancet* 309, no. 8024 (1977): 1242–243. As late as 1990 the Wistar patents were still under scrutiny in Japan, having been disputed at least twenty-five times. See M. MacKenzie, P. Keating and A. Cambrosio, "Patents and Free Scientific Information in Biotechnology: Making Monoclonal Antibodies Proprietary," *Science, Technology and Human Values* 15, no. 1 (1990): 65–83, 70–71.

23. The events surrounding the NRDC's decision not to patent Mabs are described in detail by contemporary witnesses in Tansey and Caterall, "Technology," and in Finch, *Nobel*, 238–39.

24. Interview with Lefkovits; Milstein to Koprowski, 16 Feb. 1981, MSTN, file C324; Interview with Milstein; C. Milstein, "With the Benefit of Hindsight," *Immunology Today* 8 (2000): 359–64, 360; Marks, "Story."

25. D. Secher, "The Making of Mabs," *MRC News* (1993): 26, cited in S. de Chadarevian, "The Making of an Entrepreneurial Science," *Isis* 102 (2011): 601–33.

26. D. Secher in Tansey and Caterall, "Technology," 27; Finch, *Nobel*, 238 (includes quotation); Interview with Milstein; Milstein, "Benefit," 360; de Chadarevian, *Designs*, 358; de Chadarevian, "Entrepreneurial"; Anon., "Awards to Inventors—MRC Scheme," 26 Oct. 1989; and Milstein, "Draft Memorandum on MRC Policy for Research Supported by Industry or Other External Sources," unpublished paper, 2 June 1988, MSTN, file F19.

27. Interview with Milstein; Secher and Milstein in Tansey and Caterall, "Technology," 7–8, 27–28, 29; de Chadarevian, *Designs*, 358–62; C. Milstein, "Monoclonal Antibodies," *Sci Am* 243 (1980): 66–75.

28. Secher in Tansey and Caterall, "Technology," 17.

29. Interview with David Secher; Milstein, Early manuscript of "Messing About with Isotopes," Miami Winter Symposium, 1981, MSTN, file D23. Interview

with John Jarvis; Milstein in Tansey and Caterall, "Technology," 20;
C. Milstein, "The Hybridoma Revolution: An Offshoot of Basic Research,"
BioEssays 21 (1999): 966–73, 968; G. Galfré and C. Milstein, "Preparation of
Monoclonal Antibodies: Strategies and Procedures," *Methods in Enzymology*
73 (1981): 3–46; Marks, "Story."

30. Milstein, Samples Notebook, MSTN, file C281, folder 1; Wilkinson to Milstein, 20 Jan. 1976, Milstein to Wilkinson, 29 Jan. 1976, Wilkinson to Milstein, 24 Dec. 1976, and Milstein to Wilkinson, 4 May 1977, all in MSTN, file
C285; Wilkinson to Milstein, 14 Mar. 1976, Milstein to Wilkinson, 12 Jan.
1977, and Wilkinson to Milstein, 28 Mar. 1977, all in MSTN, file C284. Another researcher who was sent an early sample apparently had no problem
growing the cells. See Van Venrooij to Milstein, 23 Jan. 1976, MSTN, file
C284.

31. Macnab to Milstein, 18 Oct. 1977, MSTN, file C285; Köhler in Tansey and
Caterall, "Technology," 20; H. Lemke, G. J. Hämmerling, C. Höhmann,
and K. Rajewsky, "Hybrid Cell Lines Secreting Monoclonal Antibody Specific for Major Histocompatibility Antigens of the Mouse," *Nature* 271, no.
5642 (1978): 248–51.

32. Kapatos to Milstein, 22 Oct. 1983, MSTN, file 301. Problems with medium
were also reported in Nabholz to Milstein, 2 Apr. 1978, MSTN, file C283, file
2; Interview with Jarvis. For tissue culture difficulties, see B. P. Lucey, W. A.
Nelson-Rees, and G. M. Hutchins, "Henrietta Lacks, HeLa Cells, and Cell
Contamination," *Archives of Pathology and Laboratory Medicine* 133, no. 9
(2009): 1463–67; D. Wilson, "The Early History of Tissue Culture in Britain:
The Interwar Years," *Social History of Medicine* 18, no. 2 (2005): 225–43.

33. Interview with Jarvis. The informality of transferring cell lines from one
laboratory to another was very common. See R. Skoot, *The Immortal Life of
Henrietta Lacks* (New York, 2010), 110–11.

34. Interview with Jarvis; Jarvis to Scott, 24 Oct. 1977; Embleton to Milstein,
11 May 1977; Scott to Jarvis, 7 Nov. 1977; all in MSTN, file C285; Kumar to
Milstein, 10 Feb. 1978, and Martin to Milstein, 16 Oct. 1978, all in MSTN,
file C283, folder 2; Gordon to Milstein, 21 June 1983, MSTN, file C308;
Maeder to Milstein, 20 July 1983, and Booth to Jarvis, 4 Aug. 1983, all in
MSTN, file C308; Booth to Jarvis, 20 Mar. 1984, MSTN, file C309; Firth to
De Bishnu, 11 Oct. 1984, MSTN, file C316; Firth to Dubey, 2 Apr. 1984, Judy
to John, 11 July 1984; Dubey to Milstein, 20 July 1984; Firth to Dubey, 31 July
1984; Dubey to M/S Olrose Freight Ltd, 9 Aug. 1984, De to Milstein, 14 Nov.
1984, all in MSTN, file C316; Wilsnack to Milstein 5 Mar. 1976, MSTN, file
C284; Capra to Milstein, 1 Apr. 1985, MSTN, file H27; Jarvis to Scott, 24 Oct.
1977 and Scott to Jarvis 7 Nov. 1977, MSTN, file C285; Firth to Kanoh, 7 Mar.
1984, MSTN, file C303; Jarvis to Trucco, 3 Oct. 1991, MSTN, file C332.

35. Volkers to Milstein, 12 Oct. 1977 and 11 Nov. 1977, MSTN, file C281, folder 1;
Booth to Jarvis, 20 Mar. 1984, MSTN, file C309; Carter to Jarvis, 16 Nov.
1983, MSTN, file C308.

36. Interview with Jarvis. Freezing temporarily interrupts cell division and metabolism. This is a well-established process in tissue culture. See Skoot, *Immortal*, 114.

37. Wilsnack to Milstein, 5 Mar. 1976, MSTN, file C284; H. Zola and D. Brocks, "Techniques for the Production and Characterization of Monoclonal Antibodies," in J. G. R. Hurrell, ed., *Monoclonal Hybridoma Antibodies: Techniques and Applications* (Boca Raton, Fla., 1982), 4–5, cited in Cambrosio and Keating, *Exquisite*, 52–53; A. Cambrosio and P. Keating, "'Going Monoclonal': Art, Science, and Magic in the Day-to-Day Use of Hybridoma Technology," *Social Problems* 35, no. 3 (1988): 244–60.

38. Jarvis to Miller, 16 Dec. 1982, MSTN, file C307. Other letters revealing the uncertainties appear in Nabholz to Milstein, 2 Apr. 1978, MSTN, file C283, folder 2; Voigt to Milstein, 20 June 1980 and Karpas to Voigt, 15 July 1980, both contained in MSTN, file C306, folder 2; Joshua to Jarvis, 1 June 1982, MSTN, file C307; and Hartman to Milstein, 29 Oct. 1982, MSTN, file C301. By 1984 cells were being sent out with detailed instructions on how they should be handled on receipt and with a request for a viability report. See guidelines for cell line NG9/9.1.21, 6 Aug. 1984, MSTN, file C294; Jarvis to Jenny, Sera-Lab, 14 Jan. 1982, MSTN, file C305.

39. EMBO, *Hybridoma Techniques*, SKMB Course 1980 Basel (Cold Spring Harbor, N.Y.), cited in Cambrosio and Keating, *Exquisite*, 53; Interview with Milstein.

40. Interview in Cambrosio and Keating, *Exquisite*, 53, 69.

41. Ibid., 57.

42. The different protocols reflected modifications made to the technique, some of which were valued and others which were rejected. The basic technique, however, remained essentially the same. See Cambrosio and Keating, *Exquisite*, 57, 62–68.

43. Interview with Clark.

44. Cambrosio and Keating, "Going Monoclonal."

45. C. Milstein and J. C. Howard, "The First "Useful" Hybridoma," *Current Contents* 14 (1993): 9; Interview with Milstein.

46. Cambrosio and Keating, *Exquisite*, 30; Milstein to Froud, 17 Sept. 1993, MSTN, file H58. Milstein originally obtained Cohn's cells from Alan Munro, who worked at the LMB after a sabbatical at the Salk Institute. The cell lines were developed by Michael Potter. See Milstein, Early Manuscript for "Messing About with Isotopes," 2, unpublished manuscript, MSTN, file D23. For the quotation, see Cohn to Milstein, 17 Jan. 1977, MSTN, file C285; see also Milstein, Samples Notebook, MSTN, file C281, folder 1.

47. For Milstein's notebook see http://www.whatisbiotechnology.org/exhibitions/milstein/world (accessed 18 Sept. 2014); Cambrosio and Keating, *Exquisite*, 15.

48. Interview with Milstein. Köhler and Milstein's allusion to the medical and industrial potential of Mabs in their *Nature* article was primarily within the

context of their value for immunoassays and passive therapy. See Milstein, "The Hybridoma Revolution," 966; Secher in Tansey and Caterall, "Technology," 17; Cambrosio and Keating, *Exquisite*, 30, 32.

49. Milstein, Samples notebook, MSTN, file C281, file 1. The interest the 1997 *Nature* article generated among scientists can be seen in Leeuwenhoekhuis to Milstein, 23 May 77, Edwards to Milstein, 12 May 1977, Embleton to Milstein, 15 Apr. 1977, Bradford to Milstein, 18 July 1977, and Jansen to Milstein, 25 Oct. 1977, MSTN, file C285.

50. The prefix "hist" comes from the Greek word "tissue." Histocompatibility denotes compatibility between tissues. The major histocompatibility complex is a group of genes that code for proteins found on the surfaces of cells that help the immune system to recognize foreign substances.

51. G. Galfré, S. C. Howe, C. Milstein, G. W. Butcher, and J. C. Howard, "Antibodies to Major Histocompatability Antigens Produced by Hybrid Cell Lines," *Nature* 266 (1977): 550–52. This paper had been cited in more than 1,490 publications by 1993. By comparison Milstein and Köhler's article in *Nature* in 1975 was cited 6,905 times. See Milstein and Howard, "First," 9; Cambrosio and Keating, *Exquisite*, 34, and "Between," 222.

52. K. I. Welsh, "News and Views: Antibody Production Made Easier," *Nature* 266 (1977): 495. Welsh was at the informal meeting between NRDC officials and Richard Batchelor, then director of the McIndoe Memorial Research Unit at the Queen Victoria Hospital in East Grinstead. The purpose of the meeting was to help NRDC officials understand the applicability of Mabs. According to Batchelor, the NRDC officials at the meeting were "hopeless" in that they were unable to understand Mabs' potential. He himself was excited about the possibilities for his specialty, transplant immunology. Interview with Richard Batchelor. This recollection was shared by Ken Welsh; see Ken Welsh, emails to Lara Marks, 28 July 2011 and 30 July 2011.

53. Welsh, "News and Views."

54. Editorial, "Spin-Off from Cell Fusion," *Lancet* 309, no. 8024 (1977): 1242–43.

55. I. A. F. Williams, G. Galfré, and C. Milstein, "Analysis of Cell Surfaces by Xenogeneic Myeloma-Hybrid Antibodies: Differentiation Antigens of Rat Lymphocytes," *Cell* 12, no. 3 (1977): 663–73. By 1993, this paper had been cited 660 times. See also Milstein and Howard, "First." For Milstein's work with Williams, see Chapter 4. See also Interview with Milstein. Capturing the enthusiasm generated by the paper, one biologist wrote, "Your cell paper . . . is beautiful." Capechhi to Milstein, 19 Apr. 1978, MSTN, file C283.

56. E. Haber, "Introduction," in E. Haber and R. M. Krauser, eds., *Antibodies in Human Diagnosis and Therapy* (New York, 1977), 1–6.

57. Ibid., 3.

58. Milstein to Tridgell, 7 Mar. 1979, MSTN, file C325; Judy to Bronwen, 11 July 1984, MSTN, file C316.

59. Dowding to La Placa, Bologna, 14 Jan. 1981, MSTN, file C306.

60. Milstein to Stanley, 6 July 1983, MSTN, file C308; Firth to Campbell, 2 May 1984, MSTN, file C299.

61. Ken Welsh, emails to Lara Marks, 28 July 2011 and 30 July 2011.

62. T. Lloyd, *Dinosaur and Co.: Studies in Corporate Evolution* (London, 1984), 53–54.

63. Murray to Milstein, 23 Mar. 1977; Hamlyn to Milstein, 2 May 1977; Milstein to Murray, 4 May 1977; Murray to Milstein, 6 May 1977; Murray to Milstein, 19 July 1977; all in MSTN, file F13. Volkers to CM, 22 Sept. 1977; Volkers to Milstein, 12 Oct. 1977; Volkers to Milstein, 16 Dec. 1977; Milstein to Volkers, 17 Feb. 1978; all in MSTN, file C281. Murray to Vittery, 7 Nov. 1977; Note from Pat Webb, Feb. 1978; Murray, "An Important Addition to the Sera-Lab Product Range," n.d; all in MSTN, file F13. For information relating to the contract, see Vittery to Murray, 3 May 1978; Murray to Vittery, 5 May 1978; Vittery to Murray, 4 July 1978; Milstein to Vittery, 17 July 1978; Milstein to Vittery, 18 Oct. 1978; all in MSTN, file F13.

64. Milstein to Nicholls, 20 Apr. 1978, MSTN, file C281; Murray to Milstein, 25 Apr. 1978, MSTN, file F14; Murray to Milstein, 27 Nov. 1980; Kemp to Jarvis, 5 Dec. 1980; Murray to Milstein, 7 May 1981; Jarvis to Jenny, 14 Jan. 1982; "Agreement between MRC and Sera-Lab Ltd," 30 June 1983; all in MSTN, file C305. In 1980 MRC received £2,014 out of the £11,065 income that Sera-Lab had made as part of the distribution agreement for the LMB and a laboratory in Oxford. Handwritten note, n.d., MSTN, file C305, folder 1; F. W. Matthews, "Draft Distribution of Research Reagents," 20 Jan. 1983, MSTN, file C326; Murray to Milstein, 21 July 1980, MSTN, file F15.

CHAPTER 3. BREAKTHROUGHS AT THE BENCH

1. J. M. Davie, "Hybridomas: A Revolution in Reagent Production," *Pharmaceutical Review* 34 (1982): 115–18; A. S. Rabson in *The Cancer Letter* 8, no. 3 (1982); A. Cambrosio and P. Keating, *Exquisite Specificity: The Monoclonal Antibody Revolution* (Oxford, Eng., 1995), 86–90.

2. P. Keating and A. Cambrosio, *Biomedical Platforms: Realigning the Normal and the Pathological in Late Twentieth Century Medicine* (London, 2003), 172; C. Milstein, "With the Benefit of Hindsight," *Review: Immunology Today* 21, no. 8 (2000): 359–64; Milstein lecture, MRC conference celebrating Mabs 25th anniversary, unpublished paper, MSTN, file D65; Celltech publication, n.d., MSTN, file E11.

3. Williams to Milstein, 3 Jan. 1986, MSTN, file H149; Milstein's penciled note on "Notes for Lecture(s) for Japan," unpublished ms., MSTN, file D38.

4. C. Milstein, "From the Structure of Antibodies to the Diversification of Antibodies of the Immune System," Nobel Lecture, 8 Dec. 1984, repr. *EMBO J* 4, no. 5 (1985): 1083–92, 1086; Interview with Steven Sacks.

5. C. Milstein, "Notes for Plenary Lecture at Cytology Workshop," n.d., unpublished ms., MSTN, file D66; Milstein, "Notes on Lecture(s) for Japan"; C. Milstein, "The Impact of Monoclonal Antibodies on Studies of Differenti-

ation of Lymphocytes," in A. Bernard et al., *Leucocyte Typing: Human Leuco-cyte Differentiation Antigens Detected by Monoclonal Antibodies* (Berlin, 1984), 3–8.

6. Cambrosio and Keating, *Exquisite,* 120; Milstein, "From the Structure of Antibodies," 1086; Interview with César Milstein.

7. Interview with Claudio Cuello; A. C. Cuello, "Augusto Claudio Guillermo Cuello," in L. R. Squire, *The History of Neuroscience in Autobiography,* vol. 3 (London, 2001), 168–213; Milstein to the Registrar, Oxford University, 13 Sept 1982, MSTN, file H45.

8. Interview with Cuello; A. C. Cuello, G. Galfré, and C. Milstein, "Detection of Substance P in the Central Nervous System by a Monoclonal Antibody," *PNAS* 76, no. 7 (1979): 3532–36; J. T. Hughes, "The Neuroanatomy of the Spinal Cord," *Paraplegia* 27 (1989): 90–98, esp. 92; L. Osenfeld, "A Golden Age of Clinical Chemistry: 1948–1960," *Clin Chem* 46 (2000): 1705–14.

9. J. C. Howard, "The Future of Immunology," British Pharmaceutical Society Conference, Newcastle, 19 Nov. 1980, unpublished ms., 8–9, MSTN, file H78

10. A. Fagraeus and N. R. Bergquist, "The Raison D'être of Standards in Indi-rect Immunofluorescence," *Annals of New York Academy of Sciences* 254, no. 1 (1975): 69–76.

11. The guinea-pig serum had been developed by Cuello's Japanese colleague Ichiro Kanazawa; Cuello and his team's work offered the first most compre-hensive "neuroanatomical mapping of a neuroactive peptide with transmitter -like characteristics." It also demonstrated that such peptides were not stored at random or in any cell, but rather in defined neuronal systems and as such had their own unique properties. Interview with Cuello; A. C. Cuello, J. M. Polak, and A. Pearse, "Substance P: A Naturally Occurring Transmitter in Human Spinal Cord," *Lancet* 2 (1976): 1054–56; A. C. Cuello and I. Kanazawa, "The Distribution of Substance P Immunoreactive Fibers in the Rat Central Nervous System," *Journal of Comparative Neurology* 178 (1978): 129–56; Cuello, "Augusto," 189; Cuello, Galfré, and Milstein, "Detection"; Hughes, "Neuroanatomy," 92.

12. Cuello, "Augusto," 195, 199; Interview with Cuello; E. P. Pioro, J. T, Hughes, and A. C. Cuello, "Demonstration of Substance P Immunoreactivity in the Nucleus Dorsalis of Human Spinal Cord," *Neuroscience Letter* 51 (1984), 61–65; J. K. Mai, P. H. Stephens, A. Hopf, and A. C. Cuello, "Substance P in the Human Brain," *Neuroscience* 17 (1986): 709–39.

13. Cuello to Milstein, 31 July 1981, MSTN, file H44; A. Consolazione, C. Milstein, B. Wright, and A. C. Cuello, "Immunocytochemical Detection of Serotonin with Monoclonal Antibodies," *Journal of Histochemistry and Cyto-chemistry* 29, no. 12 (1981): 1425–30; P. Somogyi et al., "Synaptic Connections of Enkephalin-Immunoreactive Nerve Terminals in the Neostriatum: A Corre-lated Light and Electron Microscopic Study," *Journal of Neurocytology* 11 (1982): 779–807; A. C. Cuello, J. V. Priestly, and C. Milstein, "Immunocytochemistry

with Internally Labelled Monoclonal Antibodies," *PNAS* 79, no. 2 (1982): 665–69; D. Boorsma, A. C. Cuello, and F. W. Van Leeuwen, "Direct Immunocytochemistry with Horseradish Peroxidase Conjugated with Monoclonal Antibody against Substance P," *Journal of Histochemistry and Cytochemistry* 30 (1982): 1211–16; A. C. Cuello, C. Milstein, and J. V. Priestley, "Use of Monoclonal Antibodies in Immunocytochemistry with Special Reference to the Central Nervous System," *Brain Research Bulletin* 5 (1980): 575–78; A. C. Cuello and C. Milstein, "Hybridoma Technology in Immunocytochemistry," *BioEssays* 1, no. 4 (1984): 178–79; Cuello, "Augusto," 196, 200–201.

14. Haber, "Introduction"; Cuello, Priestly, and Milstein, "Immunocytochemistry"; Cuello, "Augusto," 196; A. C. Cuello et al., "Development and Application of a Monoclonal Rat Peroxidase Antiperoxidase (PAP) Immunocytochemical Reagent," *Histochemistry* 80 (1984): 257–61; C. Milstein, M. R. Clark, G. Galfré, and A. C. Cuello, "Monoclonal Antibodies from Hybrid Myelomas," in M. Fougereau and J. Dausset, eds., *Fourth International Congress of Immunology, 80: Progress in Immunology*, vol. 4 (London, 1980), 17–33, 29; Cuello and Milstein, "Hybridoma."

15. Milstein, "Notes on Lecture(s) for Japan," 11; C. Milstein and A. C. Cuello, "Hybrid Hybridomas and the Production of Bi-Specific Monoclonal Antibodies," *Immunology Today* 5, no. 10 (1984): 299–304. For details on the many ways in which bispecifics were used for immunodiagnosis, see M. A. Ritter and H. M. Ladyman, *Monoclonal Antibodies: Production, Engineering and Clinical Application* (Cambridge, Eng., 1995), 132. While Milstein and Cuello were the first to demonstrate the possibility to make bispecific Mabs, they were unable to patent the method because a scientist based at the University of Texas had already taken out a patent based on a theoretical experiment. Crawley to Bush, 19 Sept. 1984, MSTN, file C326; Interview with Milstein.

16. Jones to Milstein, 10 Nov. 1981, MSTN, file H44; E. S. Jaffe, "Classification of Lymphoid Neoplasms: The Microscope as a Tool for Disease Discovery," *Blood* 112, no. 12 (2008): 4384–99.

17. E. Wilander, "Letter to the Editor," *Lancet;* A. C. Cuello, C. A. Wells, C. Milstein, "Letter to the Editor," *Lancet*, sent 16 June 1982; both in MSTN, file H45. The suggestion to use the Mab against serotonin for diagnosing carcinoid tumors appeared first in Consolazione et al., "Immunocytochemical Detection of Serotonin with Monoclonal Antibodies"; Vice President of Research and Development, Cytogen, in "Speakers at Battelle '82 Bearish on Market Future, Medical Uses of Monoclonals," *McGraw-Hill's Biotechnology Newswatch* 2, no. 14 (1982): 6, cited in Cambrosio and Keating, *Exquisite*, 109; D. E. Yelton and M. D. Scharff, "Monoclonal Antibodies: A Powerful New Tool in Biology and Medicine," *Annual Review of Biochemistry* 50 (1981): 657–80.

18. Interview with Michael Clark; A. Cambrosio and P. Keating, "A Matter of FACS: Constituting Novel Entities in Immunology," *Medical Anthropology Quarterly* 6, no. 4 (1992): 362–84; P. Keating and A. Cambrosio, "'Ours Is

an Engineering Approach': Flow Cytometry and the Constitution of Human T-Cell Subsets," *J Hist Biol* 27, no. 3 (1994): 449–79, esp. 454; D. J. Arndt-Jovin and T. M. Jovin, "Automated Cell Sorting with Flow Systems," *Annual Review of Biophysics and Bioengineering* 7 (1978): 527–58; F. Traganos, "Flow Cytometry: Principles and Applications, II," *Cancer Investigation* 2, no. 3 (1984): 239–58.

19. R. G. Miller et al., "Usage of the Flow Cytometer-Cell Sorter," *J Immunol Methods* 47 (1981): 13–24; Arndt-Jovin and Jovin, "Automated," 536; Keating and Cambrosio, *Biomedical,* 119–22; L. A. Herzenberg and L. A. Herzenberg, "Genetics, FACS, Immunology and Redox: A Tale of Two Lives Intertwined," *Ann Rev Immunol* 22 (2004): 1–31, 16; L. A. Herzenberg et al., "The History and Future of Fluorescence Activated Cell Sorter and Flow Cytometry: A View from Stanford," *Clin Chem* 48, no. 10 (2002): 1819–27; Keating and Cambrosio, "Ours"; L. A. Herzenberg, S. C. De Rosa, and L. A. Herzenberg, "Monoclonal Antibodies and the FACS: Complementary Tools for Immunobiology and Medicine," *Review: Immunology Today* 21, no. 8 (2000): 383–90; Anon., "Herzenberg, Inventor of Cell Sorter, Wins Kyoto Prize," *Stanford Report,* 9 June 2006.

20. Milstein, unpublished paper for Cytology Workshop, n.d., MSTN, file D66; Herzenberg and Herzenberg, "Genetics," 16; C. Milstein and L. Herzenberg, "T and B Cell Hybrids," in E. Sercarz, L. Herzenberg, and C. F. Fox, eds., *Immune System: Genetics and Regulation, ICN-UCLA Symposia on Molecular and Cellular Biology,* vol. 6 (New York, 1977), 273–75; V. T. Oi, P. P. Jones, J. W. Goding, and L. A. Herzenberg, "Properties of Monoclonal Antibodies to Mouse Ig Allotypes, H-2 and Ia Antigens," *Current Topics in Microbiology and Immunology* 81 (1978): 115–20.

21. Arndt-Jovin and Jovin, "Automated"; Traganos, "Flow," 239; A. Cambrosio and P. Keating, "A Matter of FACS: Constituting Novel Entities in Immunology," *Medical Anthropology Quarterly,* 6, no. 4 (1992): 362–84; Keating, Cambrosio, " 'Ours," 454.

22. C. Milstein, "Monoclonal Antibodies," *Sci Am* 243 (1980): 56–65. In the early 1970s many immunologists were debating the function of B and T cells and their relationship with other leukocyte subsets. See Keating and Cambrosio, *Biomedical,* 159–66.

23. Keating and Cambrosio, *Biomedical,* ch. 4.

24. Ibid., 89; Milstein, "Benefit," 359; Milstein, "The Hybridoma Revolution: An Offshoot of Basic Research," *BioEssays* 21, no. 11 (1999): 966–73, esp. 970. Early discoverers of differentiation antigens were perplexed about the function of such entities, believing that the presence of a distinctive surface molecule was inadequate for explaining the ways that cells recognized each other. See Keating and Cambrosio, *Biomedical,* 101.

25. Williams, unpublished recollections, ca. 1986, MSTN, file H149; R. J. Morris and A. F. Williams, "Antigens on Mouse and Rat Antiserum against Rat Brain: The Quantitative Analysis of a Xenogeneic Antiserum," *EJI* 5 (1975):

274–81; R. Morris, "Thy-1, the Enigmatic Extrovert on the Neuronal Surface," *BioEssays* 14, no. 10 (1992): 715–22.

26. Williams, unpublished recollections.

27. C. Milstein, Cytology Workshop paper.

28. Milstein, "Hybridoma," 969; Milstein, "Monoclonal"; Interview with Milstein; Williams, recollections; M. J. Crumpton, "Alan Frederick Williams," *Biographical Memoirs of the Fellows of the Royal Society* 50 (2004): 351–66.

29. Milstein, "Hybridoma," 969; Milstein, "Monoclonal"; C. Milstein, "Inspiration from Diversity in the Immune System," *New Sci* (21 May 1987): 54–58.

30. A. F. Williams, G. Galfré, and C. Milstein, "Analysis of Cell Surfaces by Xenogeneic Myeloma-Hybrid Antibodies: Differentiation Antigens of Rat Lymphocytes," *Cell* 12 (1977): 663–73; Milstein, "Inspiration," 58.

31. C. J. Barnstable et al., "Production of Monoclonal Antibodies to Group A Erythrocytes, HLA and Other Human Cell Surface Antigens—New Tools for Genetic Analysis," *Cell* 14 (1978): 9–20; Milstein, "Hybridoma," 969; Interview with Andrew McMichael. For more on Askonas, see Chapter 1.

32. Interview with McMichael.

33. Ibid.

34. Ibid.; A. J. McMichael et al., "A Human Thymocyte Antigen Defined by a Hybrid Myeloma Monoclonal Antibody," *EJI* 9, no. 3 (1979): 205–10; Milstein, "Monoclonal Antibodies" and "Hybridoma Revolution," 970; M. S. Neuberger and B. A. Askonas, "César Milstein CH. 8 October 1927–24 March 2002," *Biographical Memoirs of the Fellows of the Royal Society* 51 (2005): 267–89, 277.

35. Keating and Cambrosio, *Biomedical*, 171; Keating and Cambrosio, "Ours," 471–73; Interview with McMichael; C. Milstein and L. A. Herzenberg, "T and B Cell Hybrids: Regulatory Genetics of the Immune System," repr. *Regulatory Genetics of the Immune System, ICN-UCLA Symposia on Molecular and Cellular Biology* 6 (1977): 273–75; Cambrosio and Keating, *Exquisite*, 92–93. Williams discussed the utility of Mabs just before the *Cell* publication with Schlossman at the Third International Congress of Immunology, Sydney, in July 1977, disclosing the techniques to develop Mabs against rat T-cells and how Mabs could be produced against human antigens. Williams, unpublished recollections.

36. Keating and Cambrosio, *Biomedical*, 171; G. Goldstein, "Monoclonal Antibody Specificity: Orthoclone OKT3 T-Cell Blocker," *Nephron* 46, supp. 1 (1987): 5–11; E. Shorter, *The Health Century* (New York, 1987), 254–55.

37. P. Kung et al., "Monoclonal Antibodies Defining Distinctive Human T Cell Surface Antigens," *Science* 206, no. 4416 (1979): 347–39; E. L. Reinherz et al., "Discrete Stages of Human Intrathymic Differentiation: Analysis of Normal Thymocytes and Leukemic Lymphoblasts of T-Cell Lineage," *PNAS* 77, no. 3 (1980): 1588–92; Goldstein, "Monoclonal"; Shorter, *Health*, 254–55; Keating and Cambrosio, *Biomedical*, 171–74. Schlossman took out a patent on these Mabs. Milstein found this striking, since he and Williams did not ap-

ply for patents for the rat antigens they had developed. Interview with Milstein.

38. Keating and Cambrosio, *Biomedical,* 171, 173, 399; Shorter, *Health,* 255.
39. Interview with McMichael; Milstein, "Inspiration," 58.
40. Keating and Cambrosio, "Ours," 468; Cambrosio and Keating, *Exquisite,* 93–98.
41. Interviews with Robert Tindle, Kelly Sapsford, and Jane Pelly; Murray to Milstein, 7 May 1981, MSTN, file F16.
42. Milstein to Vittery, 5 May 1978; Appendix to "Contract with Sera-Lab," n.d; Trucco to Murray, 23 Oct. 1978; all in MSTN, file F13. Murray to Milstein, 25 Apr. 1979; Appendix to "Contract with Sera-Lab," 1979; Cox to Williams, 7 Aug. 1979; Appendix attached to letter from Cox to Murray, 15 Aug. 1979; all in MSTN, file F14. Murray to Loder, 22 Feb. 1980, MSTN, file F15; McMichael to Milstein, 24 Mar. 1980, MSTN, file H108. Hamlyn to Cuello, 4 Dec. 1981; Hamlyn to Murray, 18 Dec. 1981; and Hamlyn to Milstein, 18 Dec. 1981; all in MSTN, file F16. Murray to Milstein, 12 Feb. 1982, MSTN, file F17; Interviews with Tindle, Sapsford, and Pelly.
43. Chapters 1 and 2; Cohn to Milstein, 9 June 1977, MSTN, file C285; Cambrosio and Keating, *Exquisite,* 99–100; A. Cambrosio and P. Keating, "Monoclonal Antibodies: From Local to Extended Networks," in A. Thackray, *Private Science: Biotechnology and the Rise of the Molecular Sciences* (Philadelphia, 1998), 165–81, 175.
44. B. E. Kirsop, *Bacteria* (Cambridge, Eng., 1991), 39; Cambrosio and Keating, *Exquisite,* 97–103.
45. Kirsop, *Bacteria,* 39; Cambrosio and Keating, *Exquisite,* 97–103.
46. Cambrosio and Keating, *Exquisite,* 94–95 and *Biomedical,* 171–72.
47. Milstein to Rajewsky, 21 May 1979, MSTN, file H116; Interview with McMichael; Cambrosio and Keating, *Exquisite,* 93–94, 135–36.
48. J. Klein, "Feuilleton: The New Shylocks," *Immunogenetics* 15 (1982): 109–10.
49. Klein, "Letter to the Editor," *Immunogenetics* 16 (1982): 100–101; J. Klein, "Publishing a Controversial Essay," online talk, Aug. 2005, available at http://www.webofstories.com/play/15878?o=MS (accessed 19 Sept. 2014).
50. Leonard Herzenberg and Leonore Herzenberg, "Letter to the Editor," *Immunogenetics* 16 (1982): 99–100.
51. Cambrosio and Keating, "Monoclonal," 176.
52. Interview with McMichael; A. Bernard, L. Boumsell, and C. Hill, "Joint Report of the First International Workshop on Human Leucocyte Differentiation Antigens by the Investigators of the Participating Laboratories," in A. Bernard et al., eds., *Leucocyte Typing: Human Leucocyte Differentiation Antigens Detected by Monoclonal Antibodies* (Berlin, 1984), 9–14; Milstein, Clark, Galfré, and Cuello, "Monoclonal," 20.
53. E. Thorsby, "A Short History of HLA," *Tissue Antigens* 74 (2009): 101–16; N. K. Mehra, *The HLA Complex in Biology and Medicine: A Resource Book* (New Dehli, 2010), 45–46, 50–51. The workshops continue to be held every three years. Interview with Richard Batchelor.

54. Bernard, Boumsell, and Hill, "Joint," 9–14; J. Dausset, "Introductory Remarks," in Bernard et al., *Leucocyte Typing,* 1–2.

55. H. Zola et al., "Human Leucocyte Differentiation Antigen Nomenclature: Update on CD Nomenclature: Report of IUIS/WHO Subcommittee," *J Immunol Methods* 275 (2003): 1–8; H. Zola and B. Swart, "The Human Leucocyte Differentiation Antigens (HLDA) Workshops: The Evolving Role of Antibodies in Research, Diagnosis and Therapy," *Cell Research* 15 (2005): 691–4; Keating and Cambrosio, *Biomedical,* 184–98.

56. T. A. Springer, "César Milstein, the Father of Modern Immunology," *Nat Immunol* 3, no. 6 (2002): 501–503.

57. Interview with McMichael; H. Zola, "CD Molecules 2005: Human Cell Differentiation Molecules," *Blood* 106, no. 9 (1 Nov. 2005): 3123–26; A. G. Dagleish et al., "The CD4 (T4) Antigen Is an Essential Component of the Receptor for the AIDS Retrovirus," *Nature* 312 (1984): 763–67; P. J. Maddon, "The T4 Gene Encodes the AIDS Virus Receptor and Is Expressed in the Immune System and the Brain," *Cell* 47, no. 3 (1986): 333–48.

58. Interview with Tim Bernard.

59. Ibid. Mabs became less important to the research carried out in the HLDA workshops once molecular biological tools, such as gene cloning, became more adept at identifying unidentified proteins. The HLDA objectives also changed with the establishment of the Human Genome Project. See D. Mason et al., "CD Antigens 2002," *Blood* 99 (2002): 3877–80; Zola, "CD Molecules 2005: Human Cell Differentiation Molecules"; M. Vidal-Laliena, X. Romero, and P. Engel, "Report of the VII International Workshop of Human Leukocyte Differentiation Antigens," *Immunologia* 24, no. 4 (2005): 374–77.

CHAPTER 4. THE FIRST MEDICAL APPLICATIONS

1. Milstein, "Notes for lecture(s) for Japan," unpublished ms., MSTN, file D38; Interview with Michael Clark.

2. Granner to Milstein, 15 Feb. 1978; Lessard and Akeson to Milstein, 6 Apr. 1978; Davies to Milstein, 14 Apr. 1978; Beavo to Milstein, 27 Sept. 1978; Lecomte to Milstein, 14 Apr. 1980; Oram to Milstein, 8 Dec. 1978; all in MSTN, file C283; Koprowski to Milstein, 19 Nov. 1976; Koprowski to Milstein, 22 Apr. 1977; both in MSTN, file C284; Fambrough to Milstein, 12 May 1977; Hilgers to Milstein, 23 May 1977; Hudson to Milstein, 14 July 1977; Howell to Milstein, 5 Oct. 1977; Jansen to Milstein, 25 Oct. 1977; Ruddle to Milstein, 27 Oct. 1977; Rees Smith to Milstein, 16 Nov. 1977; all in MSTN, file C285. Stephenson to Milstein, 24 Apr. 1979, MSTN, file C295; Oikawa to Milstein, 12 Dec. 1979, MSTN, file C296; C. Milstein, "Monoclonal Antibodies," *Sci Am* 243 (1980): 66–75.

3. Pereira to Milstein, 11 Jan. 1978, MSTN, file C283.

4. Milstein, "Monoclonal"; D. C. Burke, "Early Days with Interferon," and I. Gresser, "Interferon: An Unfolding Tale," both in *Journal of Interferon and Cytokine Research* 27 (2007): 91–96, 447–52; S. Pestka, "The Interferons:

50 Years after Their Discovery, There Is Much More to Learn," *J Biol Chem* 282, no. 28 (13 July 2007): 20047–51; Anon., "Bonanza of Interferon Antibody Springs from a Single Cell," *New Sci* (3 July 1980): 24; K. Cantell, "Is Natural Human Leukocyte Interferon Still Needed?" *Journal of Interferon Research* 7 (1987): 597–601; F. Hauptfuhrer, "Will Interferon Kill Cancer?" *People* 12, no. 1 (2 July 1979); I. Löwy, *Between Bench and Bedside: Science, Healing and Interleukin-2 in a Cancer Ward* (Cambridge, Mass., 1996), 122.

5. T. Taniguchi, Y. Fujii-Kuriyama, and M. Muramatsu, "Molecular Cloning of Human Interferon cDNA," *PNAS* 77, no. 7 (1980): 4003–4006; T. Taniguchi, "Aimez-Vous Brahms? A Story Capriccioso from the Discovery of a Cytokine Family and Its Regulators," *Nature Immunol* 10, no. 5 (2009): 447–49; P. Fitzgerald-Bocarsly, "The History of Interferon: An Interview with Sid Pestka," *ISICR Newsletter* 4, no. 2 (2004), available online at http://www.cytokines-interferons.org/PDFS/ICIS/newsletter/isicr4.2.pdf (accessed 6 Oct. 2014); A. Kornberg, *The Golden Helix: Inside Biotech Ventures* (Sausalito, Calif., 1995), 112–13; Löwy, *Between*, 122, 124–25; T. Peters, *Interferon: The Science and Selling of a Miracle Drug* (London, 2005), 143–44.

6. D. S. Secher and D. C. Burke, "A Monoclonal Antibody for Large-Scale Purification of Human Leukocyte Interferon," *Nature* 285 (1980): 446–50; Fitzgerald-Bocarsly, "History."

7. Interview with César Milstein; Interview with David Secher; Secher and Burke, "Monoclonal," 448–49.

8. Milstein to Paucker, 4 Oct. 1977, MSTN, file C283; Interview with Secher; Secher and Burke, "Monoclonal," 448–49; D. S. Secher, "Monoclonal Antibodies by Cell Fusion," *Immunology Today* (July 1980): 22–26.

9. D. S. Secher, "Development of NK2-Sepharose," 30 Jan. 1981, MSTN, file E15; International Patent Application PCT/GB81/00067, filed 13 Apr. 1981, MSTN, file C326; G. H. Fairtlough, "Strategy for Anti-Interferon," 25 Aug. 1981, MSTN, file E14.

10. Interview with Secher; Secher in E. M. Tansey and P. Caterall, "Technology Transfer in Britain: The Case of Monoclonal Antibodies," in E. M. Tansey et al., eds., *History of Twentieth Century Medicine Witness Seminars, 1993–1997*, vol. 1 (Apr. 1997): 27; C. Milstein, "With the Benefit of Hindsight," *Immunology Today* 21, no. 8 (2000): 359–63, esp. 361.

11. Interview with Secher; Secher evidence in Tansey and Catterall, "Technology," 27; Patent PCT/GB81/00067; Celltech, "Report on Progress against Objectives and Highlights of Period 25 March to 23 April," MSTN, file E13.

12. S. de Chadarevian, "The Making of an Entrepreneurial Science," *Isis* 102 (2011): 601–33; Interview with Secher.

13. Anon., "Strategic Issues in Relation to Celltech Products," unpublished paper for Celltech's Scientific Council Meeting, 24 Mar. 1981, MSTN, file E13.

14. Milstein to Brenner and Stoker, 14 Apr. 1981, MSTN, file E16.

15. Milstein to Brenner, 27 Apr. 1981; Brenner to Kirkman, 29 Apr. 1981; Brenner, memo, 29 Apr. 1981; all in MSTN, file E16; Milstein, "An Assessment of

MRC-Celltech Collaboration," unpublished paper, MSTN, file E17; de Chaderevian, "Making."

16. Fitzgerald-Bocarsly, "History"; Interview with Theo Staehelin.

17. Interview with Staehelin.

18. Ibid.

19. Ibid.; emails from T. Staehelin and I. Lefkovits to Lara Marks, March 2012; T. Staehelin et al., "Production of Hybridomas Secreting Monoclonal Antibodies to the Human Leukocyte Interferons," *PNAS* 78, no. 3 (1981): 1848–52.

20. Interview with Staehelin; Fitzgerald-Bocarsly, "History"; S. Smith-Hughes, *Genentech: The Beginnings of Biotech* (Chicago, 2011), 142–46; emails from Staehelin and Lefkovits.

21. Fitzgerald-Bocarsly, "History"; T. Staehelin et al., "Purification and Characterization of Recombinant Human Leukocyte Interferon (IFLrA) with Monoclonal Antibodies," *J Biol Chem* 256, no. 18 (1981): 9750–54.

22. Interview with Staehelin.

23. Interviews with Secher and Staehelin; Secher in Tansey and Catterall, "Technology," 27; Board of Patent Appeals and Interferences, Patent and Trademark Office, Staehelin et al. v. Secher et al., Patent Interference no. 101,597, 28 Sept. 1992, 24 U.S.P.Q.2d 1513, 1517, available online at http://ipmall.info/hosted_resources/BPAI_Decisions/BPAI_Appeal_101597.asp (accessed 19 Sept. 2014). Interestingly, Celltech explored collaborating with Roche in 1981 to develop Secher and Burke's Mab. See Anon., "Anti interferon," n.d., MSTN, file E15.

24. S. G. Sandler and M. M. Abedalthagafi, "Historic Milestones in the Evolution of the Crossmatch," *Immunohematology* 25, no. 4 (2009): 147–51.

25. Ibid., 147–48; N. C. Hugh-Jones, "Monoclonal Antibodies in Haematology," *Blood Reviews* 3 (1989): 3, 53–58.

26. Sandler and Abedalthagafi, "Historic," 147–48; Hughes-Jones, "Monoclonal," 54. Today thirty blood groups have been identified.

27. E. Lennox and S. H. Sacks, "Monoclonal Antibody," patent application filed 17 Nov. 1986, granted 26 July 1988, U.S. Patent 4760026; Sandler and Abedalthagafi, "Historic," 148.

28. S. Sacks, "Hybridomas: A Potent New Source of Blood Typing Reagents," unpublished paper, n.d., 2–4, kindly supplied by Sacks; D. Voak et al., "Monoclonal Anti-A and Anti-B: Development as Cost-Effective Agents," *Medical Laboratory Sciences* (1982): 39, 109–122.

29. Voak et al., "Monoclonal Anti-A."

30. Sacks, "Hybridomas," 2–3; Voak et al., "Monoclonal Anti-A."

31. Sacks, "Hybridomas," 2; Voak et al., "Monoclonal Anti-A," 110; Lennox and Sacks, "Monoclonal Antibody."

32. C. Milstein, "Inspiration from the Diversity in the Immune System," *New Sci* (21 May 1987): 54–58; interview with Milstein; Anon., "Hybrid Cells Are a Good Source of Antibody," *New Sci* (27 July 1978): 271.

33. Voak et al., "Monoclonal Anti-A," 110. Interview with Sacks; Sacks, "Hybrid-omas," 3–4.
34. Sacks, "Hybridomas," 5.
35. Ibid.; T. Downs, "Transfusion Service Automation," *Advance* 19, no. 9 (2010): 31.
36. Interview with Sacks; E. Lennox, D. Voak, and S. Sacks, "Monoclonal Anti-bodies as New Blood Typing Reagents," in S. B. Rosalki, ed., *New Approaches to Laboratory Medicine* (Düdingen, Switz., 1981), 105–12.
37. Voak et al., "Monoclonal Anti-A," 120.
38. Ibid.; Lennox, Voak, and Sacks, "Monoclonal," 110.
39. Interview with Milstein; Anon., "Britain's Biotechnologists Put Monoclonals on the Market," *New Sci* (20 Jan 1983): 158; G. H. Fairtlough, "Exploitation of Biotechnology in a Smaller Company," *Phil Trans R Soc Lond* (1989): B 324, 589–97.
40. Anon., "Monoclonals by the Million," *New Sci* (28 July 983): 271; J. R. Birch, R. Boraston, and L. Wood, "Bulk Production of Monoclonal Anti-bodies in Fermenters," *Trends in Biotechnology* 3, no. 5 (1985): 162–66.
41. Fairtlough, "Exploitation," 592; Anon., "Monoclonals by the Million"; Birch, Boraston, and Wood, "Bulk," 162–66; W. R. Arathoon and J. R. Birch, "Large-Scale Cell Culture in Biotechnology," *Science* 232 (13 June 1986): 1390–95; G. Kretzmer, "Industrial Processes with Animal Cells," *Applied Microbiology and Biotechnology* 59 (2002): 135–42; O. W. Merten, "Introduc-tion to Animal Cell Culture—Past, Present and Future," *Cytotechnology* 50 (2006): 1–7.
42. K. Zoon, P. J. Bridgen, and M. E. Smith, "Production of Human Lympho-blastoid Interferon by Namalwa Cells Cultured in Serum-Free Media," *Jour-nal of General Virology* 44 (1979): 227–29; Interview with James Christie. After some bruising patent battles, Genentech acquired Wellcome's manu-facturing process, which it advanced for deep cell cultures of 10,000 liters. Genentech leveraged the technology for its commercialization of tissue plas-minogen activator, which is used for blood clotting, and its subsequent de-velopment of Mab drugs.
43. Birch, Boraston, and Wood, "Bulk," 163; Anon., "Monoclonals by the Mil-lion"; Arathoon and Birch, "Large-Scale," 1394; Fairtlough, "Exploitation," 593.
44. Birch, Boraston, and Wood, "Bulk"; D. Voak, "Monoclonal Antibodies as Blood Grouping Reagents," *Baillière's Clinical Haematology* 3, no. 2 (Apr. 1990): 219–42.
45. P. Rouger, F. Noizat-Pirenne, and P. Y. Le Pennec, "Advances in the Use of Monoclonal Antibodies for Blood Group Testing," *Transfusion Clinique et Biologique* 4 (1997): 345–49, esp. 346.
46. Milstein, "Inspiration."
47. Prior to the development of treatment, approximately 1 percent of all British newborns suffered from hemolytic disease and it was responsible for one

death in every 2,200 births. In 1976 the new treatment was estimated to save between 3,000 and 4,000 U.S. perinatal deaths per year. F. S. Rosen, "On the Prevention of Rh Hemolytic Disease of the Newborn by Hyperimmune Anti-Rh Globulin with Comments on the IgG Effector Site for Oposonic Activity," in E. Haber and R. M. Krauser, eds., *Antibodies in Human Diagnosis and Therapy* (New York, 1977), 359–63; NICE, "Pregnancy (Rhesus Negative Women)—Routine Anti-D," NICE Technology Appraisal (Aug. 2008), available online at http://www.nice.org.uk/guidance/ta156 /resources/pregnancy-rhesus-negative-women-routine-antid-draft-scope2 (accessed 2 Oct. 2014).

48. D. Bron et al., "Production of Human Monoclonal IgG Antibodies against Rhesus (D) Antigen," *PNAS* (May 1984): 3214–17; K. M. Thompson et al., "Production of Human Monoclonal IgG and IgM Antibodies with Anti-D (Rhesus) Specificity Using Heterohybridomas," *Immunology* 58 (1986): 157–60.

49. Bron et al., "Production"; Thompson et al., "Production"; Voak, "Blood Grouping," 227–28; Rouger et al., "Advances," 347.

50. Voak, "Blood Grouping," 237, 239; Rouger et al., "Advances," 348.

51. S. Sheldon and K. Poulton, "HLA Typing and Its Influence on Organ Transplantation," *Transplantation Immunology* 33 (2006): 157–74.

52. J. Colombani et al., "HLA Typing with Monoclonal Antibodies," *Tissue Antigens* 34, no. 2 (1989): 97–110; N. S. Hakim and G. M. Danovitch, eds., *Transplantation Surgery* (London, 2001), 43–45.

CHAPTER 5. JOY, DISAPPOINTMENT, DETERMINATION

1. M. Goldberg, *Cell Wars: The Immune System's Newest Weapons against Cancer* (New York, 1989), 19.

2. J. L. Marx, "Monoclonal Antibodies in Cancer," *Science* 216, no. 4543 (1982): 283–85, esp. 283.

3. Ibid., 283.

4. D. Pressman, "The Development and Use of Radiolabelled Antitumor Antibodies," *Cancer Research* 40 (1980): 2960–64; F. H. DeLand, "A Perspective of Monoclonal Antibodies: Past, Present, and Future," *Seminars in Nuclear Medicine* 19, no. 3 (1989): 158–65; S. Wolf, *Brain, Mind and Medicine: Charles Richet and the Origins of Physiological Psychology* (New Brunswick, N.J., 1993), 80–81; T. A. Oelschlaeger, "'Bacteria as Tumor Therapeutics?' *Bioengineered Bugs* 1, no. 2 (2010): 146–47; S. S. Hall, *A Commotion in the Blood* (London, 1998), chs. 1–5.

5. D. Pressman and G. Keighley, "The Zone of Activity of Nephritoxic Use of Radioactive Tracers: The Antibodies as Determined by the Antikidney Serum," *JI* 59 (1948): 141–46; Pressman, "Development"; D. Thomson, "Immunodiagnosis of Cancer," *Proceedings of the Royal Society of Medicine* 65 (1975): 635–36.

6. Thomson, "Immunodiagnosis"; J. Y. Douillard et al., "Pharmacokinetic Study of Radiolabelled Anti-Colorectal Carcinoma Monoclonal Antibodies in

Tumor-Bearing Nude Mice," *European Journal of Nuclear Medicine* 11 (1985): 107–13; Marx, "Monoclonal," 283.

7. R. Vaughan, *Listen to the Music: The Life of Hilary Koprowski* (New York, 2000), 138; Goldberg, *Cell Wars*, 46–47.

8. H. Koprowski, Z. Stepleswki, S. Herlyn, and M. Herlyn, "Study of Antibodies against Human Melanoma Produced by Somatic Cell Hybrids," *PNAS* 75, no. 7 (1978): 3405–409; M. Herlyn et al., "Colorectal Carcinoma-Specific Antigen: Detection by Means of Monoclonal Antibodies," *PNAS* 76 (1979): 1438–42.

9. Marx, "Monoclonal," 283.

10. J. D. Minna et al., "Methods for Production of Monoclonal Antibodies with Specificity for Human Lung Cancer Cells," *In Vitro* 17, no. 12 (1981): 1058–70; Marx, "Monoclonal," 283.

11. Herlyn et al., "Colorectal," 1439, 1441.

12. Vaughan, *Listen*, 187–88; Herlyn et al., "Colorectal"; Z. Stepleswki, M. Herlyn, D. Herlyn, W. H. Clark, and H. Koprowski, "Reactivity of Monoclonal Anti-Melanoma Antibodies with Melanoma Cells Freshly Isolated from Primary and Metastatic Melanoma," *EJI* 9 (1979): 94–96; T. H. Chang, Z. Steplewski, H. F. Sears, and H. Koprowski, "Detection of Monoclonal Antibody-Defined Colorectal Carcinoma Antigen by Solid-Phase Binding Inhibition Radioimmunoassay," *Hybridoma* 1, no. 1 (1981): 37–45; H. Koprowski, M. Herlyn, Z. Steplewski, and H. Sears, "Specific Antigen in Serum of Patients with Colon Cancer," *Science*, n.s. 212, no. 4490 (1981): 53–55; H. F. Sears et al., "Ex Vivo Perfusion of Human Colon with Monoclonal Anticolorectal Cancer Antibodies," *Cancer* 49, no. 6 (1982): 1231–35; M. Herlyn, H. F. Sears, Z. Stepleswki, and H. Koprowski, "Monoclonal Antibody Detection of a Circulating Tumor-Associated Antigen in Presence of Antigen in Sera of Patients with Colorectal, Gastric, and Pancreatic Carcinoma," *J Clin Immunology* 2, no. 2 (1982): 135–40; H. Sears, M. Herlyn, B. Del Villano, Z. Steplewski, and H. Koprowski, "Monoclonal Antibody Detection of a Circulating Tumor-Associated Antigen, II: A Longitudinal Evaluation of Patients with Colorectal Cancer," *J Clin Immunology* 2, no. 2 (1982): 141–48; Goldberg, *Cell Wars*, 30–32.

13. D. Herlyn, Z. Steplewski, M. Herlyn, and H. Koprowski, "Inhibition of Growth of Colorectal Carcinoma in Nude Mice by Monoclonal Antibody," *Cancer Research* 40 (1980): 717; H. F. Sears et al., "Phase-I Clinical Trial of Monoclonal Antibody in Treatment of Gastrointestinal Tumors," *Lancet* (3 Apr. 1982): 762–65; H. F. Sears, D. Herlyn, Z. Steplewski, and H. Koprowski, "Effects of Monoclonal Antibody Immunotherapy on Patients with Gastrointestinal Adenocarcinoma," *J Biological Response Modifiers* 3 (1984): 138–50, 140–41; Vaughan, *Listen*, 188.

14. Interview with Jeff Mattis; H. F. Sears, "Phase-I Clinical Trial of Monoclonal Antibody in Treatment of Gastrointestinal Tumors," *Lancet* (1982): 762–65; Goldberg, *Cell Wars*, 9.

15. Sears et al., "Effects," 144; Goldberg, *Cell Wars*, 114.

16. Vaughan, *Listen*, 187–89; Interview with Zenon Steplewski.

17. Goldberg, *Cell Wars*, 117, 121.

18. H. Koprowski et al., "Human Anti-Idiotype Antibodies in Cancer Patients: Is the Modulation of the Immune Response Beneficial for the Patient?," *PNAS* 81 (1984): 216–19; Goldberg, *Cell Wars*, 67.

19. G. T. Stevenson and F. K. Stevenson, "Antibody to a Molecularly-Defined Antigen Confined to a Tumour Cell Surface," *Nature* 254 (1975): 714–16; F. K. Stevenson, E. V. Elliott, and G. T. Stevenson, "Some Effects on Leukaemic B Lymphocytes of Antibodies to Defined Regions of Their Surface Immunoglobulin," *Immunology* 3 (1977): 54–59; G. T. Stevenson and F. K. Stevenson, "Treatment of Lymphoid Tumors with Anti-Idiotype Antibodies," *Springer Seminars Immunopathology* 6 (1983): 99–115.

20. Stevensons, "Antibody." The anti-idiotype antibodies were created by injecting sheep with purified idiotype determinants on leukemic cells taken from the guinea pigs.

21. F. K. Stevenson, L. E. Mole, C. M. Raymont, and G. T. Stevenson, "A λ Bence-Jones Protein in Guinea Pigs," *Biochemistry* 151 (1975): 751–53; Stevenson et al., "Some Effects"; D. W. Hough et al., "Anti-Idiotype Sera Raised against Surface Immunoglobulin of Human Neoplastic Lymphocytes," *JEM* 144 (1976): 960–69; T. J. Hamblin et al., "Preliminary Experience in Treating Lymphocytic Leukemia with Antibody to Immunoglobulin Idiotype on the Cell Surfaces," *British Journal of Cancer* 42 (1980): 495.

22. Interview with Martin Glennie; M. Glennie and G. T. Stevenson, "Univalent Antibodies Kill Tumor Cells in Vitro and in Vivo," *Nature* 295 (1982): 712–14.

23. Chapters 1 and 2; J. P. Mach et al., "*In Vivo* Localisation of Radiolabelled Antibodies to Carcinoembryonic Antigen in Human Colon Carcinoma Grafted into Nude Mice," *Nature* 248 (1974): 704–706; interviews with Ron Levy and Ivor Royston; B. Azar, "Profile of Ronald Levy," *PNAS* 107, no. 29 (2010): 12745–46, esp. 12745; R. Levy, J. Dilley, R. I. Fox, and R. Warnke, "A Human Thymus-Leukemia Antigen Defined by Hybridoma Monoclonal Antibodies," *PNAS* 76, no. 12 (1979): 6552–56.

24. Interview with Levy; R. Levy and J. Dilley, "The *In Vitro* Antibody Response to Cell Surface Antigens, I: The Xenogeneic Response to Human Leukemia Cells," and "The In Vitro Antibody Response to Cell Surface Antigens, II: Monoclonal Antibodies to Human Leukemia Cells," both in *JI* 119, no. 2 (1977): 387–400; R. Levy, R. Wartnke, R. Dorfman, and J. Haimovich, "The Monoclonality of Human B-Cell Lymphomas," *JEM* 145 (1977): 1014–28; Levy et al., "Human"; S. Brown, J. Dilley, and R. Levy, "Immunoglobulin Secretion by Mouse x Human Hybridomas: An Approach for the Production of Anti-Idiotype Reagents Useful in Monitoring Patients with B Cell Lymphoma," *JI* 125 (1980): 1037–43.

25. Interview with Levy; R. A. Miller and R. Levy, "Response of Cutaneous T Cell Lymphoma to Therapy with Hybridoma Monoclonal Antibody," *Lancet*

(1 Aug. 1981): 226–29; R. A. Miller, D. G. Maloney, R. Warnke, and R. Levy, "Treatment of B Cell Lymphoma with Monoclonal Anti-Idiotype Antibody," *NEJM* 306 (1982): 517–22; Anon., "Mouse Cells Help Send Cancer into Remission," *Modesto Bee* (18 Sept. 1981); K. Hobson, "Cancer's Natural Enemy," *U.S. News & World Report* (4 July 2004).

26. Interview with Levy; Azar, "Profile."

27. Anon., "Two Doctors Win $50,000 Each for Work on a Cancer Drug," *New York Times* (4 Dec. 1982); M. Roth, "Guided Missile against Tumors," *Pittsburgh Gazette* (21 Oct. 1985); R. Levy and R. A. Miller, "Biological and Clinical Implications of Lymphocyte Hybridomas: Tumor Therapy with Monoclonal Antibodies," *Annual Review of Medicine* 34 (1983): 107–16.

28. A. Kraft, "Atomic Medicine: The Cold War Origins of Biological Research," *History Today* 59, no. 11 (2009); A. Kraft, "Manhattan Transfer: Lethal Radiation, Bone Marrow Transplantation, and the Birth of Stem Cell Biology, ca. 1942–1961," *Historical Studies in the Natural Sciences* 39, no. 2 (Spring 2009): 171–218; H. Waldmann, G. Hale, and S. Cobbold, "The Immunobiology of Bone Marrow Transplantation," in A. J. McMichael et al., eds., *Leukocyte Typing, III: White Cell Differentiation Antigens* (Oxford, Eng., 1987): 932–37; V. T. Ho and R. J. Soiffer, "The History and Future of T-Cell Depletion as Graft-Versus-Host Disease Prophylaxis for Allogeneic Hematopoietic Stem Cell Transplantation," *Blood* 98, no. 12 (2001): 3192–204; N. Brown, A. Kraft, and P. Martin, "The Promissory Pasts of Blood Stem Cells," *BioSocieties* 1 (2006): 329–48.

29. Interview with Herman Waldmann.

30. Ibid.

31. Y. Reisner, N. Kapoor, R. J. O'Reilly, and R. A. Good, "Allogeneic Bone Marrow Transplantation Using Stem Cells Fractionated by Lectins, VI: In Vitro Analysis of Human and Money Bone Marrow Cells Fractionated by Sheep Red Blood Cells and Soybean Agglutin," *Lancet* 2 (20–27 Dec. 1980): 1320–24; G. Hale et al., "Removal of T cells from Bone Marrow for Transplantation: A Monoclonal Anti-Lymphocyte Antibody That Fixes Human Complement," *Blood* 62 (1983): 873–82.

32. T. W. Chang, P. Kung, S. P. Gingas, and G. Goldstein, "Does OKT3 Monoclonal Antibody React with Antigen-Recognition Structure on Human T Cells?" *PNAS* 78, no. 3 (1981): 1805–808; A. Filipovich et al., "Pretreatment of Donor Bone Marrow with Monoclonal Antibody OKT3 for Prevention of Acute Graft-Versus-Host Disease in Allogeneic Histocompatible Bone Marrow Transplantation," *Lancet* (5 June 1982): 1266–69; H. G. Prentice, H. A. Blacklock, G. Janossy, et al., "Use of the Anti-T Monoclonal Antibody OKT3 for Prevention of Acute Graft Versus Host Disease (GVHD) in Allogeneic Bone Marrow Transplantation for Acute Leukemia," *Lancet* (27 Mar. 1982): 700–703; S. M. Granger et al., "Elimination of T Lymphocytes from Human Bone Marrow with Monoclonal Anti-T Antibodies and Cytolytic Complement," *British Journal of Haematology* 50, no. 2 (1982): 367–74.

33. D. A. Vallera, C. C. B. Soderling, G. J. Carlson, and J. H. Kersey, "Bone Marrow Transplantation across Major Histocompatibility Barriers in Mice: Effect of Elimination of T Cells from Donor Grafts by Treatment with Monoclonal Thy-1 2 Plus Complement or Antibody Alone," *Transplantation* 31 (1981): 218–22; Granger et al., "Elimination"; Hale, "Removal," 873; G. Hale and H. Waldmann, "From Laboratory to Clinic: The Story of Campath-1," in A. J. Y. George and C. E. Urch, ed., *Diagnostic and Therapeutic Antibodies* (New York, 2000): 243–66, 244; Waldmann et al., "Immunobiology," 933.

34. Hale and Waldmann, "Laboratory," 244–45; Interviews with Michael Clark.

35. Hale and Waldmann, "Laboratory," 245; M. Clark, "Mike's Campath Story," available online at http://www.path.cam.ac.uk/~mrc7/campath/campath .html (accessed 19 Sept. 2014); H. Waldmann, "A Personal History of the Campath-1H Antibody," *Medical Oncology* 19 supp. (2002): S3–S9.

36. M. Clark, S. Cobbold, G. Hale, and H. Waldmann, "Advantages of Rat Monoclonal Antibodies," *Immunology Today* 4, no. 4 (1983): 100–101. Clark, "Mike's"; Waldmann, "Personal."

37. Hale, "Removal"; Hale and Waldmann, "Laboratory."

38. Hale and Waldmann, "Laboratory."

39. Hale, "Removal"; ibid., 246; Waldmann, "Personal"; L. Marks, "The Life Story of a Biotechnology Drug: Alemtuzumab," available online at www .whatisbiotechnology.org/exhibitions/campath (accessed 19 Sept. 2014).

40. Interview with Waldmann.

41. In due course, the experience gained from treating the Hammersmith patient led to further studies applying Campath antibodies in aplastic anemia. Ibid.; H. Waldmann and G. Hale, "Campath: From Concept to Clinic," *Phil Trans R Soc Lond B* 360, no. 1461 (29 Sept. 2005): 1707–11.

42. H. Waldmann et al., "Elimination of Graft-Versus-Host-Disease by In-Vitro Depletion of Alloreactive Lymphocytes with Monoclonal Rat Anti-Human Lymphocyte Antibody (Campath-1)," *Lancet* (1 Sept. 1984): 483–86; Email from Slavin to Marks, 3 Oct. 2013.

43. Interview with Waldmann; Waldmann et al., "Elimination"; G. Hale, S. Cobbold, and H. Waldmann, "T Cell Depletion with Campath-1 in Allogeneic Bone Marrow Transplantation," *Transplantation* 45 (1988): 753–59; Waldmann and Hale, "Campath"; S. P. Cobbold, G. Martin, S. Qin, and H. Waldmann, "Monoclonal Antibodies to Promote Marrow Engraftment and Tissue Graft Tolerance," *Nature* 323 (1986): 164–66.

44. S. Cobbold, G. Martin, and H. Waldmann, "Monoclonal Antibodies for the Prevention of Graft-Versus-Host Disease and Marrow Graft Rejection," *Transplantation* 42, no. 3 (1986): 239–47; S. P. Cobbold, G. Martin, S. Qin, and H. Waldmann, "Monoclonal Antibodies to Promote Marrow Engraftment and Tissue Graft Tolerance," *Nature* 323 (1986): 164–66; Hale and Waldmann, "Laboratory," 248; Waldmann, "Personal," S5–S6.

45. Hale and Waldmann, "Laboratory," 248–49.

46. Ibid., 249.
47. Interview with Waldmann; Waldmann and Hale, "Campath," 1708–709; Waldmann et al., "Immunobiology," 933–35.
48. Waldmann et al., "Immunobiology," 933–35; G. Hale et al., "Meeting Report: Campath-1 Antibodies in Stem-Cell Transplantation," *Cytotherapy* 3, no. 3 (2001): 145–64. See Chapter 9 for a discussion of what constitutes a humanized Mab.
49. Interviews with Steplewski, Levy, Geoff Hale, and Jenny Phillips.
50. Interview with Phillips.
51. Ibid.
52. Interviews with Steplewski, Hale, and Waldmann; Hale and Waldmann, "Laboratory," 254.
53. Hale and Waldmann, "Laboratory," 254.
54. Interviews with Steplewski, Hale, and Phillips; J. Phillips et al., "Manufacture and Quality Control of Campath-1 Antibodies for Clinical Trials," *Cytotherapy* 3, no. 3 (2001): 233–42.
55. Interview with Hale.
56. Phillips et al., "Manufacture."
57. Ibid.

CHAPTER 6. THE WILD WEST OF ANTIBODY COMMERCIALIZATION

1. S. Smith Hughes, *Genentech: The Beginnings of Biotech* (Chicago, 2011).
2. Interview with Jenny Murray.
3. Ibid.
4. Ibid.; T. Lloyd, *Dinosaur and Co.: Studies in Corporate Evolution* (London, 1984): 42–44, 47–48.
5. Interview with Murray; Lloyd, *Dinosaur,* 47–48.
6. Ibid.; D. Murray, untitled and undated document sent with letter to Vittery, 29 July 1977, MSTN, file F13.
7. Interview with Murray; Lloyd, *Dinosaur,* 50–51, 57.
8. For details on this chance encounter, see Chapter 2.
9. Murray, document to Vittery.
10. Ibid.
11. Ibid.
12. Lloyd, *Dinosaur,* 54–55.
13. Ibid., 55. Factoring is where a business sells its invoices to a third party.
14. Ibid., 55–56.
15. Interviews with Jane Pelly and Murray; Murray to Milstein, 21 July 1980, MSTN, file F15.
16. Lloyd, *Dinosaur,* 54; Murray to Milstein, 21 July 1980.
17. Murray to Milstein, 21 July 1980.
18. Sera-Lab, *Catalogue* (1982).
19. Murray to Milstein, 21 July 1980.
20. Ibid.; Sera-Lab, *Catalogues* (1981, 1989).

21. G. Fjermedal, *Magic Bullets* (New York, 1984): ch. 7; M. P. Jones, "Biotech's Perfect Climate: The Hybritech Story," Ph.D. diss., University of California, San Diego, 2005, ch. 6.

22. Interviews with Howard Birndorf (1) and (2) and Ivor Royston; Jones, "Biotech's," 371–74. For more on Klinman, Levy, and Herzenberg, see Chapters 1, 3, and 5.

23. Jones, "Biotech's," 372–74; Interviews with Royston and Birndorf (1).

24. Interview with Birndorf (1); Fjermedal, *Magic*, 93.

25. Interviews with Royston and Birndorf (1).

26. Fjermedal, *Magic*, 95; Interview with Birndorf (1); Jones, "Biotech's," 413.

27. Interviews with Birndorf (1) and Royston, 26; Jones, "Biotech's," 405–407.

28. Jones, "Biotech's," 408–11.

29. Ibid., 409–11.

30. Interview with Royston, 25–28; Ibid., 432.

31. Interview with Brook Byers; C. Robbins-Roth, *From Alchemy to IPO: The Business of Biotechnology* (Cambridge, Mass., 2000): 51; Jones, "Biotech's," 382, 419; 434–48, 457–64, 471–74; Interviews with Birndorf (1) and Byers, 24; Fjermedal, *Magic*, 96.

32. Jones, "Biotech's," 468–70.

33. Greene's interest in Mabs had been initially sparked as the result of his attendance of a conference in the autumn of 1978 where Bill Dryer, a Caltech biology professor, ditched his presentation on fluorescent tagging of conventional antibodies to talk about Milstein and Köhler's technique, which he declared to be the "greatest breakthrough in the history of . . . antibody technology." Jones, "Biotech's," 511–29, esp. 524, 533; Interview with Ted Greene.

34. Jones, "Biotech's," 509–10, 527–28, 576.

35. Ibid., 529–37, 539–40; 550–51.

36. Ibid., 552–53, 624–25, 658, 727; R. Teitelman, *Gene Dreams: Wall Street, Academia and the Rise of Biotechnology* (New York, 1991), 77.

37. R. Vaughan, *Listen to the Music: The Life of Hilary Koprowski* (Berlin, 2000), 179.

38. Ibid., 179; Centocor, *Centocor Oncogene Research Partners LP*, 9 June 1984, HS-PP; Interview with Hilary Koprowski.

39. M. A. Wall and E. C. Allen, "Investment Prospectus: Medical Diagnostic Business," date unknown, 34–35, HS-PP.

40. Interviews with Holveck (1) and (2), Ann McKenzie, Paul Schoemaker, and Paul Brock.

41. Interviews with McKenzie and Schoemaker.

42. Interview with Vincent Zurawski; V. R. Zurawski et al., "Antibodies of Restricted Heterogeneity Directed against the Cardiac Glycoside Digoxin," *JI* 121 (1978): 121–29.

43. Centocor, *Annual Report* (1982); Interviews with Zurawski and Tony Evnin.

44. Wall and Allen, "Investment"; A. Hedin et al., "A Monoclonal Antibody— Enzyme Immunoassay for Serum Carcinoembryonic Antigen with

Increased Specificity for Carcinomas," *PNAS* 80 (June 1983): 3470–474; M. Fleisher et al., "Roche RIA and Abbott EIA Carcinoembryonic Antigen Assays Compared," *Clin Chem* 30, no. 2 (1984): 200–205.

45. Wall and Allen, "Investment," 37.

46. Interviews with Evnin and Zurawski; L. F. Rothschild et al., *Centocor Inc.: Prospectus for Public Offering* (22 July 1983), 16–17, HS-PP; Anon., "A Medical Marvel Goes to Market," *Business Week* (11 Apr. 1983): 56; Anon., "Biotechnologists Are Ready to Market Another Trick," *Economist* (7 Feb. 1981): 87; Anon., "Smart Bombs of Biology," *Newsweek*, U.S. ed. (22 June 1981): 59.

47. Wall and Allen, "Investment," 30. Interview with David Holveck (2); Vaughan, *Listen*, 179, 186; Interviews with Koprowski and Michael Dougherty.

48. Interview with Evnin; Rothschild et al., *Centocor Inc.*, 21; R. Teitelman, "Searching for Serendipity: Centocor Combs University Labs for Technology," *Forbes* (6 May 1985): 80.

49. W. Muraskin, *The War against Hepatitis B: A History of the International Task Force on Hepatitis B Immunization* (Philadephia, 1995), 3–4.

50. Ibid., 3–4; Wall and Allen, "Investment," 40; Centocor, *Annual Report* (1983): 2, HS-PP.

51. Interview with Byers, 20–21; Robbins-Roth, *Alchemy*, 51; Jones, "Biotech's," 382, 434–48, 457–64, 471–74; M. Mackenzie, A. Cambrosio, and P. Keating, "The Commercial Application of a Scientific Discovery: The Case of the Hybridoma Technique," *Research Policy* 17 (1988): 155–70, fn18, 162; Jones, "Biotech's," 591; Teitelmann, *Gene*, 114–20.

52. A. Cambrosio and P. Keating, *Exquisite Specificity: The Monoclonal Antibody Revolution* (Oxford, Eng., 1995): 143–44; Jones, "Biotech's," 590–91.

53. Interview with Byers, 20–21; Robbins-Roth, *Alchemy*, 51; Jones, "Biotech's," 382, 434–48, 457–64, 471–74.

54. Centocor, *Prospectus* (14 Dec. 1982): 16, HS-PP; Cambrosio and Keating, *Exquisite*, 144–45, 152–53; Mackenzie, Cambrosio, and Keating, "Commercial," 165; J. R. Wands and V. R. Zurawski, "Process for Producing Antibodies to Hepatitis Virus and Cell Lines Therefor" (filed 22 Oct. 1979, issued 2 June 1981), U.S. Patent 4,271,145; J. R. Wands and V. R. Zurawski, "High Affinity Monoclonal Antibodies to Hepatitis B Surface Antigen (HBsAg) Produced by Somatic Cell Hybrids," *Gastroenterology* 80, no. 2 (1981): 225–32; J. R. Wands et al., "Immunodiagnosis of Hepatitis B with High-Affinity IgM Monoclonal Antibodies," *PNAS* 78, no. 2 (1981): 1214–18; Centocor, *Prospectus* (14 Dec. 1982): 17; H. J. P. Schoemaker, J. R. Wands, B. L. Westrick, and V. R. Zurawski, "Immunoassay for Multi-Determinant Antigens Using High-Affinity," filed Apr. 24 1984, issued June 6 1989, U.S. Patent 4,837,167.

55. Centocor, *Annual Report* (1983): 14; Anon., "FDA Approved the First Hepatitis-B Monoclonal Assay," *Chemical Week* (27 June 1984): 96.

56. Interview with Holveck (2). Centocor's partners included Warner-Lambert to cover the United States, Toray/Fujizoki for Japan, and Byk-Mallinckroft for Europe; see Centocor, *Annual Report* (1983): 2, 14, 18, and (1985): 15, 27.

57. Jones, "Biotech's," 579–87.

58. Ibid., 649, 652. Interview with Greene.

59. B. Ritter, "Hybritech Cancer-Testing Product," *Los Angeles Times* (3 Jan. 1985); J. S. Nisselbaum et al., "Comparison of Roche RIA, Roche EIA, Hybritech EIA and Abbott EIA Methods for Measuring Carcinoembryonic Antigen," *Clin Chem* 34, no. 4 (1988): 761–64; F. B. Dunn, "Value of Prostrate-Specific Antigen: Are Higher Levels Meaningful?" *Journal of the National Cancer Institute* 94, no. 6 (2002): 415–16; M. Baker, "Is PSA Test a Lifesaver or of Little Use?," *Stanford Report* (9 Mar. 2005), http://news.stanford.edu/news/2005/march9/med-prostate-030905.html; Anon., "PSA Test: Don't Do It, Say Angry Men," *Los Angeles Times Blogs* (4 Aug. 2008), available online at atimesblogs.latimes.com/booster_shots/2008/08/psa-test-dont-d.html (accessed Jan. 2013). One critic highlighted that PSA screening cost the United States at least $3 billion a year, most of it paid by Medicare and the Veterans Administration. The article points out that while American men have a 16 percent chance of receiving a diagnosis of prostate cancer, only 3 percent have a chance of dying from it. R. J. Ablin, "The Great Prostrate Mistake," *New York Times* (9 Mar. 2010), available online at http://www.nytimes.com/2010/03/10/opinion/10Ablin.html (accessed 19 Sept. 2014).

60. S. A. Leavitt, "'A Private Little Revolution': The Home Pregnancy Test in American Culture," *Bulletin for the History of Medicine* 80, no. 2 (2006): 317–45. One of the disadvantages of the Hybritech test was that it involved the user going through multiple steps to get the result. In 1988 Unilever introduced an improved version of Clearblue. All this required was a woman holding the test sampler in her morning urine stream and then waiting for the result, which took three minutes to appear. K. May, "Home Tests to Monitor Fertility," *American Journal of Obstetrics and Gynecology* 165, no. 6, pt. 2 (1991): 2000–2002; G. Jones and A. Kraft, "Corporate Venturing: The Origins of Unilever's Pregnancy Test," *Business History* 46, no. 1 (2004): 100–22.

61. Anon., "Monoclonal Antibodies Inc Wins Patent Infringement Lawsuit Brought by Hybritech Inc," *Biotechnology Law Report* 302 (Oct. 1985); Jones, "Biotech's," 726–32, 824–27, 834. Lilly paid between $350 to $480 million for the acquisition of Hybritech. For the court's judgment in the dispute in 1985, see U.S. Northern District of California, "Hybritech Inc vs. Monoclonal Antibodies," No.C-84-0930, SC Findings of Fact and Conclusions of Law, 28 Aug. 1985, MSTN, file C306; M. MacKenzie, P. Keating, and A. Cambrosio, "Patents and Free Scientific Information in Biotechnology: Making Monoclonal Antibodies Proprietary," *Science, Technology, & Human Values* 15, no. 1 (1990): 65–83.

62. Jones, "Biotech's," 34–35, 877; Chapter 10.

63. Letter from Murray to Lichtman, 4 July 1989, David Murray's personal papers; P. Marsh, "City Split over Porton's Promise of Success," *Financial Times* (8 Dec. 1988). The initial product the company hoped to market was a treatment for herpes. For details on this project, see Letters to *BMJ* 300 (16 June

1990): 1583–84. By the late 1990s Haydon-Baillie had ceased to have control of Porton International, having been accused of personal enrichment at the expense of the company. A multimillionaire, Haydon-Baillie suffered a mental breakdown and was near bankruptcy. K. Dovkants, "My Doomed Love Affair with England's Greatest House," *Evening Standard* (16 Feb. 2007), available online at http://smart-grid.tmcnet.com/news/2007/02/16/2344743 .htm (accessed 19 Sept. 2014). In 1994 Porton sold Sera-Lab's business to Harlan Laboratories, an American company specializing in laboratory animals and contract research services. Interview with Murray.

64. Celltech brochure, MSTN, file E9; Murray to Milstein, 21 July 1980; Tridgell to Murray, 5 Aug. 1980; Hay to Murray, 5 Aug. 1980; all in MSTN, file F15. For the confusion about Sera-Lab, see Interview with Royston, 26, and Jones, "Biotech's," 410, fn13.

65. Murray to Milstein, 17 Sept. 1982, MSTN, file F17; Author unknown, "Draft: Research Monoclonals," 28 Apr. 1981, MSTN, file E15.

66. Interviews with Ed Bernard, Tim Bernard, and Lisa Mynheer; Morphosys press statement, 12 Jan. 2006, available online at http://www.morphosys .com/pressrelease/morphosys-acquires-serotec-group-strengthen-global-research-antibody-business (accessed 19 Sept. 2014).

67. S. X. Yu, "Antibody Reagent Market 2012," *BioAstrum* (2012), available online at http://www.bioastrum.com/home/sites/docs/Antibody-reagent -market-2012.pdf (accessed 19 Sept. 2014).

68. Centocor, *Annual Report* (1992), (1993), 12; Interview with Holveck (1).

69. Interview with Zurawski; H. M. Davis, T. L. Klug, and V. R. Zurawski, "Method of Isolating CA 125 Antigen" (filed 24 Nov. 1986, issued 22 Oct. 1991), U.S. patent 5,059,680; R. C. Bast et al., "A Radioimmunoassay Using a Monoclonal Antibody to Monitor the Course of Epithelial Ovarian Cancer," *NEJM* 309 (1983): 883; T. L. Klug et al., "A Monoclonal Antibody Immunoradiometric Assay for an Antigenic Determinant (CA 125) Associated with Human Epithelial Ovarian Carcinomas," *Cancer Research* 44 (1984): 1048.

70. Interviews with Holveck (1) and (2), 4–35; D. Fishlock, "Why Centocor Gets the 20% It Asks For: The 'Intel of Biotechnology' Stakes Its Claim," *Financial Times* (24 Oct. 1983), 14; D. Dickinson, "Biotech's Centocor Jockeys for Position in Drug Field," *Scientist* 4 (1990) 1–5, esp. 3; Centocor, *Annual Report* (1983): 14, (1990): 14; B. Momich, "Building Something Significant at Centocor," *Pennsylvania Technology* (2nd quarter, 1990): 25–31; Centocor Press Release, "Centocor Receives FDA Panel Recommendation to Approve Ovarian Cancer Test," 3 Nov. 1986, HS-PP; L. Thompson, "New Test for Ovarian Cancer Detects Residual Cells in the Blood," *Washington Post* (16 June 1987); Interview with Zurawski; Anon., "TWST Names Award Winners Biotechnology," *Wall Street Transcript* 97, no. 11 (14 Dec. 1987).

71. Mackenzie, Cambrosio, and Keating, "Commercial," 158; J. Marx, *A Revolution in Biotechnology* (Cambridge, Eng., 1989), 145, 147.

72. BCC Research, "Monoclonal Therapeutics and Companion Diagnostic Products," Report BIoo16G, Jan. 2008, available online at http://www.bccre search.com/report/monoclonal-therapeutics-products-bioo16g.html (accessed 19 Sept. 2014).

CHAPTER 7. THE CHALLENGE OF MONOCLONAL ANTIBODY DRUGS

1. Z. An, ed., *Therapeutic Monoclonal Antibodies: From Bench to Clinic* (Hoboken, N.J., 2009), ch. 1.
2. G. Goldstein et al., "OKT3: Monoclonal Antibody Plasma Levels during Therapy and the Subsequent Development of Host Antibodies to OKT3," *Transplantation* 42 (Nov. 1986): 507–11; D. Abramowicz and M. Goldman, "Anaphylactic Shock after Retreatment with OKT3 Monoclonal Antibody," *NEJM* 3 (Sept. 1992): 736; K. J. Palevliet and P. T. Schellekens, "Monoclonal Antibodies in Renal Transplantation: A Review," *Transplant International* 5, no. 4 (Sept. 1992): 234–46; C. Sgro, "Side-Effects of a Monoclonal Antibody, Muromonab CD3/Orthoclone OKT3: Bibliographic Review," *Toxicology* 105, no. 1 (Dec. 1995): 23–29; S. L. Smith, "Ten Years of Orthoclone OKT3 (muromonab-CD3): A Review," *Journal of Transplant Coordination* 6, no. 3 (Sept 1996): 109–19; M. I. Wilde and K. L. Goa, "Muromonab CD3: A Reappraisal of Its Pharmacology and Use as Prophylaxis of Solid Organ Transplant Rejection," *Drugs* 51, no. 5 (May 1996): 865–94; A. F. LoBuglio et al., "Mouse/Human Chimeric Monoclonal Antibody in Man: Kinetics and Immune Response," *PNAS* 86 (June 1989): 4220–24.
3. G. Kretzmer, "Industrial Processes with Animal Cells," *Applied Microbiology and Biotechnology* 59 (2002): 135–42; G. Bylinsky, "Coming: Star Wars Medicine," *Fortune* (27 Apr. 1987); Interview with Renato Fuchs.
4. Centocor, *Annual Report* (1983): 2.
5. Centocor, *Annual Report* (1985): 11; Bylinsky, "Coming"; Interview with Stelios Papadopolous, 22.
6. Centocor, *Annual Report* (1983): 2, (1984): 16, (1990): 7; Centocor, *Investment Prospectus*, 14 Dec. 1982; PaineWebber, *Centocor Common Stock*, 13 Dec. 1985, 4, 6, 34; PaineWebber, *Tocor II and Centocor Prospectus*, 21 Jan. 1992; all in HS-PP; A. Pollack, "The Next Wave of Diagnostics," *New York Times* (28 Aug. 1989).
7. Centocor, *Investment Prospectus*, 14 Dec. 1982, 17; Centocor, *Annual Report* (1983): 2, (1988). Interviews with Fuchs and Jeffrey Mattis.
8. Interview with Fuchs; Centocor, *Annual Reports* (1988): 4, (1990): 7; Anon., "Centocor's Myoscint Imaging Agent Backed in USA," *Pharmaletter* (5 Feb. 1996), available online at http://www.thepharmaletter.com/file/25880 /centocors-myoscint-imaging-agent-backed-in-usa.html (accessed 19 Sept. 2014).
9. BCC Research, "Antibodies for Therapeutic and Diagnostic Imaging Applications," Report BIoo16D, Feb. 2000, available online at http://www.bccre search.com/market-research/biotechnology/BIOo16D.html, and BCC

Research, "Dynamic Antibody Industry," Report BIO016F, Aug. 2005, available online at http://www.bccresearch.com/market-research/biotechnology/BIO016F.html (both accessed 2 Oct. 2014); R. Wolf, "Centocor Makes a Deal on Product Marketing," *Philadelphia Inquirer* (7 Dec. 1987).

10. Cetus was the only other biotechnology company that had managed to develop more human antibodies at this stage. Centocor, *Annual Reports* (1983): 6 18, 28; (1985) 2; (1986); Rothschild, *Centocor Inc* (1983): 47; Interview with Stephen Evens-Freke; Bylinsky, "Coming."

11. Interviews with Pedro Tetteroo, Bruce Peacock, and Erik and Kathleen Schoemaker; PaineWebber, *Centocor Common Stock*, 13 Dec. 1985, 4, 6, 34. Centocor, *Annual Report* (1988): 8; P. Pfeiffer Chambers, "Two Area Firms Ready for Biotech Boom," *Focus* (15 July 1987): 17–19.

12. Interviews with Tetteroo and James Christie.

13. Interview with Christie; Kretzmer, "Industrial."

14. Centocor, *Annual Reports* (1988): 3, (1989): 8, (1990): 2.

15. Interview with Tetteroo. Email from Jacques Fonteyne to Anne Faulkner Schoemaker, 8 Nov. 2005, HS-PP; Centocor, *Annual Reports* (1986): 17; (1988): 5; S. Dickinson, "Biotech's Centocor Jockeys for Position in Drug Field," *Scientist* 4 (14 May 1990): 1–5, 2.

16. Centocor, *Annual Report* (1986): 2. Genentech was one of the first biotechnology companies to use R&D partnerships, in 1982, using it to develop human growth hormone and gamma interferon drugs. R&D partnerships had tax benefits and potentially higher returns than equity investments. Interview with Evens-Freke.

17. Centocor, *Annual Report* (1985): 29, (1988): 2, 12; Interviews with Fuchs, Richard McCloskey, Denise McGinn, David Holveck (1), and Vincent Zurawski; B. E. Kreger, D. E. Craven, P. C. Carling, and W. R. McCabe, "Gram-Negative Bacteremia, III: Reassessment of Etiology, Epidemiology and Ecology in 612 Patients," *American Journal of Medicine* 68 (1980): 332–43; R. C. Bone, "Gram-Negative Sepsis: Background, Clinical Features and Intervention," *Chest* 100 (1991): 802–808.

18. W. R. McCabe, B. E. Kreger, and M. Johns, "Type-Specific and Cross-Reactive Antibodies in Gram-Negative Bacteremia," *NEJM* 287 (1972): 261–67; E. J. Ziegler et al., "Treatment of Gram-Negative Bacteremia and Shock with Human Anti-Serum to a Mutant Escherichia Coli," *NEJM* 307 (1982): 1225–30; K. F. Bayston and J. Cohen, "Bacterial Endotoxin and Current Concepts in the Diagnosis and Treatment of Endotoxaemia," *Journal of Medical Microbiology* 31 (1990): 73–83; E. J. Ziegler et al., "Treatment of Gram-Negative Bacteremia and Septic Shock with HA-1A Human Monoclonal Antibody against Endotoxin: A Randomized, Double-Blind, Placebo-Controlled Trial. The HA-1A Sepsis Study Group," *NEJM* 324 (1991): 429–36; A. Cometta, J. D. Baumgartner, and M. P. Glauser, "Polyclonal Intravenous Immune Globulin for Prevention and Treatment of Infections in Critically Ill Patients," *Clinical and Experimental Immunology* 97 (1994): 69–72.

19. D. Shaw, "A Bruising Battle over Two Lifesaving Drugs," *Philadelphia Inquirer* (5 Nov. 1991); N. N. Teng et al., "Protection against Gram-Negative Bacteremia and Endotoxemia with Human Monoclonal IgM Antibodies," *PNAS* 82 (1985): 1790–94; I. R. Poxton, "Antibodies to Lipopolysaccharide," *J Immunol Methods* 186 (1995): 1–15; P. J. Scannon, "Applying Lessons Learned from Anti-Endotoxin Therapy," *Journal of Endotoxin Research* 2 (1995): 217–20; B. Momich, "Building Something Significant at Centocor," *Pennsylvania Technology* (2nd quarter, 1990): 25–31.

20. Interview with Tony Evnin; R. Koenig, "Remembering Hubert," *American Enterprise Magazine* (16 May 2006). Amgen's blockbuster drugs were Epogen, approved in 1989 to treat anemia, and Neupogen, approved in 1991 to help cancer patients receiving chemotherapy avoid infections.

21. Centocor, *Annual Reports* (1986): 16, (1988); Dickinson, "Biotech's"; R. Longman, "The Lessons of Centocor," *In Vivo: The Business and Medicine Report* (May 1992); 23–27; R. Winslow, "Centocor's New Drug Clears FDA Panel, Xoma's Put on Hold: Both Stocks Go Wild," *Wall Street Journal* 217 (5 Sept. 1991): 47; Interview with Peacock; Interview with Sandra Faragalli, Ray Heslip and Patty Durachko; Interviews with Paul Touhey and Pat D'Antonio.

22. Centocor, *Annual Report* (1989): 3–4.

23. C. J. Zimmerman et al., "Initial Evaluation of Human Monoclonal Anti-Lipid A Antibody (HA-1A) in Patients with Sepsis Syndrome," *Critical Care Medicine* (1990): 18, 1311–15; Ziegler et al., "Treatment of Gram-Negative Bacteremia and Septic Shock"; S. A. Syed, "Successful Use of Monoclonal Anti-Lipid-A IgM in Infant with Meningococcal Sepsis," *Lancet* (22 Feb. 1992): 339, 496.

24. Anon., "Centocor Inc," *Wall Street Transcript* (27 May 1991): 111; J. M. Luce, "Introduction of New Technology into Critical Care Practice: A History of HA-1A Human Monoclonal Antibody against Endotoxin," *Critical Care Medicine* 21, no. 8 (1993): 1233–40; Winslow, "Centocor's New Drug Clears FDA Panel"; Anon., "Centocor's Drug Is Ruled Safe," *New York Times* (5 Sept. 1991); Anon., "Centocor, Inc.," *Times Magazine* (25 Feb. 1991).

25. "Xoma Sues Centocor on Patent Infringement," *Biotechnology Law Report* 90 (1990): 90, no. 2; Centocor, *Annual Report* (1991): 38–39; Shaw, "Bruising"; Longman, "Lessons," 24; L. L. Valerino, "Centocor Stock Slides on News of Drug Snag," *Wall Street Journal* (20 Feb. 1992); L. M. Fisher, "Centocor and Xoma Settle Patent Fight," *New York Times* (30 July 1992); Winslow, "Centocor's New Drug Clears FDA Panel"; Centocor, *Annual Report* (1991): 38–39; Interviews with Bernie Schaffer, Holveck (1), Faulkner Schoemaker and Papadopoulos; Quezado et al., "Controlled"; D. N. Leff, "Animal Study Showed Mortality with HA-1A," *BioWorld Today* 1993 (1991): 5.

26. J. D. Baumgartner et al., "Association between Protective Efficacy of Anti-Lipopolysaccharide (LPS) Antibodies and Suppression of LPS-Induced Tumor Necrosis Factor Alpha and Interleukin 6: Comparison of Side Chain-Specific Antibodies with Core LPS Antibodies," *JEM* 171 (1990): 889–96;

J. Baumgartner, "Letter to the Editor," *NEJM* 325 (1991): 281–82; Anon., "At the Market's Edge: How a $1 Billion Drug Fell Flat," *New York Times* (Feb. 1993); F. Curie, M. D. Feher, and A. F. Lant, "How to Pay for Expensive Drugs," *BMJ* 303 (1991): 1476–78.

27. Curie et al., "How"; K. A. Schulman, H. A. Glick, and J. M. Rubin, "Cost-Effectiveness of HA-1A Monoclonal Antibody for Gram-Negative Sepsis: Economic Assessment of a New Therapeutic Agent," *Journal of the American Medical Association* 266 (1991): 3466–71; R. C. Bone, "Monoclonal Antibodies to Endotoxin: New Allies against Sepsis?" *Journal of the American Medical Association* 266 (1991): 1125–26; C. J. Hinds, "Monoclonal Antibodies in Sepsis and Septic Shock," *BMJ* 304 (1992): 132–33; G. D. Magi, "Letter to Editor," *BMJ* 303 (1991): 1477.

28. Schulman et al., "Cost-Effectiveness"; Magi, "Letter."

29. Longman, "Lessons"; Hinds, "Monoclonal"; Magi, "Letter."

30. Interview with Faragalli, Heslip and Durachko; Interviews with Holveck (1), and Anne Faulkner Schoemaker; D. Shaw, "FDA, Wall Street Brings Bad Tidings to Centocor," *Philadelphia Inquirer* 20 (1992): 11; Centocor, *Annual Report* (1986): 16; L. L. Valeriano, "Centocor Stock Slides on News of Snag," *Wall Street Journal* (1992); S. Usdin, "Wall St. Vents Frustration at Centocor," *BioWorld Today* (1992); Koenig, "Remembering"; D. Shaw, "Centocor Absorbs New Blows," *Philadelphia Inquirer* (1992); Anon., "FDA: Centoxin Data Insufficient," *BioWorld Today* 3 (1992): 1.

31. A. Newman and D. Pettit, "Biotech Stock Lead Index 0.64% Lower; Centocor Plunges on Worry over Drug," *Wall Street Journal* (20 Feb. 1992); Email from Don Drakeman to Marks, 4 May 2012; Longman, "Lessons."

32. Interview with Faragalli, Heslip and Durachko; Interviews with Papadopolous and Michael Melore. For the Weisman quotation, see R. L. Shook, *Miracle Medicines* (New York, 2007), 206.

33. Centocor, *Annual Report* (1992): 7; Interviews with Touhey, Papadopoulos, and J. P. Garnier; L. Marks, "Collaboration—A Competitor's Tool: The Story of Centocor, an Entrepreneurial Biotechnology Company," *Business History* 51, no. 4 (2009): 529–46; Anon., "Lilly to Acquire Marketing Rights to Centocor Drug"; Centocor, *Centroids;* N. Garcia, "Centocor Resumes Trials in Children," *BioWorld Today* (20 Jan. 1993); D. Shaw, "A New Round of Bad News: Unexplained Test Deaths," *Philadelphia Inquirer* (19 Jan. 1993); R. M. Enigma, "Centocor to Terminate HA-1A," Centocor press release, 15 Mar. 1993, HS-PP; N. Garcia, "But Company Kills HA-1A Trials," *BioWorld Today* 4, no. 52 (17 Mar. 1993): 1.

34. Hubert Schoemaker to David Kessler, Sept. 1992, HS-PP; Interview with Ann McKenzie.

35. Garcia, "Centocor"; Garcia, "But"; R. M. Enigma, "Centocor to Terminate HA-1A: Centocor Press Release" (1993), HS-PP; G. Kolata, "Halted at the Market's Door: How a $1 Billion Drug Failed," *New York Times* (12 Feb. 1993); Interview with Melore.

36. Interviews with Garnier and with Erik and Kathleen Schoemaker.

37. Dickinson, "Biotech's"; Longman, "Lessons"; Kolata, "Halted."

38. Interviews with George Hobbs and Papadopoulous; Amgen SEC filing: Form:10-Q, 8/10/1994, available online from Amgen and at https://www.sec. gov. B. Stavro, "George B. Rathmann Dies at 84; Co-Founder of Biotech Giant Amgen," *Los Angeles Times* (24 Apr. 2012).

39. Interviews with Bernie Schaffer, Jay Siegel, Holveck (1), Papadopolous, and Faulkner Schoemaker; Usdin, "Wall"; Shaw, "FDA, Wall Street Bring Bad Tidings to Centocor"; Anon., "FDA Snag and Loss Hurt Centocor Stock," *New York Times* (20 Feb. 1992); Valeriano, "Centocor"; Newman and Pettit, "Biotech"; Longman, "Lessons"; J. P. Siegel, "Biotechnology and Clinical Trials," *J Infect Dis* 185 (2002) 52–57.

40. Interview with Siegel; H. J. P. Schoemaker and A. F. Schoemaker, "The Three Pillars of Bioentrepreneurship," *Nat Biotechnol* 16 (1998): 13–15; R. C. Bone et al., "Severe Sepsis Study Group: Sepsis Syndrome; a Valid Clinical Entity," *Critical Care Medicine* 17 (1989): 389–93; K. C. Fang, "Monoclonal Antibodies to Endotoxin in the Management of Sepsis," *Western Journal of Medicine* 158 (1993): 393–99; E. F. Mammen, "Perspectives for the Future," *Intensive Care Medicine* 19 (1993): 29–34; R. P. Wenzel et al., "Current Understanding of Sepsis," *Clin Infect Dis* 22 (1996): 407–12; N. C. Riedemann, R. F. Guo, and P. A. Ward, "The Enigma of Sepsis," *J Clin Invest* 112 (2003): 460–67.

41. Interviews with Siegel and Thomas Schaible; Siegel, "Biotechnology"; D. A. Sweeney, et al., "Once is Not Enough: Clinical Trials in Sepsis," *Intensive Care Medicine* 34 (2008): 1955–60.

42. Interview with Peacock.

43. Interview with Holveck (1).

44. Garcia, "But"; B. Derkx, J. Wittes, R. McCloskey, and European Pediatric Meningococcal Septic Shock Trial Study Group, "Randomized, Placebo-Controlled Trial of HA-1A, a Human Monoclonal Antibody to Endotoxin, in Children with Meningococcal Septic Shock," *Clin Infect Dis* 28 (1999): 770–77.

45. Interview with Harlan Weisman; J. C. Marshall, "Sepsis: Rethinking the Approach to Clinical Research," *Journal of Leukocyte Biology* 83 (2008): 471–78.

46. Anon., "Lilly to Acquire."

47. For more on chimeric Mabs, see Chapter 9.

48. Interviews with Weisman and McGinn; B. S. Coller, "Blockade of Platelet GPIIb/IIIa Receptors as an Antithrombotic Strategy," *Circulation* 92 (1995): 2373–80; D. M. Knight et al., "The Immunogenicity of the 7E3 Murine Monoclonal Fab Antibody Fragment Variable Region Is Dramatically Reduced in Humans by Substitution of Human for Murine Constant Regions," *Molecular Immunology* 32 (1995): 1271–81.

49. Interview with McGinn.

50. Ibid. Keaven Anderson was senior director at Centocor from 1991 to 2003.

51. Interviews with McGinn, Melore, and Schaible.
52. Interview with McGinn.
53. D. B. Mark et al., "Economic Assessment of Platelet Glycoprotein IIb/IIIa Inhibition for Prevention of Ischemic Complications of High-Risk Coronary Angioplasty," *Circulation* 94 (1996): 629–35; C. F. Farrell, S. Elliot Barnathan, and H. F. Weisman, "The Evolution of ReoPro Clinical Development," in K. Disembowel and P. Staler, eds., *Novel Therapeutic Proteins: Selected Case Studies* (Hoboken, N.J., 2001).
54. Centocor, *Annual Report* (1996): 5.

CHAPTER 8. ANTIBODY ENGINEERING

1. C. Milstein, "Monoclonal Antibodies from Hybrid Myelomas," *Proceedings of the Royal Society of London* 211 (1981): 393–412, 409.
2. M. B. Khazaeli, R. M. Conry, and A. F. LoBuglio, "Human Immune Response to Monoclonal Antibodies," *Journal of Immunotherapy* 15 (1994): 42–52.
3. K. M. Thompson et al., "The Efficient Production of Stable, Human Monoclonal Antibody-Secreting Hybridomas from EBV-Transformed Lymphocytes Using the Mouse Myeloma X63-Ag8.653 as a Fusion Partner," *J Immunol Methods* 94, nos. 1–2 (Nov. 1986): 7–12; J. L. Marx, "Antibodies Made to Order," *Science* 229 (2 Aug. 1985): 455–56; G. P. Winter, "Antibody Engineering," *Phil Trans R Soc Lond B* 324 (1989): 537–47, esp. 539; N. Lonberg, "Transgenic Approaches to Human Monoclonal Antibodies," in M. Rosenberg and G. P. Moore, eds., *The Pharmacology of Monoclonal Antibodies* (Berlin, 1994), 49–101, esp. 50; Emails from Michael Neuberger to author, 31 July 2012, and 5 Aug. 2012.
4. Milstein, "Monoclonal," 409; M. S. Neuberger and B. Askonas, "César Milstein," *Biographical Memoirs of the Fellows of the Royal Society* 51 (2005): 267–89, 278.
5. Interview with Michael Neuberger. Marx, "Antibodies," 455; Winter, "Antibody," 540.
6. N. Hozumi and S. Tonegawa, "Evidence for Somatic Rearrangement of Immunoglobulin Genes Coding for Variable and Constant Regions," *PNAS* 73, no. 10 (1976): 3628–32; Marx, "Antibodies," 455; Interview with Neuberger.
7. Interview with Neuberger; Emails from Neuberger.
8. D. Rice and D. Baltimore, "Regulated Expression of an Immunoglobulin Kappa Gene Introduced into a Mouse Lymphoid Cell Line," *PNAS* 79, no. 24 (1982): 7862–65; S. L. Morrison, V. T. Oi, "Transfer and Expression of Immunoglobulin Genes," *Ann Rev Immunol* 2 (1984): 239–56.
9. M. S. Neuberger, G. T. Williams, and R. O. Fox, "Recombinant Antibodies Possessing Novel Effector Functions," *Nature* 312, no. 5995 (1984): 604–608; M.S. Neuberger et al., "A Hapten-Specific Chimaeric IgE Antibody with Human Effector Function," *Nature* 314 (1985): 268–70; S. L. Morrison et al., "Chimeric Human Antibody Molecules: Mouse Antigen-Binding

Domains with Human Constant Region Domains," *PNAS* 81 (1984): 6851–55; G. Boulianne, N. Hozumi, and M. J. Shulman, "Production of Functional Chimaeric Mouse/Human Antibody," *Nature* 312 (13 Dec. 1984): 643–46.

10. C. Zeller, "The Spatial Innovation Biography of a Successful Monoclonal Antibody," *Espace* 5 (20 Jan. 2008): 1–42.

11. Interview with Gregory Winter; Emails from Neuberger; S. Cabilly et al., "Generation of Antibody Activity from Immunoglobulin Polypeptide Chains Produced in *Escherichia coli*," *PNAS* 81 (1984): 3273–77; M. A. Boss, J. H. Kenten, C. R. Wood, and J. S. Emtage, "Assembly of Functional Antibodies from Immunoglobulin Heavy and Light Chains Synthesised in *E. coli*," *Nucleic Acids Research* 12, no. 9 (1984): 3791–806; Winter, "Antibody," 540; E. Waltz, "Industry Waits for Fallout from Cabilly," *Nature* 25, no. 7 (2007): 699–700; R. L. Teskin, "It Lives for 29 Years," *Legal Times* 26, no. 44 (2004): 1–2.

12. W. R. Gombotz and S. J. Shire, "Introduction," in S. J. Shire et al., eds., *Current Trends in Monoclonal Antibody Development and Manufacturing* (New York, 2009), 3.

13. C. A. Hutchison and M. H. Edgell, "Genetic Assay for Small Fragments of Bacteriophage φX174 Deoxyribonucleic Acid", *Journal of Virology* 8, no. 2 (1971): 181–89; H. Schott and H. Kössel, "Synthesis of Phage Specific Deoxyribonucleic Acid Fragments, I: Synthesis of Four Undecanucleotides Complementary to a Mutated Region of the Coat Protein Cistron of fd Phage Deoxyribonucleic Acid," *Journal of the American Chemical Society* 95, no. 11 (1973): 3778–85; C. A. Hutchison, S. Phillips, M. H. Edgell, S. Gillham, P. Jahnke, and M. Smith, "Mutagenesis at a Specific Position in a DNA Sequence," *J Biol Chem* 253, no. 18 (1978): 6551–60; N. Kresge, R. D. Simoni, and R. L. Hill, "The Development of Site-Directed Mutagenesis by Michael Smith," *J Biol Chem* 281 (2006): e31–e33; Anon., "Michael Smith," online biography available online at http://www.science.ca/scientists/scientistprofile .php?pID=18&pg=1 (accessed 20 Sept. 2014).

14. Interviews with Neuberger and Winter; Email from Gregory Winter to Marks, 20 Jan. 2013; G. Winter et al., "Redesigning Enzyme Structure by Site-Directed Mutagenesis: Tyrosyl tRNA Synthetase and ATP Binding," *Nature* 299 (1982): 756–58; Hutchison et al., "Mutagenesis"; Winter, "Antibody," 537.

15. Interview with Winter.

16. Ibid.; E. Kabat et al., *Sequences of Proteins of Immunological Interest*, 5th ed. (Bethesda, Md., 1991); G. Hale, "Therapeutic Antibodies—Delivering the Promise," *Advanced Drug Delivery Reviews* 58 (2006): 633–39.

17. Interview with Winter; Winter, "Antibody," 540.

18. Interviews with Neuberger and Winter; P. T. Jones et al., "Replacing the Complementarity-Determining Regions in a Mouse Antibody with Those from a Mouse," *Nature* 321 (29 May 1986): 522–25; Gombotz and Shire, "Introduction," 3.

19. Interview with Michael Clark; R. J. Benjamin, S. Cobbold, M. R. Clark, and H. Waldmann, "Tolerance to Rat Monoclonal Antibodies: Implications for Serotherapy," *JEM* 163 (June 1986): 1539–52; L. Riechmann, M. Clark, H. Waldmann, and G. Winter, "Reshaping Human Antibodies for Therapy," *Nature* 332 (24 Mar. 1988): 323–24; G. Hale and H. Waldmann, "From Laboratory to Clinic: The Story of Campath-1," in A. J. Y. George and C. E. Urch, eds., *Diagnostic and Therapeutic Antibodies* (New York, 2000), 243–66, 250; M. Clark, "Mike's Campath Story," available online at http://www.path .cam.ac.uk/~mrc7/campath/campath.html (accessed 20 Sept. 2014).

20. G. Hale, "Remission Induction in Non-Hodgkin Lymphoma with Reshaped Human Monoclonal Antibody CAMPATH-1H," *Lancet* 2 (1988): 1394–99; Email from Herman Waldmann to Marks, 16 July 2012; L. Marks, "The Life Story of a Biotechnology Drug: Alemtuzumab," http://www.whatisbiotechnology.org/exhibitions/campath (accessed 20 Sept. 2014).

21. L. R. Helms and R. I. Wetzel, "Destabilizing Loop Swaps in the CDRs of an Immunoglobulin V_L Domain," *Protein Science* 4 (1995): 2073–81; C. Queen et al., "A Humanised Antibody That Binds to the Interleukin 2 Receptor," *PNAS* 86 (1989): 10029–33; M. S. Co, M. Deschamps, R. J. Whitley, and C. Queen, "Humanised Antibodies for Antiviral Therapy," *PNAS* 88 (1991): 2869–73; S. Dübel, *Handbook of Therapeutic Antibodies*, vol. 1 (Hoboken, N.J., 2007), 122; J. W. Saldanha, "Humanization of Recombinant Antibodies," in M. Little, ed., *Recombinant Antibodies for Immunotherapy* (Cambridge, Eng.), 3–11.

22. R. Olandi, D. H. Güssow, P. T. Jones, and G. Winter, "Cloning Immunoglobulin Variable Domains for Expression by Polymerase Chain Reaction," *PNAS* 86 (1989): 3833–37; Mercer to Dunston, 24 Oct. 1989, MSTN, file F19.

23. Interview with Winter; Mercer to Dunston, 24 Oct. 1989; Notes on meeting at LMB, 19 Oct. 1989, MSTN, file F19; S. de Chadarevian, "The Making of an Entrepreneurial Science: Biotechnology in Britain, 1975–1995," *ISIS* 102, no. 4 (2011): 601–33, fn84, 629.

24. Email from Winter; J. Finch, *A Nobel Fellow on Every Floor: A History of the Medical Research Council Laboratory of Molecular Biology* (Cambridge, Eng., 2008), 242; de Chadarevian, "Making," 628.

25. J. Mcafferty, A. D. Griffiths, G. Winter, and D. J. Chiswell, "Phage Antibodies: Filamentous Phage Displaying Antibody Variable Domains," *Nature* 348 (1990): 552–54; S. J. Russell, M. B. Llewelyn, and R. E. Hawkins, "The Human Antibody Library," *BMJ* 304 (1992): 585–86.

26. H. R. Hoogenboom and G. Winter, "By-Passing Immunisation: Human Antibodies from Synthetic Repertoires of Germline VH Gene Segments Rearranged *in Vitro*," *J Mol Biol* 227 (1992): 381–88; A. Nissim et al., "Antibody Fragments from a 'Single Pot' of Phage Display Library as Immunochemical Reagents," *EMBO J* 13, no. 3 (1994): 692–98; J. D. Marks et al., "By-Passing Immunization: Human Antibodies from V-Gene Libraries Displayed on Phage," *J Mol Biol* 222 (1991): 581–97; A. D. Griffiths et al., "Human Anti-Self

Antibodies with High Specificity from Phage Display Libraries," *EMBO J* 12, no. 2 (1993): 725–34; H. R. Hoogenboom, "Designing and Optimizing Library Selection Strategies for Generating High-Affinity Antibodies," *Tibtech* 15 (1997): 62–70; Russell, Llewelyn, and Hawkins, "Human."

27. Interview with Neuberger; Finch, *Nobel*, 249–50. The first transgenic mouse was created in 1974 by Rudolf Jaenisch, a biologist based at Massachusetts Institute of Technology, to study cancer and neurological disease.

28. F. W. Alt, T. K. Blackwell, and G. D. Yancopopulos, "Immunoglobulin Genes in Transgenic Mice," *Trends Genetics* (Aug. 1985): 231–36; Lonberg, "Transgenic," 60; Interview with Neuberger.

29. Emails from Neuberger; Lonberg, "Transgenic," 68.

30. Emails from Neuberger; D. T. Burke, G. F. Carle, and M. V. Olson, "Cloning of Large Segments of Exogenous DNA into Yeast by Means of Artificial Chromosome Vectors," *Science* 236 (1987): 806–12; M. Goodhardt et al., "Rearrangement and Expression of Rabbit Immunoglobulin κ Light Chain Gene in Transgenic Mice," *PNAS* 84 (1987): 4229–33; G. Buttin, "Exogenous Ig Gene Rearrangement in Transgenic Mice: A New Strategy for Human Monoclonal Antibody Production," *Trends in Genetics* 3, no. 8 (1987): 205–6; M. Brüggeman et al., "A Repertoire of Monoclonal Antibodies with Human Heavy Chains from Transgenic Mice," *PNAS* 86 (1989): 6709–13.

31. Emails from Neuberger; C. Zeller, "The Expectations on Mice—Rivalry and Collaboration in an Emerging Technological Arena," *ESPACE, Economics in Space—Working Papers in Economic Geography* (10 Jan. 2008): 1–31, 12.

32. S. L. Mansour, K. R. Thomas, and M. R. Capecchi, "Disruption of the Proto-Oncogene Int-2 in Mouse Embryo-Derived Stem Cells: A General Strategy for Targeting Mutations to Non-Selectable Genes," *Nature* 336 (1988): 348–52; M. Zilstra et al., "Germ-Line Transmission of a Disrupted Beta 2-Microglobulin Gene Produced by Homologous Recombination in Embryonic Stem Cells," *Nature* 342 (1989): 435–38; P. L. Schwartzberg S. P. Goff, and E. J. Robertson, "Germline Transmission of a c-abi Mutation Produced by Targeted Gene Disruption in ES Cells," *Science* 246 (1989): 799–803.

33. Emails from Neuberger; Interview with Nils Lonberg; Schwartzberg, Goff, and Robertson, "Germline."

34. Interview with Lonberg; A. Weintraub, "Crossing the Gene Barrier," *Business Week*, 3967 (15 Jan. 2006): 72.

35. Ibid.; A. N. Houghton et al., "Mouse Monoclonal Antibody Detecting GD3 Ganglioside: A Phase I Trial in Patients with Malignant Melanoma," *PNAS* 82 (1985): 1242–46; S. Vadhan-Raj et al., "Phase I Trial of a Mouse Monoclonal Antibody Against GD3 Ganglioside in Patients with Melanoma: Induction of Inflammatory Responses at Tumor Sites," *Journal of Clinical Oncology* 6, no. 10 (1988): 1636–48.

36. GenPharm International v. Japan Tobacco, "Complaint for Monopolization," case no. C96–0487 CW, Northern District Court of California, Oakland, 18, 21–22, 33; Interview with Lonberg; G. Stix, "The Mice That Warred," *Sci Am*

(June 2001): 34–35; Zeller, "Expectations," 13–14; S. D. Wagner et al., "Antibodies Generated from Human Immunoglobulin Miniloci in Transgenic Mice," *Nucleic Acids Research* 22, no. 8 (1994): 1389–93; S. D. Wagner et al., "The Diversity of Antigen-Specific Monoclonal Antibodies from Transgenic Mice Bearing Human Immunoglobulin Gene Miniloci," *EJI* 24, no. 11 (1994): 2672–81; N. Lonberg et al., "Antigen-Specific Human Antibodies from Mice Comprising Four Distinct Genetic Modifications," *Nature* 368 (1994): 856–59; L. D. Taylor et al., "Human Immunoglobulin Transgenes Undergo Rearrangement, Somatic Mutation and Class Switching in Mice That Lack Endogenous IgM," *International Immunology* 6, no. 4 (1994): 579–91; L. L. Green et al., "Antigen-Specific Human Antibodies from Mice Engineered with Human Ig Heavy and Light Chain YACs," *Nature Genetics* 7 (1994): 13–21; S. L. Morrison, "Success in Specification," *Nature* 368 (1994): 812–13.

37. Emails from Neuberger to Marks; Interview with Lonberg.

38. P. Chames et al., *British Journal of Pharmacology* 157 (2008): 220–33, 225; L. J. Holt et al., "Domain Antibodies: Proteins for Therapy," *Trends in Biotechnology* 21, no. 11 (2003): 484–90.

39. E. S. Ward et al., "Binding Activities of a Repertoire of Single Immunoglobulin Variable Domains Secreted from *Escherichia coli*," *Nature* 341 (1989): 544–46; R. Krelle, "Winter's Way: Why Domantis Still Leads in Antibody Technology," *Australian Life Scientist* (7 May 2004); P. Holliger and P. J. Hudson, "Engineered Antibody Fragments and the Rise of Single Domains," *Nat Biotechnol* 23, no. 9 (2005): 1126–36, esp. 1127.

40. Holliger and Hudson, "Engineered," 1127. Domantis was financed by seed capital from Peptech (£10 million) and MVM (£1 million). G. Winter, "Past, Present and Future of Antibody Therapeutics," paper presented to EAPB and EUFEPS Workshop, Amsterdam, Apr. 2007; Ward et al., "Binding;" Krelle, "Winter's."

41. M. Clark, "Antibody Humanization: A Case of the "Emperor's New Clothes?" *Immunology Today* 21, no. 8 (2000): 397–402; G. Hale, "Therapeutic Antibodies—Delivering the Promise," *Advanced Drug Delivery Reviews* 58 (2006): 633–39, esp. 636; Emails from Neuberger.

42. Interview with Lonberg.

43. Emails from Neuberger to Marks.

44. A. L. Nelson and J. M. Reichert, "Development Trends for Therapeutic Antibody Fragments," *Nat Biotechnol* 27, no. 4 (2009): 331–37, esp. 332.

45. Hale, "Therapeutic"; K. Eichmann, *Köhler's Invention* (Basel, 2005), 91; J. Van Brunt, "The Monoclonal Maze," *Signals Magazine* (30 Nov. 2005); C. Zeller, "From the Gene to the Globe: Extracting Rents Based on Intellectual Property Monopolies," *Review of International Political Economy* 15, no. 1 (2008): 86–115; Emails from Don Drakeman to Marks, 19 and 31 July 2012.

46. GenPharm, "Complaint"; Emails from Neuberger; Zeller, "Expectations"; Stix, "Mice"; A. Jakobovits et al., "From XenoMouse Technology to

Panitumumab, the First Fully Human Antibody Product from Transgenic Mice," *Nat Biotechnol* 25, no. 10 (2007): 1134–43.

47. Emails from Neuberger; Interview with Lonberg.

48. Nelson and Reichert, "Development," 332.

49. In the GenPharm and Kirin Brewery case, the mice were created from cross-breeding a GenPharm transgenic mouse with another created by Kirin Brewery. Zeller, "Expectations."

50. A. L. Nelson, E. Dhimolea, and J. M. Reichert, "Development Trends for Human Monoclonal Antibody Therapeutics," *Nat Rev Drug Discov* 9 (2010): 767–74; Emails from Drakeman.

51. Nelson, Dhimolea, and Reichert, "Development"; Interview with Lonberg.

52. De Chadarevian, "Making," 622.

53. C. Milstein, "Draft paper," 2 June 1988 attached to "Awards to Inventors— MRC Scheme," 26 Oct. 1989, MSTN, file F19; "Policy Statement by the Secretary of State for Education and Science: The Exploitation of Research Council Funded Inventions," 25 Mar. 1985, MSTN, file F21; Finch, *Nobel*; de Chadarevian, "Making," 623–24.

54. Finch, *Nobel*, 241; de Chadarevian, "Making," 623–24. The principle of broadly licensing out the technology was also pursued by companies.

55. Emails from Neuberger; de Chadarevian, "Making," 623–24, 627; Finch, *Nobel*, 241.

56. Emails from Neuberger; Winter, "Past," slide 29; de Chadarevian, "Making," 623–24. In 2006 BTG reported receiving £3.4 million in gross revenue from the MRC's humanization IP portfolio. The company reported £4.1 million such revenue for 2007, £6.3 million for 2008, and then £5.1 million for 2009. BTG, *Annual Reports* (2008), (2011).

57. A. Fazackerley, "Royalties Coup Boosts Science," *Times Higher Education* (28 Oct. 2005); House of Commons Science and Technology Committee, Research Council for Knowledge Transfer, *Third Report of Session 2005–06*, vol. 2 (15 Mar. 2006), 87; MRC News, "Sir Gregory Winter Wins Prestigious Prince of Asturias Award," 1 June 2012, available online at http://www.mrc .ac.uk/news-events/news/sir-gregory-winter-wins-prestigious-prince-of-asturias-award (accessed 2 Oct. 2014).

58. De Chadarevian, "Making," fig. 4, 630; LMB, "New Building," available online at http://www2.mrc-lmb.cam.ac.uk/about-lmb/new-building (accessed 20 Sept. 2014).

CHAPTER 9. BLOCKBUSTER MAB DRUGS

1. Anon., "First Launch of Wellcome's Panorex," *PharmaLetter*, 13 Mar. 1995; P. A. Baeuerie and D. Ruettinger, "EpCam's Renaissance," *Drug Discovery and Development* (4 Sept. 2009). Two murine antibodies were approved for non-Hodgkin's lymphoma (NHL) in 2002 and 2003 (iritumomab tiuxetan and tositumomab). These drugs contained radiolabels, the potency

of which helped reduce the amount of antibody given, thereby limiting their potential immunogenicity. See Riechert et al., "Monoclonal."

2. K. Stein, "FDA-Approved Monoclonal Antibody Products," unpublished paper in possession of Lara Marks, 2010; J. M. Reichert, "Marketed Therapeutic Antibodies Compendium," *mAbs* 4, no. 3 (2012): table 1, 414.

3. R. L. Shook, *Miracle Medicines: Seven Lifesaving Drugs and the People Who Created Them* (New York, 2007), 192.

4. L. M. Nadler and W. C. Roberts, "Lee Marshall Nadler, MD: A Conversation with the Editor," *Baylor University Medical Center Proceedings* 20, no. 4 (2007): 381–89; Nadler and Roberts, "Lee"; P. Stashenko et al., "Characterisation of a Human B Lymphocyte-Specific Antigen," *JI* 125, no. 4 (1980): 1678–85.

5. M. E. Reff, "The Discovery of Rituxan," in C. G. Smith and J. T. O'Donnell, eds., *The Process of New Drug Discovery and Development* (New York, 2006), 565–84, esp. 573; C. Zeller, "The Spatial Innovation Biography of a Successful Monoclonal Antibody," *Espace* 5 (2008): 1–42, esp. 17.

6. Stashenko et al., "Characterisation."

7. See Chapter 6.

8. P. Bofetta, "Epidemiology of Adult Non-Hodgkin Lymphoma," *Annals of Oncology* 22, no. 4 (2011): iv27–iv31.

9. Reff, "Discovery," 578; Email from R. Levy to Marks, 10 Jan. 2013.

10. Reff, "Discovery," 578; R. O. Dillman, "Magic Bullets at Last! Finally— Approval of a Monoclonal Antibody for the Treatment of Cancer!!!," *Cancer Biotherapy and Radiopharmaceuticals* 12, no. 4 (1997): 223–25, esp. 225.

11. Reff, "Discovery," 573; Zeller, "Spatial," 17; O. W. Press et al., "Monoclonal Antibody I F5 (Anti-CD2O) Serotherapy of Human B Cell Lymphomas," *Blood* 69, no. 2 (1987): 584–91; M. E. Reff et al., "Depletion of B cells in Vivo by a Chimeric Mouse Human Monoclonal Antibody to CD20," *Blood* 83, no. 2 (1994): 435–45.

12. A. J. Grillo-López et al., "Rituximab: The First Monoclonal Antibody Approved for the Treatment of Lymphoma," *Current Pharmaceutical Biotechnology* 1 (2000): 1–9, esp. 2.

13. Reff, "Discovery," 570. Idec subsequently licensed out its expression system to other companies such as Genentech, Chugai Pharmaceutical of Japan, and Boehringer Ingelheim of Germany to use in the manufacture of Mab therapeutics. The system was also used on a contract basis to help supply specific cell lines for other firms, such as F. Hoffmann–La Roche and Pharmacia & Upjohn, which was an important source of revenue. Zeller, "Spatial," 19.

14. Reff, "Discovery," 570–72, 577.

15. Grillo-López et al., "Rituximab," 1–2.

16. Reff, "Discovery," 575.

17. Email from Levy to Marks; D. G. Maloney et al., "IDEC-C2B8 (Rituximab) Anti-CD20 Monoclonal Antibody Therapy in Patients with Relapsed

Low-Grade Non-Hodgkin's Lymphoma," *Blood* 90, no. 6 (1997): 2188–95; Grillo-López et al., "Rituximab," 5–6.

18. S. M. Davis and R. King, "Cases in Strategic-Systems Auditing: Idec Pharmaceuticals Corporation," KPMG/University of Illinois Business Measurement Case Development and Research Programme (1999), 12; Interview with Ron Levy.

19. Interview with Levy; Davis and King, "Cases," 2; Zeller, "Spatial," 20.

20. D. G. Maloney et al., "IDEC-C2B8 (Rituximab) Anti-CD20 Monoclonal Antibody Therapy in Patients with Relapsed Low-Grade Non-Hodgkin's Lymphoma," *Blood* 90, no. 6 (1997): 2188–95; Grillo-López et al., "Rituximab," 5–6.

21. Idec Pharmaceuticals, *Annual Report* (2002): 8; Grillo-López et al., "Rituximab," 3.

22. Email from Levy to Marks; P. McLaughlin et al., "Rituximab Chimeric Anti-CD20 Monoclonal Antibody Therapy for Relapsed Indolent Lymphoma: Half of Patients Respond to a Four-Dose Treatment Program," *Journal of Clinical Oncology* 16, no. 8 (1988): 2825–33.

23. Dillman, "Magic Bullets at Last!"

24. K. A. Nyberg, "A New Kind of Cancer Warfare Agent: Next Generation Monoclonal Antibodies," *Oncology Business Review* (Nov 2007): 36–43, esp. 39.

25. Reff, "Discovery," 578, 581.

26. Ibid., 579; Davis and King, "Cases in Strategic-Systems Auditing," 12; R. Siegel, D. Naishadham, and A. Jemal, "Cancer Statistics, 2012," *A Cancer Journal for Clinicians* 62 (2012): 10.

27. A. Thomas, "Joe Burchenal and the Birth of Combination Chemotherapy," *British Journal of Haematology* 133, no. 5 (2006): 493–503; Anon., "FDA Approves Rituximab Plus CHOP for First Line Treatment of Diffuse Large B-Cell NHL," *HemOnc Today* (1 Mar. 2006).

28. A. Molina, "A Decade of Rituximab: Improving Survival Outcomes in Non-Hodgkin's Lymphoma," *Annual Review of Medicine* 59 (2008): 237–50.

29. Reff, "Discovery," 579; A. Protheroe et al., "Case Report: Remission of Inflammatory Arthropathy in Association with Anti-CD20 Therapy for Non-Hodgkin's Lymphoma," *Rheumatology* 38 (1998): 1150–52.

30. G. S. Alarcón, "Methotrexate Use in Rheumatoid Arthritis: A Clinician's Perspective," *Immunopharmacology* 47, nos. 2–3 (2000): 259–71; J. C. Edwards and G. Cambridge, "Hypothesis: Rheumatoid Arthritis: The Predictable Effect of Small Immune Complexes in Which Antibody Is Also Antigen," *British Journal of Rheumatology* 37 (1998): 126–30; J. C. W. Edwards, M. J. Leandro, and G. Cambridge, "B-Lymphocyte Depletion Therapy in Rheumatoid Arthritis and Other Autoimmune Disorders," *Biochemical Society Transactions* 30 (2002): 824–28; J. C. W. Edwards and J. Cambridge, "Is Rheumatoid Arthritis a Failure of B Cell Death in Synovium?," *Annals of Rheumatic Diseases* 54 (1995): 696–700; J. C. W. Edwards, G. Cambridge,

and V. M. Abrahams, "Do Self-Perpetuating B Lymphocytes Drive Human Autoimmune Disease?," *Immunology* 97 (1999): 188–96.

31. J. C. W. Edwards and G. Cambridge, "Sustained Improvement in Rheumatoid Arthritis Following a Protocol Designed to Deplete B Lymphocytes," *Rheumatology* 40 (2001): 305–11; M. J. Leandro, J. C. W. Edwards, and G. Cambridge, "Clinical Outcome in 22 Patients with Rheumatoid Arthritis Treated with B Lymphocyte Depletion," *Annals of Rheumatic Diseases* 61 (2002): 883–88; G. Cambridge et al., "Serologic Changes Following B Lymphocyte Depletion Therapy for Rheumatoid Arthritis," *Arthritis Rheum* 48, no. 8 (2003): 2146–54; J. C. W. Edwards, "Efficacy of B-Cell Targeted Therapy with Rituximab in Patients with Rheumatoid Arthritis," *NEJM* 350 (2004): 2572–81; J. M. Tuscano, "Successful Treatment of Infliximab-Refractory Rheumatoid Arthritis with Rituximab," *Arthritis Rheum* 46 (2002): 3420, LB11.

32. P. Peck, "FDA Approves Rituxan for Refractory Rheumatoid Arthritis," *MedPage Today*, 1 Mar. 2006; Roche, Media Release, 1 Mar. 2006, available online at http://www.medpagetoday.com/Rheumatology/Arthritis/2766 (accessed 2 Oct. 2014).

33. D. Symmons, C. Mathers, and B. Pfleger, "The Global Burden of Rheumatoid Arthritis in the Year 2000," *Global Burden of Disease, 2000* (15 Aug. 2006).

34. Wiki Analysis, "Arthritis Drug Market," http://www.wikinvest.com/wiki/Arthritis_Drug_Market#_note-13 (accessed 20 Sept. 2014).

35. F. Zaja, "B-Cell Depletion with Rituximab as Treatment for Immune Hemolytic Anemia and Chronic Thrombocytopenia," *Haematologica* 87 (2002): 189–95; F. Zaja et al., "The B-Cell Compartment as the Selective Target for the Treatment of Immune Thrombocytpenias," *Haematologica* 88, no. 5 (2003): 538–46; N. Walsh, "Rituximab Useful in Refractory Lupus," *MedPage Today* (6 Aug. 2010); J. T. Merrill et al., "Efficacy and Safety of Rituximab in Moderately-to-Severely Active Systemic Lupus Erythematosus: The Randomized, Double-Blind, Phase II/III Systemic Lupus Erythematosus Evaluation of Rituximab Trial," *Arthritis Rheum* 62, no. 1 (2010): 222–33; M. Eisenstein, "Approval on a Knife Edge," *Nat Biotechnol* 30 (2012): 26–29; FDA News Release, "FDA Approves Rituxan to Treat Two Rare Disorders," 19 Apr. 2011, available online at http://www.fda.gov/NewsEvents/Newsroom/Press Announcements/ucm251946.htm (accessed 20 Sept. 2014).

36. Centocor, *Annual Report* (1998): 5. While a rare condition, the annual mean medical cost of Crohn's disease in the United States was estimated to exceed $1.7 billion in 1996. See S. B. Hanaeuer et al., "Advances in the Management of Crohn's Disease: Economic and Clinical Potential of Infliximab," *Clinical Therapeutics* 20, no. 5 (1998): 1009–28, esp. 1009.

37. D. S. Stone-Wolff et al., "Interrelationships of Human Interferon-Gamma with Lymphotoxin and Monocyte Cytotoxin," *JEM* 159 (1984): 828–43; Interview with Ján Vilček; J. Vilček, "First Demonstration of the Role of TNF in

the Pathogenesis of Disease," *JI* 181, no. 1 (2008): 5–6; J. Vilček, "From IFN to TNF: A Journey into Realms of Lore," *Nat Immunol* 10, no. 6 (2009): 555–57; Cancer Research Institute, "Lloyd J. Old, M.D., Father of Modern Tumor Immunology, Dies at 78 of Prostate Cancer," 28 Nov. 2011, available online at http://www.cancerresearch.org/news/2011/november/cri-director-lloyd-old -dies-of-prostate-cancer (accessed 20 Sept. 2014).

38. Interview with Vilček.

39. By contrast, Mabs against gamma interferon had been generated easily, in part because it was easier to gain access to purified gamma interferon. In 1985 Centocor commercialized the Mabs against gamma interferon as a radioimmunoassay. The product, however, was not a success, bringing in approximately $500,000 in one year. Centocor soon lost interest in the project and later took it off the market. Interview with Vilček, 33; A. D'Andrea et al., "968 Immune-Specific Gamma Interferon (IFN) Production Correlates with Lymphocyte Blastogenesis," *Pediatric Research* 19 (1985): 272A.

40. Vilček, "From IFN to TNF," 556.

41. Interview with Vilček; Vilček, "From IFN to TNF," 556; Interview with Anne Faulkner Schoemaker; Shook, *Miracle*, 215, 218.

42. M. Feldmann et al., "Cytokine Assays: Role in Evaluation of the Pathogenesis of Autoimmunity," *Immunological Reviews* 119 (1991): 105–23; C. Q. Chu et al., "Localization of Tumor Necrosis Factor α in Synovial Tissues and at the Cartilage-Pannus Junction in Patients with Rheumatoid Arthritis," *Arthritis Rheum* 34, no. 9 (1991): 1125–32; R. O. Williams, M. Feldmann, and R. F. Maini, "Anti-Tumour Necrosis Factor Treatment Inhibits the Progression of Established Collagen-Induced Arthritis (Abstract)," *Arthritis Rheum* 24, supp. 9 (1991): S67; R. O. Williams, M. Feldmann, and R. Maini, "Anti-Tumour Necrosis Factor Ameliorates Joint Disease in Murine Collagen-Induced Arthritis," *PNAS* 89 (Oct. 1992): 9784–88; F. M. Brennan, R. N. Maini, and M. Feldmann, "TNFα—A Pivotal Role in Rheumatoid Arthritis?," *British Journal of Rheumatology* 31 (1992): 293–98; J. Keffer, L. Probert, H. Cazlaris, S. Georgopoulos, E. Kaslaris, D. Kioussis, and G. Kollias, "Transgenic Mice Expressing Human Tumour Necrosis Factor: A Predictive Genetic Model of Arthritis," *EMBO J* 10, no. 13 (1991): 4025–31.

43. European Patent Office, "Professor Mark Feldmann (UK)," available online at http://internet-i.epo.org/learning-events/european-inventor/finalists/2007 /feldmann.html (accessed 2 Oct. 2014); Albert Lasker Clinical Medical Research Award, 2003, described online at http://www.laskerfoundation.org /awards/2003_c_description.html (accessed 2 Oct. 2014); M. Elliott and R. Maini, "New Directions for Biological Therapy in Rheumatoid Arthritis," *International Archives of Allergy and Immunology* 104 (1994): 112–25, tables 1 and 2.

44. Interview with Thomas Schaible; Shook, *Miracle*, 217.

45. M. J. Elliott et al., "Treatment of Rheumatoid Arthritis with Chimeric Monoclonal Antibodies to Tumor Necrosis Factor α," *Arthritis Rheum* 36, no. 12

(1993): 1681–90; Centocor, *Annual Report* (1993); M. J. Elliott et al., "Randomised Double-Blind Comparison of Chimeric Monoclonal Antibody to Tumour Necrosis Factor A (cA2) vs. Placebo in Rheumatoid Arthritis," *Lancet* 344 (1994): 1105–10.

46. Centocor, *SEC Form*, filed 11 Mar. 1996, 27, in HS-PP; Interviews with David Holveck (1) and (2) and Rick Koenig; Shook, *Miracle*, 218–19.

47. B. Derkx et al., "Tumour-Necrosis-Factor Antibody Treatment in Crohn's Disease," *Lancet* 342 (1983): 173–74; Shook, *Miracle*, 219–20.

48. Centocor, *Annual Report* (1994); Centocor, *SEC Form 10-K for the Year Ending 31 December 1996* in HS-PP; Shook, *Miracle*, 219–20, 223.

49. Shook, *Miracle*, 222; L. Marks, "The Birth Pangs of Monoclonal Antibody Therapeutics," *mAbs* 4, no. 3 (2012): 1–10.

50. Anon., "FDA Panel Backs Centocor's Avakine for Crohn's," *The Pharma Letter* (4 June 1998); Anon., "FDA Approves Remicade for Crohn's Disease," *Doctor's Guide Publishing Limited* (24 Aug. 1998).

51. Shook, *Miracle*, 223; S. Thaul, *The Prescription Drug User Fee Act (PDUFA): History, Reauthorization in 2007, and Effect on FDA* (Washington, D.C., 2008).

52. A. Kornbluth, "Infliximab Approved for Use in Crohn's Disease: A Report on the FDA GI Advisory Committee Conference," *Inflammatory Bowel Diseases* 4, no. 4 (1998): 328–29; Shook, *Miracle*, 224.

53. Kornbluth, "Infliximab," 328.

54. Interview with Holveck (1) and (2); W. J. Sanborn and S. Hanauer, "Infliximab in the Treatment of Crohn's Disease: A User's Guide for Clinicians," *American Journal of Gastroenterology* 97, no. 12 (2002): 2962–72.

55. R. Maini et al., "Infliximab (Chimeric Anti-Tumour Necrosis Factor α Monoclonal Antibody) versus Placebo in Rheumatoid Arthritis Patients Receiving Concomitant Methotexate: a Randomised Phase III Trial," *Lancet* 354 (1999): 1932–39; P. E. Lipsky et al., "Infliximab and Methotrexate in the Treatment of Rheumatoid Arthritis," *NEJM* 343 (2000): 1594–1602.

56. Centocor, *Annual Report* (1998); Anon., "Centocor Drug Marks Milestone," *Philadelphia Business Journal* (6 Nov. 2007); Wiki, "Arthritis"; PharmaLive, "Top 500 Prescription Medicine," special report (Oct. 2011).

57. S. Abramson, "Expected Outcomes in Rheumatoid Arthritis: An Historical Perspective," *Medscape Education*, available online at http://www.medscape.org/viewarticle/464118_2 (accessed 20 Sept. 2014); P. Emery, "Treatment of Rheumatoid Arthritis," *BMJ* 332 (2006): 152–55.

58. Centocor set up a TB education program in the United States as part of its surveillance. Designed to prevent patients with TB from taking the drug, this effort also helped reduce the number of spontaneous reports of active TB in the United States more generally. Interview with Schaible; FDA, "Information for the Arthritis Advisory Committee: Remicade Efficacy and Safety Review," 4 Mar. 2003, 8, available online at http://www.fda.gov/ohrms/dockets/ac/03/briefing/3930B1_04_A-Centocor-Remicade%20.pdf (accessed 20 Sept. 2014).

59. J. M. Reichert, "Monoclonal Antibodies as Innovative Therapies," *Current Pharmaceutical Biotechnology* 9 (2008): 423–30.

60. A. Knox, "He Is Building on His Success," *Philadelphia Inquirer* (7 May 2000); J. George, "Centocor Now Bigger Than Ever," *Philadelphia Business Journal* (16 Aug. 2002).

61. Reichert, "Marketed"; J. M. Reichert and M. C. Dewitz, "Anti-Infective Monoclonal Antibodies: Perils and Promise of Development," *Nat Rev Drug Discov* 5 (2006): 191–96; J. M. Reichert, "Antibody-Based Therapeutics to Watch in 2011," *mAbs* 3, no. 1 (2011): 76–99.

62. P. A. Scolnik, "mAbs: A Business Perspective," *mAbs* 1, no. 2 (2009): 179–84, 180–81.

63. Reichert, "Monoclonal," 423–30.

64. Ibid.

65. I. Kola and J. Landis, "Can the Pharmaceutical Industry Reduce Attrition Rates?," *Nat Rev Drug Discov* 3, no. 8 (2004): 711–15; Scolnik, "mAbs," 183.

66. A. K. Pavlou and J. M. Reichert, "Recombinant Protein Therapeutics— Success Rates, Market Trends and Values to 2010," *Nat Biotechnol* 22, no. 12 (2004): 1513–19; Maggon, "Monoclonal."

67. Scolnik, "mAbs," 182; R. Leuty, "Genentech Employees to Get Big Roche Payout," *San Francisco Business Times* (13 Mar. 2009).

CHAPTER 10. A QUIET REVOLUTION

1. S. King, "The Best Selling Drugs of All Time: Humira Joins the Elite," *Forbes* (28 Jan. 2013).

2. J. M. Reichert, "Marketed Therapeutic Antibodies Compendium," *mAbs* 4, no. 3 (2012): 413–15; LMB, "MRC Millennium Medal Recognises LMB's Exceptional Research," 28 Feb. 2013, available online at http://www2.mrc-lmb .cam.ac.uk/mrc-millennium-medal-recognises-lmbs-exceptional-research (accessed 20 Sept. 2014); MD Becker Partners, "Monoclonal Antibody Companies Command Premiums," *MD Becker Partners Newsletter,* July 2010; PNS Pharma, *Global Monoclonal Antibodies Pipeline Analysis* (Jan. 2014), available online at http://www.academia.edu/7602082/Global_Monoclonal_ Antibodies_Pipeline_Analysis (accessed 11 Oct. 2014).

3. Interview with Marianne (pseud.).

4. Ibid.

5. Ibid.

6. FDA Clinical Review of BLA 98–0369, Herceptin® Trastuzumab (rhuMab HER2), date of submission 4 May 1998, date of approval 25 Sept. 1998, available online at http://www.fda.gov/downloads/Drugs/Development ApprovalProcess/HowDrugsareDevelopedandApproved/Approval Applications/TherapeuticBiologicApplications/ucm091364.pdf (accessed 11 Oct. 2014); "Trastuzumab," available online at http://www.breastcancerdead-line2020.org/breast-cancer-information/specific-issues-in-breast-cancer /trastuzumab/trastuzumab.html (accessed 2 Oct. 2014); I. E. Smith,

"Efficacy and Safety of Herceptin in Women with Metastatic Breast Cancer:
Results from Pivotal Clinical Studies," *Anticancer Drugs* 12, supp. 4 (2001):
S3–10; C. L. Vogel et al., "Efficacy and Safety of Trastuzumab as a Single
Agent in First-Line Treatment of HER2-Overexpressing Metastatic Breast
Cancer," *Journal of Clinical Oncology* 20, no. 3 (2002): 719–26; NICE,
"Guidance on the Use of Trastuzumab for the Treatment of Advanced
Breast Cancer," *Technology Appraisal* 34 (2002): 2; R. Nahta and F. J. Esteva,
"HER-2 Targeted Therapy: Lessons Learned and Future Directions," *Clinical Cancer Research* 9 (2003): 5078–84; A. Wagstaff, "Beyond the Herceptin
Hype," *Cancer World* (Mar.–Apr. 2006); Panorama TV Programme, "Herceptin: Wanting the Wonder Drug," first broadcast 5 Feb. 2006, available
online at http://bioethicsbytes.wordpress.com/2008/01/10/herceptin
-wanting-the-wonder-drug-%e2%80%93-panorama (accessed 20 Sept.
2014).

7. E. H. Romond, "Trastuzumab Plus Adjuvant Chemotherapy for Operable
HER2-Positive Breast Cancer," *NEJM* 353, no. 16 (2005): 1673–84; G. N. Hortobagyi, "Trastuzumab in the Treatment of Breast Cancer," *NEJM* 353, no. 16
(2005): 1734–36; V. Postrel, "My Drug Problem," *Atlantic* (Mar. 2009);
S. Cole, "Hope and Despair: The Funding of Herceptin," *Nathaniel Centre* 25
(2008); M. J. Piccart-Gebhart et al., "Trastuzumab after Adjuvant Chemotherapy in HER2-Positive Breast Cancer," *NEJM* 353, no. 16 (2005): 1659–
72; D. Slamon et al., "Phase III Randomized Trial Comparing Doxorubicin
and Cyclophosphamide Followed by Docetaxel (AC → T) with Doxorubicin
and Cyclophosphamide Followed by Docetaxel and Trastuzumab (AC → TH)
with Docetaxel, Carboplatin and Trastuzumab (TCH) in HER2 Positive
Early Breast Cancer Patients: BCIRG 006 Study," *Breast Cancer Research and
Treatment* 94, supp. 1 (2005): S5; H. Joensuu et al., "Adjuvant Docetaxel or
Vinorelbine with or without Trastuzumab for Breast Cancer," *NEJM* 354
(2006): 809–20; J. Baselga et al., "Adjuvant Trastuzumab: A Milestone in
the Treatment of HER-2-Positive Early Breast Cancer," *Oncologist* 11, supp. 1
(2006): 4–12.

8. S. Hall, "English Women Lose Out in Herceptin's 'Postcode Lottery',"
Guardian (10 Apr. 2006); D. Batty, "Q&A: Herceptin," *Guardian* (5 Jan.
2007); Wagstaff, "Beyond."

9. Panorama TV, "Herceptin."

10. Cole, "Hope."

11. Postrel, "My"; M. Hill, "Potential for Herceptin Treatments to Be Halved,"
available online at http://www.stuff.co.nz/national/health/7748138/Potential
-for-Herceptin-treatments-to-be-halved (accessed 20 Sept. 2014).

12. Batty, "Q&A"; A. L. Pollack, "Studies Back Length of Herceptin Cancer
Treatment," *New York Times* (1 Oct. 2012): B4.

13. H. Fortner and P. Halliquist Viale, "Health Economic Analysis of the Burden of Infusion Reactions on Patients, Caregivers and Providers," *Oncology*
23, supp. 2 (2009).

14. M. Siddiqui and S. C. Rajkumar, "The High Costs of Cancer Drugs and What We Can Do About It," *Mayo Clinic Proceedings* 87, no. 10 (2012): 935–43; A. Pollack, "Doctors Denounce Cancer Drug Prices of $100,000 a Year," *New York Times* (25 Apr. 2013).

15. A. S. A. Roy, "Stifling New Cures: The True Cost of Lengthy Clinical Drug Trials," Project FDA Report 5, *Manhattan Institute for Policy Research* (5 Apr. 2012).

16. Anon., "Monoclonal Antibody Companies Command Premiums," *MD Becker Partners Newsletter* (July 2010); G. C. Fanneau La Horie, "Making Biologic Drugs More Affordable," *Drug Discovery and Development* (10 July 2010), available online at http://www.dddmag.com/articles/2010/07/making-biologic-drugs-more-affordable (accessed 20 Sept. 2014); C. K. Schneider and U. Kalinke, "Toward Biosimilar Monoclonal Antibodies," *Nat Biotechnol* 26, no. 9 (2008): 985–89; P. Seymour, "First Monoclonal Antibody Submitted to EMA for Biosimilar Approval," Bioprocess blog (2 May 2012), available online at http://www.bioprocessblog.com/archives/409 (accessed 2 Oct. 2014).

17. S. Kingman, "Plant Factories Could Mass-Produce Antibodies," *New Sci* (11 Nov. 1989): 22; S. S. Farid, "Process Economics of Industrial Monoclonal Antibody Manufacture," *Journal of Chromatography* 848 (2007): 8–18; C. Chen, "Challenges and Opportunities of Monoclonal Antibody Manufacturing in China," *Trends in Bio/Pharmaceutical Industry* 5, no. 3 (2009): 28–33; B. Kelley, "Industrialization of mAb Production Technology," *mAbs* 1, no. 5 (2009): 443–52.

18. Farid, "Process," 9–10; Chen, "Challenges," 29; Kelley, "Industrialization."

19. Kelley, "Industrialization"; Chen, "Challenges," 29; Farid, "Process," 8, 13; D. A. Goldstein and J. A. Thomas, "Biopharmaceuticals Derived from Genetically Modified Plants," *Quarterly Journal of Medicine* 97 (2004): 705–16; A. Beck et al., "Trends in Glycosylation, Glycoanalysis and Glycoengineering of Therapeutic Antibodies and Fc-Fusion Proteins," *Current Pharmaceutical Biotechnology* 9 (2008): 482–501.

20. A. Beck et al., "Trends in Glycosylation, Glycoanalysis and Glycoengineering of Therapeutic Antibodies and Fc-Fusion Proteins," *Current Pharmaceutical Biotechnology* 9 (2008): 482–501; K. Mori et al., "Non-Fucosylated Therapeutic Antibodies: The Next Generation of Therapeutic Antibodies," *Cytotechnology* 55 (2–3): 109–14; N. Yamane-Ohnuki and M. Satoh, "Production of Therapeutic Antibodies with Controlled Fucosylation," *mAbs* 1, no. 3 (2009): 230–36.

21. Yamane-Ohnuki and Satoh, "Production"; A. Beck and J. Reichert, "Marketing Approval of Mogamulizumab: A Triumph for Glyco-Engineering," *mAbs* 4, no. 14 (2012): 1–7; Interview with Masamichi Koike.

22. Interview with Koike; A. Natsume, R. Niwa, and M. Satoh, "Improving Effector Functions of Antibodies for Cancer Treatment: Enhancing ADCC and CDC," *Drug Design, Development and Therapy* 3 (2009): 7–16; C. Liu and

A. Lee, "ADCC Enhancement Technologies for Next Generation Therapeutic Antibody," *Trends in Bio/Pharmaceutical Industry* 5, no. 3 (2009): 13–17.

23. J. M. Reichert, "Anti-Infective Monoclonal Antibodies: Perils and Promise of Development," *Nat Rev Drug Discov* 5 (2006): 191–95; J. M. Reichert, "Monoclonal Antibodies as Innovative Anti-Infective Agents," *Discovery Medicine* 5, no. 30 (2005): 544–47; A. Casadevall, "Crisis in Infectious Diseases: Time for a New Paradigm?" *Clin Infect Dis* 23 (1996): 790–94; A. Casadevall, "Antibody-Based Therapies for Emerging Infectious Diseases," *Emerging Infectious Diseases* 2, no. 3 (1996): 200–208.

24. Casadevall, "Crisis."

25. Ibid.

26. J. de Kruif et al., "A Human Monoclonal Antibody Cocktail as a Novel Component of Rabies Postexposure Prophylaxis," *Annual Review of Medicine* 58 (2007): 359–68.

27. Marasco and Sui, "Growth."

28. Ibid.

29. C. Saylor, E. Dadachova, and A. Casadevall, "Monoclonal Antibody-Based Therapies for Microbial Diseases," *Vaccine* 27, supp. 6 (2009): G38–G46; C. K. Gronvall, "Monoclonal Antibodies for Biodefense," UPMC Center for Health Security, *Clinicians Biosecurity News*, 8 Feb. 2013, available online at http://www.upmc-cbn.org/report_archive/2013/cbnreport _02082013.html (accessed 20 Sept. 2014); Reichert, "Monoclonal."

30. Reichert, "Monoclonal"; iBio Inc Press Release, 10 Apr. 2012, available online at http://in.reuters.com/article/2012/04/10/idUS115891+10-Apr-2012 +PRN201204 (accessed 2 Oct. 2014); D. Wang et al., "Immunoprophylaxis against Syncytial Virus (RSV) with Palivizumab in Children: A Systematic Review and Economic Evaluation," *Health Technology Assessment* 12, no. 36 (2008).

31. H. Zola and P. Roberts Thomson, "Monoclonal Antibodies: Diagnostic Uses," *Encyclopedia of Life Sciences* (Hoboken, N.J., 2005).

32. M. G. Scott, "Monoclonal Antibodies—Approaching Adolescence in Diagnostic Immunoassays," *Trends in Biotechnology* 3, no. 7 (1985): 170–75.

33. L. C. Goldstein and M. R. Tam, "Monoclonal Antibodies for the Diagnosis of Sexually Transmitted Diseases," *Clinics in Laboratory Medicine* 5, no. 3 (1985): 75–78; S. Chen and S. C. Silverstein, "Economic Impact of Applications of Monoclonal Antibodies to Medicine and Biology," *FASEB J* 7 (1993): 1426–32.

34. Zola and Roberts Thomson, "Monoclonal."

35. Chen and Silverstein, "Economic."

36. D. Nesterova, "Influenza Vaccine History," VRG Research Group, Information Sheet, Oct. 2012, available online at http://www.vaccination.english.vt .edu/docs/2012/updated+influenza+media+kit-4.pdf (accessed 2 Oct. 2014); P. J. Gavin and R. B. Thomson, "Review of Rapid Diagnostic Tests for Influenza," *Clinical and Applied Immunology Reviews* 4 (2003): 151–72.

37. A. M. Issa, "Personalised Medicine and the Practice of Medicine in the 21st Century," *McGill Journal of Medicine* 10, no. 1 (2007): 53–57; I. L. Ferrus et al., "Looking Back at 10 Years of Trastuzumab Therapy: What Is the Role of HER2 Testing? A Systematic Review of Health Economic Analysis," *Personalised Medicine* 6, no. 2 (2009): 194–213.

38. D. Keiger, "The Search That Paid Off—Big," *Johns Hopkins Magazine* (Apr. 2000). For more on the history of stem cells, see P. A. Martin et al., "Commercial Development of Stem Cell Technology: Lessons from the Past, Strategies for the Future," *Regenerative Medicine* 1, no. 6 (2006): 801–807.

39. NY Medical School Press Release, "Remicade Co-Inventor and NYU professor of Microbiology Ján Vilček, M.D., Ph.D. Pledge to NYU School of Medicine," 12 Aug. 2005, available online at http://communications.med.nyu.edu/news/2005/remicade-co-inventor-and-nyu-professor-of-microbiology-jan-vilcek-md-phd-pledge-to-ny (accessed 2 Oct. 2014); MRC, "Therapeutic Antibodies," 2009, available online at http://www.mrc.ac.uk/Utilities/Search/MRC003520 (accessed 2 Oct. 2014).

GLOSSARY

AFFINITY: Binding strength of an antibody. Antibodies with a high affinity have less chance of cross-reacting with other target antigens.

AGGLUTINATION: Clumping together of particles.

AMINO ACIDS: Organic compounds that combine to form proteins.

ANTIBODY: Type of protein made by the body's white blood cells (B lymphocytes) in response to a foreign substance (antigen). Some antibodies destroy antigens directly, while others make it easier for white blood cells to destroy the antigen. Each antibody is highly specific and will only bind to or destroy the antigen for which it was made.

ANTIGEN: Any substance that triggers an immune response: pollen; micro-organisms such as bacteria, viruses, fungi, or parasites; or nonliving substances such as toxins, chemicals, drugs, or foreign particles considered alien by the body.

ANTISERUM (PLURAL: ANTISERA): A part of the blood that contains antibod-ies. It is obtained from an animal or human that has been exposed to a specific antigen.

ASCITES: An abnormal accumulation of fluid in the abdominal cavity. The word "ascites" is derived from the Greek "askos," meaning bag or sac. Animals are first inoculated with solid tumors to cultivate ascites tumors, then the ascites fluid is drained from their abdomens.

AUTOIMMUNE DISEASE: A condition that arises from an abnormal response of the body against substances and tissues normally present in the body.

BIOREACTOR: Any manufactured or engineered container or system that sup-ports a biologically active environment to grow cells.

B LYMPHOCYTE (B CELL): A type of white blood cell made in the bone marrow that responds to an antigen by producing antibodies.

BONE MARROW TRANSPLANT (BMT): A therapy whereby healthy bone marrow is injected into a patient. This technique is used when a patient's bone marrow has been damaged, for example by radiotherapy.

CHIMERIC ANTIBODY: An antibody that possesses genes that are half-human and half-nonhuman.

CHROMATOGRAPHY: Chemical technique for separating the components of a mixture. During the test, a mixture dissolved in a liquid or gas is passed through a column, paper, or glass support, where the elements of the mixture are either absorbed or hindered to varying degrees and thereby become separated. The technique is used for both the purification of a mixture and the collection of components as a means of quantifying their presence in a mixture.

CLONES: Population of cells derived from a single cell.

CD: A code denoting clusters of differentiation antigens on cell surfaces.

CULTURE MEDIUM: A liquid or gel designed to aid the growth of micro-organisms or cells.

COMPLEMENT: A series of proteins made by the immune system that helps fight off bacterial and viral infections.

COMPLEMENTARITY-DETERMINING REGION (CDR): The part of the antibody structure that binds to an antigen.

CDR GRAFTING: A method for grafting the antibody-binding loops, or CDR, from a mouse antibody onto a human antibody.

CYTOKINE: A diverse group of small proteins that act as mediators between cells and help the body control infections and tumors.

DNA: Deoxyribonucleic acid, or DNA, is a complex chemical located in the cell nucleus, specifically in chromosomes. DNA provides the genetic instructions needed for an organism to develop, survive, and reproduce.

DIFFERENTIATION ANTIGENS: Molecules located on the surface of cells during sequential stages of maturation and differentiation. They are used as immunologic markers.

EFFECTOR FUNCTION: What antibodies do: activate different mechanisms of the innate immune system to respond to pathogens and antigens.

ENDPOINT (CLINICAL): A measurement used in a trial to determine a drug's efficacy. Two endpoint examples are response rates and survival. Other endpoints can be the occurrence of a disease, a symptom or sign in the patient, or a laboratory abnormality.

ENKEPHALIN: Part of the family of opioid peptides produced by the body, enkephalin occurs in the brain, spinal cord, and gastrointestinal tract. It is involved with pain perception, movement, mood, behavior, and neuroendocrine regulation.

ENZYME-LINKED IMMUNOSORBENT ASSAY (ELISA): A test that uses antibodies conjugated with a color enzyme to identify a substance.

EPITOPE: Part of the target molecule, or antigen, recognized by an antibody.

FLOW CYTOMETRY: A laser-based technique for counting and examining microscopic particles such as cells and chromosomes. The particles are suspended in a stream of fluid, which is passed through an electronic detection apparatus.

FERMENTOR: A hollow-fiber device used in the production of Mabs.

FLUORESCENCE-ACTIVATED CELL SORTING (FACS): A specialized form of flow cytometry that allows for the sorting of a heterogeneous mixture of biological cells into two or more containers. Cells are sorted according to their specific light scattering and fluorescent characteristics.

GENE EXPRESSION: Process by which a gene's information is used in the synthesis of a gene product such as proteins.

GRAFT-VERSUS-HOST DISEASE (GVHD): A potentially fatal condition that occurs when transplanted bone marrow (a graft) attacks the recipient's (or host's) organs and tissues. This condition can cause damage to the skin, liver, and gut.

GRAM-NEGATIVE BACTERIA: Bacteria that do not retain the crystal violet dye used in the Gram-staining protocol. Such bacteria can cause infections like pneumonia and sepsis and are resistant to antibiotics.

GLYCO-ENGINEERING: A technique to control the composition of carbohydrates and enhance the pharmacological properties of proteins such as antibodies.

HAPTEN: A small, separable part of an antigen that reacts specifically with an antibody but is incapable of stimulating antibody production.

HEAVY CHAIN: A long chain of amino acids that comprises one of the two building blocks of an antibody.

HISTOCOMPATIBILITY ANTIGENS: The many proteins (antigens) found on the surface of cell membranes that identify a cell as self or non-self. They help determine tissue and organ compatibility and can lead to rejection in transplantations or blood transfusions.

HUMANIZED ANTIBODY: A nonhuman-derived antibody that has had its protein sequences reengineered to make it more like a natural human antibody.

HYBRID CELL: Cell formed by the fusion of two cells of different origin.

HYBRIDOMA: A hybrid cell made in the laboratory through the fusion of an antibody-producing lymphocyte with a nonantibody-producing cancer cell, usually myeloma or lymphoma. The hybridoma proliferates and produces a continuous supply of a specific monoclonal antibody.

HAT (HYPOXANTHINE, AMINOPTERIN, THYMIDINE) MEDIUM: A medium for mammalian cell culture that is used to help promote cellular fusion.

HER2/NEU (HUMAN EPIDERMAL GROWTH FACTOR RECEPTOR 2): A protein found on the surface of tumor cells.

IDIOTYPE: A distinctive feature of an antibody's variable region that distinguishes it from other kinds of antibodies.

IMMUNOREACTION: An immune response to a particular substance.

IMMUNE SYSTEM: A biological defense system that protects the body against the invasion of foreign material (such as pollen, or invading microorganisms) and helps to prevent cancer.

IMMUNE TOLERANCE: When the immune system ignores substances or tissues in the body that have the capacity to elicit an immune response.

IMMUNOASSAY: A biochemical test measures the concentration of a specific substance in blood or a fluid sample by taking advantage of the way that an antibody binds with an antigen.

IMMUNODIAGNOSTIC: A diagnostic tool that uses the antigen-antibody reaction as a means of detection.

IMMUNOFLUORESCENCE: A technique whereby the location of an antigen (or antibody) in tissues is determined by its reaction with an antibody (or antigen) labeled with a fluorescent dye.

IMMUNOGENICITY: The ability of a particular substance to provoke an immune response.

IMMUNOGLOBULIN (IG): Also known as an antibody, this is a protein produced by the immune system to fight infection. The five primary classes of immunoglobulins are IgG, IgM, IgA, IgD, and IgE.

IMMUNOHISTOCHEMISTRY (IMMUNOCYTOCHEMISTRY): A laboratory technique that uses antibodies to detect and visualize antigens in cells and tissues.

IMMUNOLOGY: Investigation of all phenomena connected with the body's defense mechanism.

IMMUNOSUPPRESSANT: A drug given to suppress the immune system.

IMMUNOTHERAPY: A treatment designed to enhance or suppress a patient's immune response to fight a disease.

INTERFERON: A small protein messenger produced by the immune system in response to the presence of pathogens such as viruses, bacteria, parasites, or tumor cells. Interferon has two functions. It sends signals to neighboring cells to trigger their resistance mechanisms, and it activates other immune cells that then kill invading pathogens.

ISOTOPE: A variant of a particular chemical element.

IN VITRO: A process performed in a laboratory vessel or other controlled environment outside of a living organism or natural setting.

IN VIVO: A laboratory process performed in a living organism.

LEUKEMIA: A cancer of white blood cells.

LIGHT CHAIN: A short chain of amino acids that comprises one of the two building blocks of an antibody.

LEUKOPHORESIS: A technique in which a patient's white blood cells are separated from their blood sample and then returned to the patient's body.

LYMPHOCYTES: A type of white blood cell instrumental in the body's defense mechanism. The two primary types of lymphocytes are B lymphocytes (B cells) and T lymphocytes (T cells). Both originate from stem cells in the bone marrow. Those that migrate to the thymus mature into T cells, while those that remain in the bone marrow develop into B cells. Each lymphocyte has a receptor molecule on its surface that it uses to bind antigens (foreign substances) and help remove them from the body. In the presence of an antigen, B cells can differentiate into plasma cells, which secrete large quantities of antibodies.

MURINE ANTIBODY: An antibody derived from rodents like mice or rats.

MONOCLONAL ANTIBODY: An antibody produced from a single clone of cells in a laboratory.

MYCOPLASMS: Forms of bacteria that feed off live mammalian cell culture.

MYELOMA: A cancer of plasma cells, a type of white blood cell found in the bone marrow.

MYELOMA CELLS: Plasma cells that have become cancerous. Myeloma cells are an essential tool for monoclonal antibody production.

NATURAL KILLER (NK) CELLS: Type of white blood cell produced by the immune system that is instrumental to the host's rejection of both tumors and virally infected cells.

NEUROPEPTIDE: A small, protein-like substance produced and released by neurons that helps neurons communicate with each other.

NEUROTRANSMITTER: A brain chemical that relays signals between nerve cells called neurons. Neurotransmitters tell the heart to beat, the lungs to breathe, and the stomach to digest. They can also affect mood, sleep, concentration, and weight and when imbalanced can cause adverse reactions.

OKT MABS: A series of Mabs that targets various T-cells.

OLIGONUCLEOTIDES: Short single-stranded DNA or RNA molecules.

P3: A myeloma cell line developed by Michael Potter.

PATENT: A form of intellectual property rights granted by a government to an inventor or their assignee for a limited amount of time in exchange for the public disclosure of the invention. A patent provides the right to exclude all others from making, using, or selling an invention or products made by an invented process. Like any other property right, it may be sold, licensed, assigned or transferred, given away, or simply abandoned.

PHAGE DISPLAY: A research method that uses bacteriophages (viruses that infect bacteria) to connect proteins with genetic information that then encodes them. This method is used to study protein-to-protein, protein-to-peptide, and protein-to-DNA interactions.

PHAGOCYTE: A type of white blood cell that digests bacteria and other foreign invaders.

PHASES OF TRIALS: Clinical trials of drugs are commonly divided into three categories. Phase I trials are conducted with small numbers of people and are designed to test the safety of a new drug. Phase II trials may have up to one hundred people taking part and aim to test the efficacy of a new drug and determine the best dose to give patients. Phase III trials can involve thousands of patients and are designed to compare new treatments with the best currently available treatment.

PLASMID: Small, circular, double-stranded DNA molecules found in bacteria, archae, and eukaryotes that can replicate independently of chromosomal DNA. Scientists often use reengineered plasmids as vectors in molecular cloning.

POLYCLONAL: A mixed pool of antibodies, each with different binding specificities, produced by a number of different white blood cells in response to an antigen.

POLYMERASE CHAIN REACTION (PCR): A laboratory method that enables the multiple reproduction of very small samples of DNA.

RADIOIMMUNOASSAY: A test that makes use of radioactively labeled antibodies and antigens to detect and quantify important substances, such as hormone levels in the blood.

REAGENT: A chemical or biological substance used in an experiment.

RECOMBINANT DNA (RDNA): Also known as gene cloning or splicing, recombinant DNA is a technique that produces identical copies (clones) of a gene.

RHEUMATOID ARTHRITIS (RA): An autoimmune disorder that can cause chronic inflammation of the tissues and organs, primarily synovial joints. Symptoms can be disabling and painful. If left untreated, the condition can result in substantial loss of mobility and function.

SENDAI VIRUS: A virus that affects mice, hamsters, guinea pigs, rats, and sometimes pigs. It is used in research laboratories because it can induce genetically different cells to fuse.

SEPSIS (BLOOD POISONING OR SEPTICAEMIA): A potentially fatal condition caused by an overwhelming immune response to an infection.

SEROTONIN: Found in the tissues, particularly in blood platelets, the intestinal wall, and the central nervous system, serotonin is a compound thought to play a part in transmitting nerve impulses and regulating moods, temper, anxiety, depression, sleep, aggression, appetite, and sexuality.

Serotonin is also considered instrumental in regulating body temperature and metabolism.

SITE-DIRECTED MUTAGENESIS (SDM): A method used to make specific, targeted changes to the DNA sequence of a gene.

SERUM: The straw-colored liquid component of blood from which blood cells and the chemicals that cause clotting have been taken out.

SPLENIC FRAGMENT TECHNIQUE: A method that involves harvesting antibodies from the spleen of an immunized mouse and growing these antibodies in tissue culture. Once this is done, antigen is added to the culture and any antibodies produced against that particular antigen are isolated from the culture medium.

SOMATIC CELL: Any cell type in the mammalian body apart from the sperm and ova.

SOMATIC MUTATION: The alteration of DNA that occurs after conception. Such changes can happen in any of the cells of the body except germline cells (sperm and ova) and so cannot be passed on to offspring. The alteration can cause various diseases, including cancer.

SPLEEN: An organ that plays an important role in the immune system and helps in the creation of red blood cells. The spleen removes old red blood cells and recycles iron. It also synthesizes antibodies and removes from circulation antibody-coated bacteria and antibody-coated blood cells.

SUPERNATANT: The liquid part of a mixture that lies above a precipitate or settled precipitate after it has been centrifuged.

STEM CELLS: Biological cells that have the ability to divide (self-replicate) and under the right conditions can develop into cells that have the characteristic shapes and specified functions of other cells in the body, such as heart cells, skin cells, muscle cells, or nerve cells.

SUBSTANCE P (SP): A small peptide found in the spinal cord and brain that transmits pain signals from the sensory nerves to the central nervous system. It is also associated with the regulation of stress and anxiety.

T LYMPHOCYTES (T CELLS): A type of white blood cell that originates in the thymus and protects the body from infection.

TRANSGENIC: An organism that contains genetic material that has been artificially introduced from an unrelated organism.

x63: A myeloma cell line prepared by David Secher. It was derived from P3, a myeloma cell line developed by Michael Potter.

BIBLIOGRAPHY

RESEARCH METHODOLOGY

Research for this book was conducted by searching medical and scientific journals, business literature, patent applications, and papers kept in publicly accessible archives. These efforts were followed up where possible by contacting key individuals mentioned in the literature to request an interview. Those interviewed often generously shared their personal papers, which included company papers difficult to access elsewhere, and provided other useful interview contacts. All interviews were conducted with questions prepared from prior reading of the literature. Interviews were done both face-to-face and on the phone. Every person interviewed was shown drafts of chapters where their material appears.

Some background material that informs the historical insights made in this book can be found on www.whatisbiotechnology.org. See in particular the exhibitions by L. Marks titled *A Healthcare Revolution in the Making: The Story of César Milstein and Monoclonal Antibodies* and *The Life Story of a Biotechnology Drug: Alemtuzumab;* as well as the essays about David Murray and Hubert Schoemaker in the "People" section.

The sources listed below are restricted to unpublished primary material. All published material is listed in full in the Notes.

ARCHIVED PERSONAL PAPERS

César Milstein Papers (Churchill College Archives Centre, Cambridge)
Key files (beginning with MSTN): C281, C283–85, C294–96; C299, C301, C303; C305–9; C316; C324–C326; C332; C337; D23; E16; F13; F15; F17; F21; H135; H27; H44; H45; H58.

Anon. "Draft: Research Monoclonals." 28 Apr. 1981. MSTN/E15.

———. "Letter to the Editor." *Lancet*. Sent 16 June 1982. MSTN/H45.

———. "Strategic Issues in Relation to Celltech Products." Unpublished paper presented to Celltech's Scientific Council Meeting. 24 Mar. 1981. MSTN/E13.

Celltech. "Anti-IFN Market Appraisal." 19 Oct. 1981. Unpublished paper. MSTN/C326.

———. "Report on Progress against Objectives and Highlights of Period 25 March to 23 April." MSTN/E13.

Cotton, R. "The Road to Monoclonal Antibodies." Unpublished paper. MSTN/D112.

Fairtlough, G. H. "Report of the Chief Executive on Progress against Objectives for 1980/81 Adopted in December 1980 and on Other Major Matters." 26 Aug. 1981. MSTN/E14.

———. "Strategy for Anti-Interferon." 25 Aug. 1981. MSTN/E14.

Howard, J. C. "The Future of Immunology." British Pharmaceutical Society Conference. Newcastle. 19 Nov. 1980. Unpublished ms., 8–9, MSTN/H78.

International Patent Application PCT/GB81/00067. Filed 13 Apr. 1981. MSTN/C326.

Milstein, C. "An Assessment of MRC-Celltech Collaboration." N.d. Unpublished paper. MSTN/E17.

———. Milstein's notebook. MSTN/C282.

———. "Notes for Lecture(s) for Japan." Unpublished manuscript, MSTN/D38.

———. "Notes for Plenary Lecture at Cytology Workshop." N.d. Unpublished ms. MSTN/D66.

———. Title unknown. N.d. Unpublished paper for Cytology Workshop. MSTN/D66.

Murray, D. Untitled and undated document sent with letter to Vittery. 29 July 1977. MSTN/F13.

Newell, J. "Living Factories—New Drugs from Hybrid Cells." 12 Aug. 1975. Unpublished paper for BBC External Services. MSTN/A/2/A.7.

Secher, D. S. "Development of NK2-Sepharose." 30 Jan 1981. MSTN/E15.

U.S. Northern District of California. "Hybritech Inc vs Monoclonal Antibodies." No. C-84–0930 SC Findings of Fact and Conclusions of Law. 28 Aug 1985. MSTN/C306.

Williams, Alan. Unpublished recollections. 1986(?). MSTN/H149.

David Murray Papers (kept by Jenny Murray)
Murray's diaries and correspondence.
Sera-Lab, *Catalogues* (1979), (1983), (1986).

Hubert Schoemaker Papers (kept by Anne Faulkner Schoemaker)
Anon. "Hubert J. P. Schoemaker" profile article. N.d.
Castello, John L., president and CEO of Xoma, to Hubert. 16 July 1992.
Centocor. *Annual Reports*. 1982–98.

———. Centocor Oncogene Research Partners LP. 9 June 1984.

———. *CenTropics* 1, no. 4. Fall 1992.

———. *Investment Prospectus.* 14 Dec. 1982.

———. Press Release. "Centocor Receives FDA Panel Recommendation to Approve Ovarian Cancer Test." 3 Nov 1986.

———. Press Release. Untitled. 28 May 1993.

———. *Prospectus.* 22 July 1983.

Enigma, R. M. "Centocor to Terminate HA-1A: Centocor Press Release." 1993.

Executive (name unknown). Letter to Hubert. 19 July 1992.

PaineWebber. *Centocor Common Stock.* 13 Dec. 1985.

PaineWebber, Tocor II, and Centocor. *Prospectus.* 21 Jan. 1992.

Rothschild, L. F., et al. *Centocor, Inc.: Prospectus for Public Offering.* 22 July 1983.

Schoemaker, H. Letter to David Kessler, head of the FDA. Sept 1992.

———. "Wharton Talk." Unpublished paper. 17 Apr. 2000.

Scott, E Michael D, (CoMed Communications) to Hubert Schoemaker. 19 Jan. 1993.

Strauss, R. "High Profile: Schoemaker." Feb. 2001.

Wall, M., and E. C. Allen. "Investment Prospectus: Medical Diagnostics Business." n.d .

Wolf, R. "Centocor Makes a Deal on Product Marketing." *Philadelphia Inquirer* (7 Dec. 1987).

Zoon, K. (FDA). Letter to Martin Page (Centocor). 21 May 1993.

ORAL INTERVIEWS

Except where transcripts are cited, Lara Marks has recordings and accompanying notes for all the interviews she conducted listed below. Interview transcripts have been deposited at the Chemical Heritage Foundation (CHF), Philadelphia; the San Diego Technology Archive (SDTA); the Regional Oral History Office, Bancroft Library, University of California, Berkeley (UCB); and the Laboratory of Molecular Biology (LMB), Cambridge, Eng.

Interviews by Lara Marks

Ashworth, John. 19 July 2011 and 5 Oct. 2011.

Batchelor, Richard. 12 Oct. 2011.

Bernard, Ed. 18 Nov. 2011.

Bernard, Tim. 1 Dec. 2011.

Brock, Paul. 30 Jan. 2007. CHF.

Christie, James. 12 Nov. 2011 and 24 Feb. 2012.

Clark, Michael. 2 Dec. 2011 and 6 Mar. 2012.

Croce, Carlo. 10 Feb. 2012.

Cuello, Claudio. 29 Sept. 2011.

Dougherty, Michael. 23 Jan. 2007. Transcript. CHF.

Faragalli, Sandra, Ray Heslip, and Patty Durachko. 12 Sept. 2006. Transcript. CHF.

Faulkner Schoemaker, Anne. 10 July 2006. Transcript. CHF.
Fuchs, Renato. 1 July 2008.
Gerhard, Walter. 13 Mar. 2012.
Glennie, Martin. 14 Nov. 2011.
Hale, Geoff. 25 Nov. 2011 and 10 Jan. 2012.
Harrison, Roger, and Tony Dolan. 7 Sept. 2012.
Hobbs, George. 12 Sept. 2006. Notes only.
Jarvis, John. 31 Aug. 2011.
Koike, Masamichi. 2 Dec. 2013.
Lefkovits, Ivan. 12 Dec. 2010 and 17 Feb. 2011.
Levy, Ron. 18 Feb. 2012.
Lonberg, Nils. 26 July 2012.
Marianne (pseudonym). 30 Sept. 2006. Transcript. CHF.
Mattis, Jeffrey. 22 Feb. 2007.
McCloskey, Richard. 19 Jan. 2007. Transcript. CHF.
McGinn, Denise. 12 Sept. 2006. Transcript. CHF.
McMichael, Andrew. 24 Nov. 2011.
Melore, Michael. 21 May 2007. Transcript. CHF.
Murray, Jenny. 21 Sept. 2011.
Mynheer, Lisa. 1 Dec. 2011.
Neuberger, Michael. 31 Aug. 2011.
Papadopolous, Stelios. 19 Oct. 2006. Transcript, 22. CHF.
Pelly, Jane. 24 Oct. 2011.
Peacock, Bruce. 10 July 2006. Transcript.
Phillips, Jenny. 5 Apr. 2012.
Sacks, Steve. 11 Nov. 2011.
Sapsford, Kelly. 20 Oct. 2011.
Schaffer, Bernie. 11 Sept. 2006. Transcript.
Schaible, Thomas. 24 Sept. 2010.
Schoemaker, Erik, and Kathleen Schoemaker. 11 Sept. 2006. Transcript. CHF.
Secher, David. 28 June 2011.
Siegel, Jay. 20 Sept. 2010.
Staehelin, Theo. 16 Mar. 2011.
Steplewski, Zenon. 20 Feb. 2012.
Tetteroo, Pedro. Transcript. 30 June 2006. CHF.
Tindle, Robert. 1 Aug. 2011.
Vilček, Ján. Transcript. 12 July 2006. CHF.
Waldmann, Herman. 19 Nov. 2012.
Weisman, Harlan. 20 Nov. 2006. Transcript. CHF.
Winter, Gregory. 31 Aug. 2011.

Interviews by Lara Marks and Ted Everson
Evens-Freke, Stephen. 14 Sept. 2006. Transcript. CHF.
Evnin, Tony. 14 Sept 2006. Transcript. CHF.

Holveck, David (1). 14 July 2006 and 9 Sept 2009. Transcripts. CHF.
Koenig, Rick. 15 Sept 2006. Transcript. CHF.
Koprowski, Hilary. 13 July 2006. Transcript. CHF.
Touhey, Paul. 15 Sept 2006. Transcript. CHF.

Interviews by Ted Everson
D'Antonio, Pat. 2 May 2007. Transcript. CHF.
Garnier, J. P. 12 July 2006. Transcript. CHF.
McKenzie, Ann. 14 Sept. 2007. Transcript. CHF.
Schoemaker, Paul. 5 July 2006. Transcript CHF.
Zurawski, Vincent. 4 Jan. 2007. Transcript. CHF.

Other Interviews
Birndorf, Howard (1), by Mark Jones. 11 Feb. 1997. Transcript. SDTA.
Birndorf, Howard (2), by Matthew Shindell. 30 Apr. 2008. Transcript. SDTA.
Byers, Brook, by Thomas Kiley. 2002–2005. Transcript. UCB.
Greene, Ted, by Matthew Shindell. 8 Oct. 2008. Transcript. SDTA.
Holveck, David (2), by Sally Smith-Hughes. 2 Feb. 1999. Transcript. UCB.
Milstein, César, by David Secher. Transcript. LMB.
Royston, Ivor, by Mark Jones. 10 Mar. 1997. Transcript. SDTA

EMAIL CORRESPONDENCE WITH LARA MARKS
Drakeman, Don. 4 May 2012, 19 and 31 July 2012.
Fischer, Alastair. 26 Feb. 2013.
Levy, Ron. 10 Jan. 2013.
Neuberger, Michael. 31 July 2012.
Staehelin, Theophil, and Lefkovits, Ivan. Mar. 2012.
Waldmann, Herman. 16 July 2012.
Welsh, Ken. 28 July 2011 and 30 July 2011.
Winter, Gregory. 20 Jan. 2013.

OTHER UNPUBLISHED SOURCES
Jones, M. P. "Biotech's Perfect Climate: The Hybritech Story." Ph.D. diss., UCSD. 2005.
Stein, K. "FDA-Approved Monoclonal Antibody Products." Paper. 2010.

INDEX